HYPERTHERMIA

Edited by **Nagraj Huilgol**

Hyperthermia
http://dx.doi.org/10.5772/2993
Edited by Nagraj Huilgol

Contributors

Andras Szasz, Nora Iluri, Oliver Szasz, Mario Francisco Jesús Cepeda Rubio, Arturo Vera Hernández, Lorenzo Leija Salas, El-Sayed El-Sherbini, Ahmed El-Shahawy, Mansour Lahonian, Ragab Hani Donkol, Ahmed Al Nammi, Timothy A. Okhai, Cedric J. Smith, Angelika Moder, Heidi Dobias, Markus Ritter, Iustin V. Tabarean

Published by InTech

Janeza Trdine 9, 51000 Rijeka, Croatia

Publishing Process Manager Oliver Kurelic
Technical Editor InTech Prepress, Novi Sad
Cover InTech Design team

Additional hard copies can be obtained from orders@intechopen.com

Hyperthermia, Edited by Nagraj Huilgol
p. cm.
ISBN 978-953-51-1129-0

For EU product safety concerns:
IN TECH d.o.o., Prolaz Marije Krucifikse Kozulić 3, 51000 Rijeka, Croatia,
info@intechopen.com or visit our website at intechopen.com.

Meet the editor

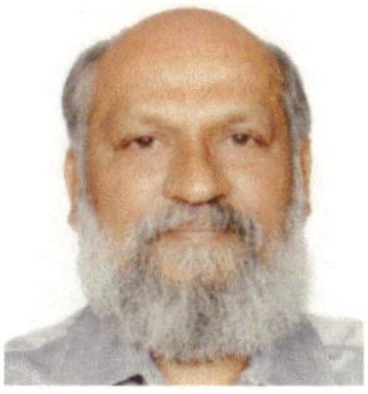

Dr. Nagraj G. Huilgol, Chief, Division of Radiation Oncology at Nanavati Hospital finished his diploma in Gynecology and Obstetrics in Mumbai. He then finished his M.D. in Radiation Oncology from All Indian Institute of Medical Sciences, New Delhi. He joined Tata Memorial Hospital as Senior Registrar after which he worked briefly as assistant professor at Kidwai Memorial Institution of Oncology at Banglore. He later Joined Nanavati Hospital as Chief of Radiation Oncology. He has served on various government bodies including Atomic Energy Regulatory Board for licensing radiation equipments. He is founder member of Society for Cancer Research and Communication. He is also the member of American Therapeutic Radiation Oncologist, Radiation Research Society, USA, and European Society for Hyperthermic Oncology. He is the President of Indian Association of Hyperthermic Oncology and Medicine and Joint Secretary of Indian Society of Oncology. He has nearly 100 published papers published in national and international journals and, edited three books related to cancer. He has been elected Fellow of the Indian Academy of Sciences. He is involved in clinical research and bench research in collaboration with the Indian Institute of Technology, Powai as well as the Bhaba Atomic Research Centre Bombay. He is currently investigating the role of hyperthermia in the treatment of head & neck cancer & HIV. The trials are being supported by Indian council of medical research.

Contents

Chapter 1

Local Hyperthermia in Oncology – To Choose or not to Choose?

Andras Szasz, Nora Iluri and Oliver Szasz

Additional information is available at the end of the chapter

http://dx.doi.org/10.5772/52208

1. Introduction

1.1. Historical way – To go or not to go?

Hyperthermia means the overheating of the living object completely (systemic) or partly (regionally or locally). If overheating can be identical with higher temperature then a/the question arises: could overheating be identical with higher temperature or could "higher temperature" be caused only by "overheating"?

Hyperthermia is one of the most common therapies in "house" applications. It is applied according to unwritten traditions in every culture and in every household. It can be applied simply to prevent the common cold but it is also good for its treatment moreover it is effective against various pains (joints, muscle-spasms, etc.), it can be applied for better overall conditions and simply for relaxation, or sometimes for spiritual reasons. The various heat therapies are commonly used complementary with natural drugs (teas, herbs, oils, aromas, etc.) or with natural radiations (sunshine, red-hot iron radiation, etc.) This popular medicine is sometimes connected with ritual, cultural and social events (ritual hot bath cultures), or ancient healing methods (like special spa treatments, hot-spring natural drinks, etc.).

Hyperthermia has two certainly different fields in medicine: hyperthermia as a treatable disease or as a therapeutic method for various diseases (see Figure 1.)

The source of whole body temperature increase as a disease can be internal, having fever by reaction to infections [1] or pyrogens [2] or malignant hyperthermia [3] as well. These whole-body "heating" processes differ also in their systemic reaction. The natural fever is induced by the living system [4], while the system works against the compulsory metabolic heating and tries to keep the temperature normal. Whole-body hyperthermia can be induced by external heating as well [5]. This happens in hot environments when the body is not able to cool itself down, although the system fights against the increase of its temperature. This whole-body heating can be unwanted, mainly accidental from environmental sources, and it might be accelerated by additional heavy muscular work or by extra metabolic activity. This is a life-threatening situation with the danger of a heat-stroke [6]. Hyperthermia requests definite and effective medical treatment when it appears as a disease, having elevated body temperature and the patient suffers from its serious consequences. This medical intervention applies therapies to reestablish the normal temperature of the body keeping the healthy homeostasis (overall stability) and handling the consequences of the unwanted high body temperature.

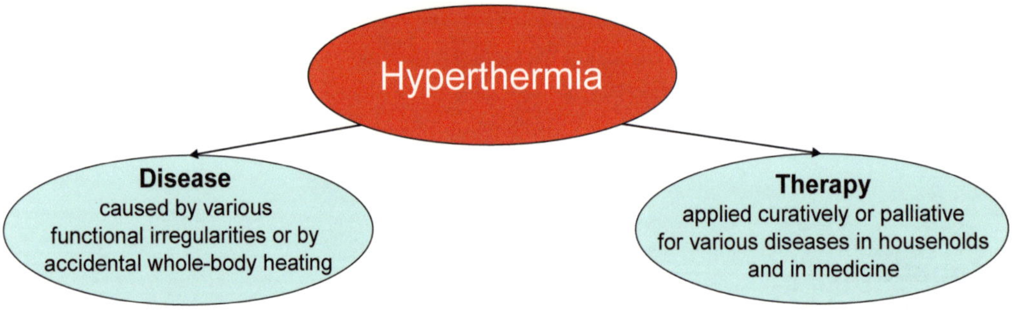

Figure 1. Main categories of hyperthermia

The popular heat-treatment applications are types of "kitchen medicine": the old recipes are "sure", the patient follows them, and is cured when everything is done according to the auricular traditional regulations. The meaning of "kitchen medicine" is: do it like in the kitchen, reading the process from the cookery-book: "heat it on the prescribed temperature for the prescribed time and the success is guaranteed". This type of thinking has its origin in the ancient cultures, when the Sun - the fire, the heat - was somehow in the centre of the religious beliefs and philosophical focus.

This idea of "take it for sure" is the disadvantage of the popular wisdom. It interprets this heating method as a simple causal process, "do it, get it", however, hyperthermia is not as simple as traditions interpret it.

1.2. Medical history of hyperthermia in oncology

Hyperthermia is really an ancient tradition of human medicine. It is one of the very first known medical therapies, more than 5000 years old, [7].It has been historically recognized that malignant and infectious diseases can be successfully treated by raising the body temperature.

It has been historically recognized that malignant and infectious diseases can be successfully treated by raising the body temperature. The first known oncotherapy by heat was made by an Egyptian priest/physician, Imhotep, in the 5th century BC. He exposed the tumors to "natural heat" (fever) before surgically removing them, which was in fact the very first immune approach as well.

Many ancient cultures used heat to treat diseases and to maintain health. The thermal baths for their curative properties were used by the Greeks, the pre-Christian Jews and the Romans too [8]. The Chinese treated many diseases including syphilis and leprosy by hot spring baths [9]. Taking regular, extremely hot baths from infancy is the block of developing rheumy, according to the ancient Japanese medical notes.

Naturally, this treatment had a sacral meaning in historic times, regarding the Sunlight, the fire and the heat as parts of the leading spiritual object in all ancient religions. This belief was behind when the heat was applied to locally affected parts of the body and to its entirety by means of hot water, steam, hot sand and hot mud baths. Natural hot air caverns connected with volcanic sources were also used. By the development of the medical knowledge, more and more heat applications were applied in practice. Later Hippocrates documented it [10], and he was convinced of its overall efficacy, telling when hyperthermia (fire) does not help, then the disease has to be declared as incurable. Hippocrates said: "Give me the power to produce fever and I will cure all diseases". His followers in line were Aurelius Cornelius Celsus and Rufus of Ephesus, who believed in the curative effect of fever. The progress continued in the Middle Ages [11], when the ablation techniques (burn out the tumor) and hot-bathes dominated the hyperthermia practices, while the temperature measurement was worked out step by step.

- The first clinical thermometer was introduced only later by Sir Clifford Allbutt in 1868. This was the start of the modern history of heat-therapies. The controllable era of hyperthermia was started. The temperature measurement made it possible to control the homogeneous heating and to make correlations with various physiological changes, like:
- Increased rate of nerve conduction,
- Elevation of pain threshold, altering muscle strength,
- Possible changes in enzyme reactions,
- Increased soft tissue extensibility,
- Increased heat- and field-stress reactions (mainly the developments of heat-shock-proteins),
- Increased venous and lymphatic flow,
- Changes in physical properties of tissues,
- Increased tissue extensibility,
- Supporting muscular relaxation, reduced muscle spasm,
- Lymphedema reduction,
- Superficial wound healing,
- Treatment of venous ulcers,
- Assistance in removal of cellular debris and toxins,
- Alteration of diffusion rate across the cell membrane,
- Increased intramuscular metabolism,
- Relieving pain, analgesia,

- Increased metabolic rate of contracted joints using heat and stretch techniques,
- Need of stretching during and/or immediately following the treatment,
- Alterations of collagen properties, allowing it to elongate,
- Increased rate of phagocytosis,
- Increased ATP activity (assisting wound regeneration),
- Psycho-feedback (pleasant sensing) [positive placebo effect],
- Ability to control the chronic infection by increasing the circulation,
- Heat increases the extensibility of fibrous tissues such as tendons, joint capsules and scars.

It was applied for many various diseases like:

- rheumy,
- gout,
- pain-management,
- arthritis,
- some dermatological disorders,
- muscle spasms,
- supportive therapies in sport,
- some gynecological disorders,
- some allergies,
- rhinitis, common cold,
- pediatric ear diseases,
- wound healing,
- supporting the general rehabilitation process.

A Nobel Prize was also granted for hyperthermia in Physiology & Medicine in 1927 "for his discovery of the therapeutic value of malaria inoculation in the treatment of dementia paralytica" to Julius Wagner-Jauregg, (1857-1940, Austria).

The application of heat in oncology has been restarted with huge intensity. Among the first modern curative applications in oncology, Busch [12] and Coley [13] were successful at the end of the 19th century with artificial fever generated by infection and toxins, respectively. These systemic applications were soon followed by local and regional heating by Westermark F. [14], Westermark N. [15], and Overgaard K. [16]. The leading German surgeon at that time, Bauer KH's opinion in his monograph "Das Krebsproblem" about the oncologic hyperthermia is typical: "All of these methods impress the patient very much; they do not impress their cancer at all." However, very early, in 1912, a controlled Phase II clinical study was published, 100 patients showing the benefit of the thermo-radiation therapy [17]. Tremendous number of publications were prepared in the first quarter of the 20th century, expecting fantastic development in the topic, [18], [19], [20], [21], [22], [23], [24], [25], [26], [27], [28], [29], [30], [31], [32], [33], [34], [35], [36], [37], [38], [39], [40], [41], [42], [43], [44], [45], [46], [47], [48], [49].

1.3. Heating methods – local and systemic

As it was shown before, there are two, basically different hyperthermia processes: the systemic (heats the complete body, whole-body treatment), and the local/regional heating (heats only a part of the organism). The two basic kinds of the heating methods also differ in their physiological limitations: the systemic treatment, of course, modifies the entire physiology of the organism, and that could limit the applied energy-absorption and body-temperature. There is a possibility to absorb energy in large volume equally or having a layer-by-layer changing front (heat-diffusion, heat-flow flux) depending on the penetration depth of the actually applied energy. Nevertheless, the old direct heating methods (hot solids or liquids in the area or in the nearest body cavity) were not effective enough for local deep heating without skin injury.

Thermodynamically the systemic and local/regional treatments differ by their energy-intake. The whole body treatment is based on the blood-heating (mostly heats up the subcutaneous capillary bed, or heats the mainstream of the blood directly with extracorporeal heater), while the local hyperthermia is definitely a tissue heating approach. This difference drastically divides the two methods from thermal point of view. In whole body treatment the blood is a heating media, it delivers the heat to the tumor and heats it up; while in local treatment, the blood remains on body temperature during the local heating, so it is a cooling media (heat-sink) for the locally heated tumor, (see Figure **3**).

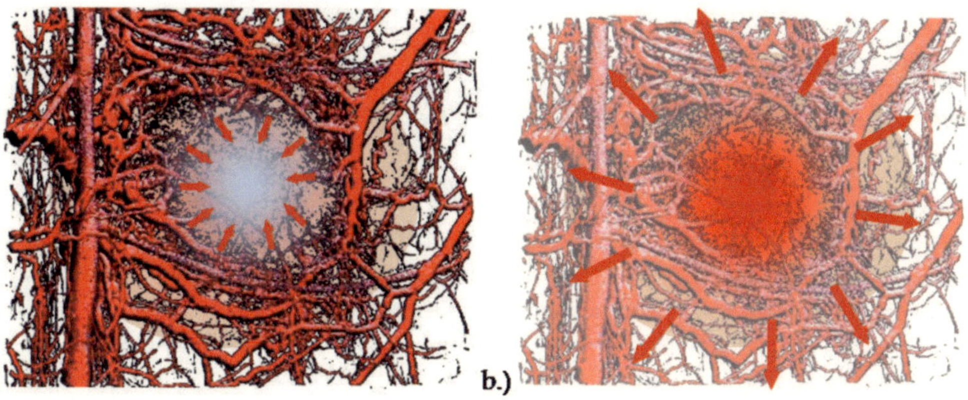

Figure 2. Opposite thermodynamic mechanisms of whole-body, systemic (a) and local (b) heating methods. The blood-heated tumor in whole body treatment reaches thermal equilibrium after a certain time, while the local treatment is always in non-equilibrium state, because the body temperature is lower than the heated tissue, creating intensive heat-flow from the target to the neighborhood.

The systemic (whole-body) treatment uses the blood-circulation to heat-up the body. (see Figure **3**.)

The artificially elevated body-temperature is the source of heating in fever inducing methods. Fever inducing can be solved with various drugs [50], as well as with special inflammation-inducing toxins.

The oldest whole body heating was the contact method, immersing the patient into the hot bath, but due to its numerous disadvantages of this method, it is rarely in use any more. Mainly two direct methods are available in the modern medicine to make systemic hyperthermia. The less frequently used is the extracorporeal (the blood is heated outside the body), or the intracorporeal (the blood is heated in-situ in the body). In most cases the capillary bed of the subcutane area is heated by conductive (e.g. hot-bath) or radiative (e.g. infrared) way, using extra-corporal blood-heating. This method takes out the blood from the continuous flow by a definite arterial outlet and the outside heated hot blood is pumped back to the patient.

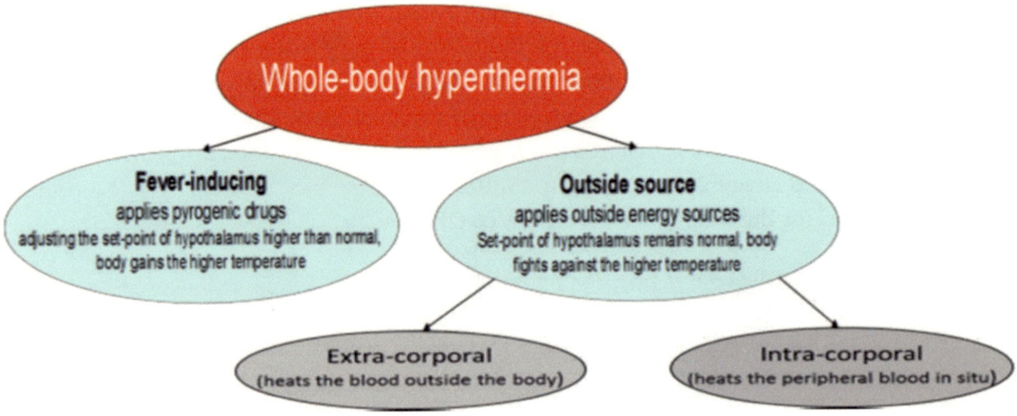

Figure 3. Categories of whole-body hyperthermia

The whole-body heating could be solved in various ways, like steam, water or radiation heating (see Figure 4.). There are other possibilities as well (e.g. wax heating, hot-air heating, etc.) but the limited possible heat-flux and the poor technical realizations hinder these solutions. By all of these whole-body heating forms the patient's safety has to be seriously considered. These are based on the blood-heating in the subcutaneous capillary bed, and the physiological reactions (vasodilatation and sweating) work well against the huge heat-flux into the body. The long heating time is also challenging (over an hour) moving the body away from the healthy homeostasis. The heat-flux through the skin is limited by the heat injuries (~1 W/cm^2 is the limit) so the contact heating with steam and water has definite problems. The radiation heating can be solved by special infrared wave (Infrared A) which penetrates deeper (~1-2 mm) into the subcutaneous layer, and can manage higher energy-flux without burn injuries. The method has many early descriptions [51], [52], [53], [54]; but the dominant systemic hyperthermia method is based on the infra-red radiation by multi-reflecting filtering [55], [56] or by water-filtering [57], [58], [59], [60].

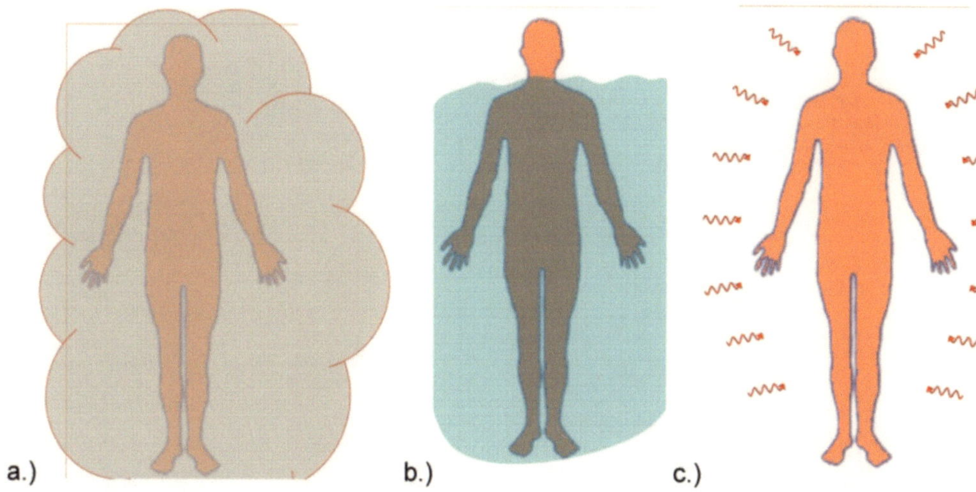

Figure 4. Various main methods of the whole-body heating: (a) steam, (b) water, (c) electromagnetic radiation

When the whole body is systemically heated, it has a strict physiological limit: 42 ºC in humans. The thermal distribution till this level is homogeneous and well controllable. No hot-spots exist, no question arises about the isotherms; the physiologically extreme temperature can be fixed all over the body. Suppressing the risk; a decreased treatment temperature (moderate WBH/whole-body fever-range thermal-therapy) is also applied. The application of lower temperatures for longer time period (fever-therapy, or mild-hyperthermia) also showed surprisingly good efficacy for whole-body hyperthermia treatments [61], [62], [63], [64]. The whole body hyperthermia and even its fever-range versions mean effective immune support, [65], [66], [67], [68], which might be a very important factor for patients with weak immune-system.

The local/regional hyperthermia has also large categories (see Figure 5.) and various technical choices (see Figure 6.). The widely applied technical solutions were available only after the discovery of the electromagnetic heating. The electromagnetic waves can penetrate deeply into the body. Dominantly, the local/regional systems work by radiative [69], [70], [71], or by capacitive [72], [73], [74] technical solutions.

Both heating categories form large groups of treating options having special subcategories, which are involved in different physiological actions and support different reaction mechanisms in the organism.

Technically, a huge variety of heating can be applied by heat therapies. Its energy-production, its selectivity, locality, kind of energy-delivery, invasivity control, frequency of the electromagnetic waves, as well as their medical applications and combination with other methods make the heat-therapies different, (see Figure 7.).

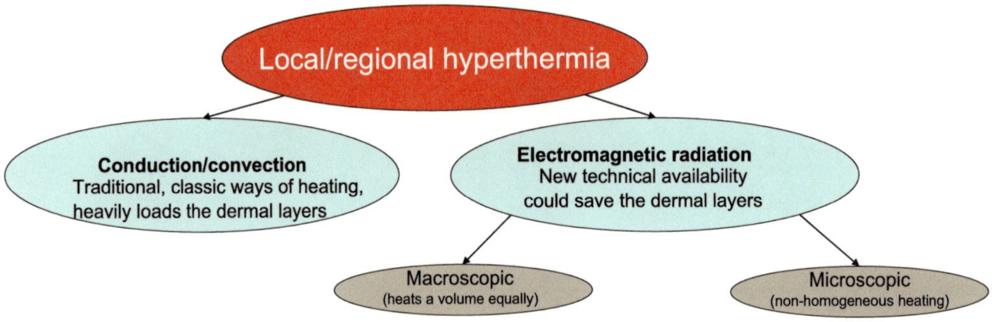

Figure 5. Categories of local heat-treatments

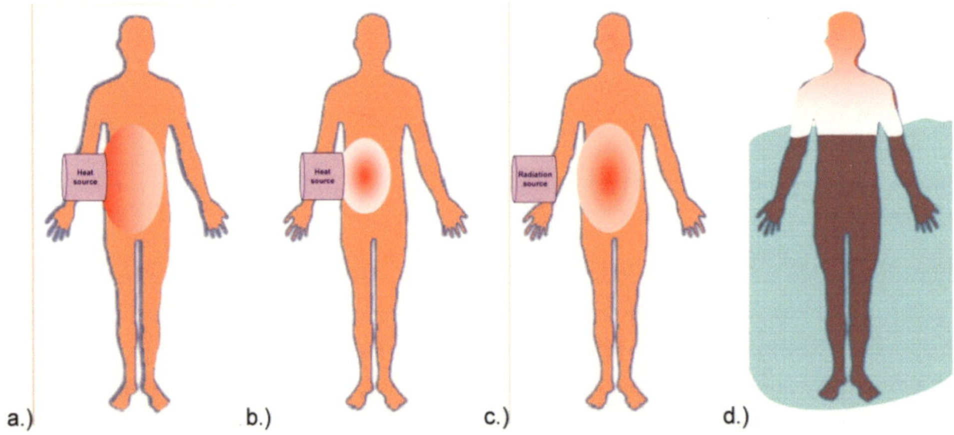

Figure 6. Main technical solutions of local heating: (a) contact heat, (b) deep-heating, (c) radiative heating, (d) immersing a part of the body in hot water

These combinations involve more than a hundred solutions of hyperthermia used as treatment, which make the therapy indefinite in its applications. This emphasizes the reason why the present review tries to summarize the main categories.

The thermodynamic situation, and in consequence of the physiological effects of the systemic and local/regional heating modalities are entirely different. There is a definite difference between the temperature of the blood and the inter-capillary volume in the microscopic structure of the target: the blood-arteries are hot-sources in case of systemic treatment, they deliver the heat. However, in case of local/regional hyperthermia it is entirely the opposite: the blood is relatively cold (remaining on unchanged body temperature), the arteries are heat-sinks which are cooling the tumor down, in fact, these work against the local heating.

One question automatically arises: when the heat, the energy-flow has a central role in hyperthermia, then what does the temperature do in the living systems?

The temperature as the average of kinetic energy in the system has a double role in the control of the heat-absorption. It characterizes the heat-absorption, when the heating is homogeneous, and its gradients (non-homogeneities) are the driving forces of the dynamic processes in case of microscopic (non-homogeneous) heating. The average temperature does not inform us about the distribution of the real energy-absorption (see Figure 8.).

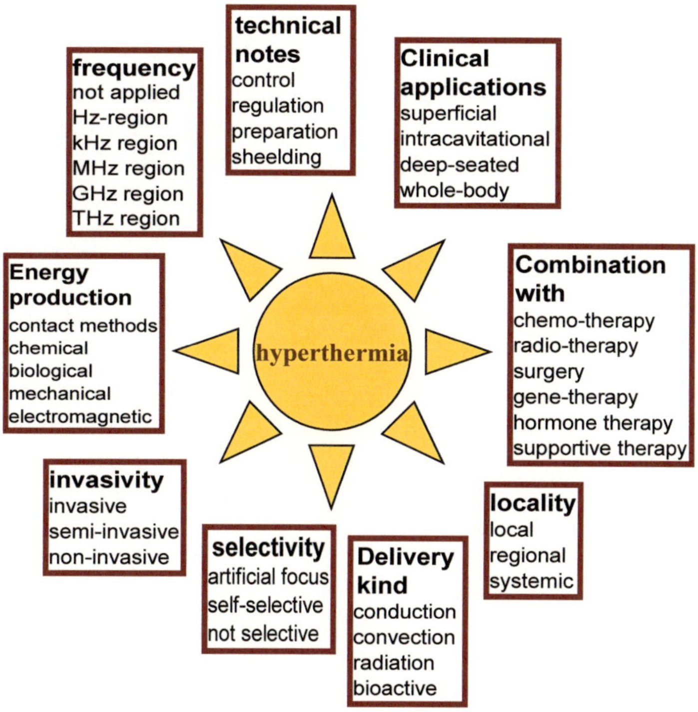

Figure 7. Categories of the possible hyperthermia methods. A few hundred of healing processes have been introduced

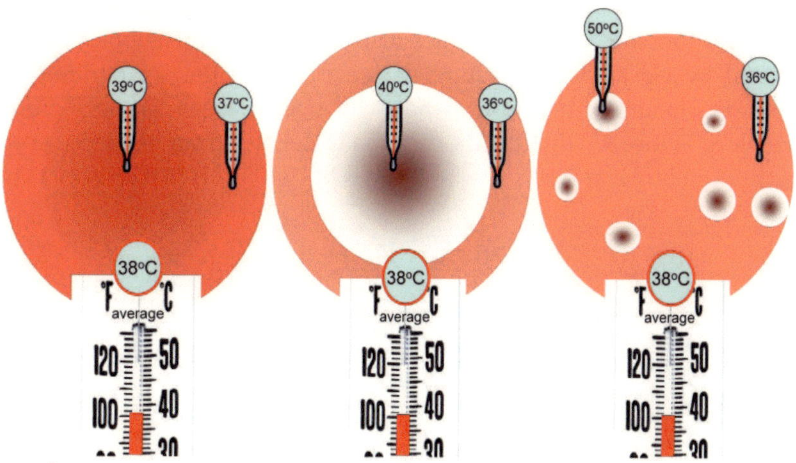

Figure 8. The average temperature cannot characterize the thermodynamic situation. The internal temperature differences can serve as driving forces of various processes on the same average temperature of the system

Herewith we do not discuss the extreme temperature facilities in local treatments, the ablative techniques with high temperature (heat-ablation, [75]) or low-temperature (cryo-ablation, [76]).

1.4. Technical history of local hyperthermia in oncology

Despite the hyperthermia was among the very first medical treatments in human medicine, this approach has ambivalent evaluation as a therapy. While it is popular in households to "treat" many diseases like common cold, pain, various orthopedic problems, etc., it is on the periphery of the serious medical therapies. This frustration characterizes the complete history of hyperthermia in medicine, and explains why hyperthermia has no well- deserved place in the medical armory to treat various diseases.

At the end of the 19th century, energy delivery by electromagnetic fields became possible; but the real technical revolution of the heat therapies was when the modern microwave heating was developed, and applied in medicine from the middle of the 20th century. This focused, temperature-based deep heating became one of the line (focused local/regional heating), while the other was the whole body heating with various methods. In local heating, the paradigm is to reach the appropriate temperature locally.

Nevertheless, the intensive use of hyperthermia in oncology began in the last third of the 20th century. The first symposium on oncological hyperthermia was held in Washington DC, USA in 1975; and the second one in Essen, Germany in 1977. Both conferences were supported by the local scientific communities. We may consider the birth of the modern oncological hyperthermia from this time on, and take it as a strong candidate and a member of the acknowledged tumor therapies.

The original idea of the hyperthermia was the "fire by fire" concept: set a controlled contra-fire depleting the possible fire-supply, blocking the coming large bush-fire endangering a house. The heated tumor is forced to higher metabolism; high metabolic rate of the cancer lesion is gained by elevated temperature. However, when the surrounding is intact, it delivers the same amount of nutrients as before, it does not deliver more glucose for the forced metabolism Figure **9**. The tumor very quickly deflates from nutrients, empties all its energies, suffers and burns away.

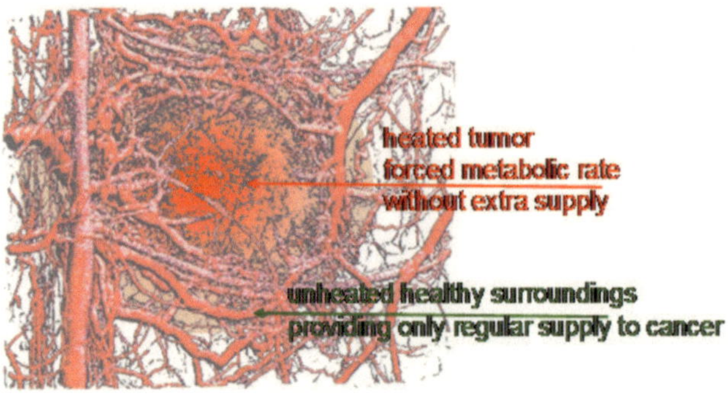

Figure 9. The focused local heating situation, expecting the locality for longer time

Indeed, there are many factors showing the validity of this assumption, but the breakthrough to accept the method widely hasn't been reached in the long historic period. The appropriate temperature selectively administered in the tumor still cannot be reached. This fact forms a lot of questions in the published literature:

- Is the community of radiation oncologist ready for clinical hyperthermia? [77];
- What happened to hyperthermia and what is its current status in cancer treatment? [78];
- Where there's smoke, is there fire? [79];
- Should interstitial thermometry be used for deep hyperthermia? [80];
- If we can't define the quality, can we assure it? [81];
- Is there a future for hyperthermia in cancer treatment? [82];
- What is against the acceptance of hyperthermia? [83];
- Progress in hyperthermia? [84];
- Prostate cancer: hot, but hot enough? [85];
- Is heating the patient a promising approach? [86];
- Hyperthermia: has its time come? [87].

Many of the researchers evaluating the capabilities of oncological hyperthermia share the opinion expressed in the editorial comment of the European Journal of Cancer in 2001: the biological effects are impressive, but physically the heat delivery is problematic. The hectic results are repulsive for the medical community. The opinion, to blame the "physics" (means technical insufficiency) for inadequate treatments is general in the field of oncological hyperthermia, formulated the following statement: "The biology is with us, the physics are against us [82]. In the latest oncological hyperthermia consensus meeting the physics was less problematic. However, in accordance with the many complex physiological effects, a modification was proposed: "The biology and the physics are with us, but the physiology is against us" [88].

The most problematic issues have always been technical: how to heat in depth, locally focused, being selective for malignant cells, and the other side: how to control it and how to measure the efficacy of the treatment? Even when the local treatment is focused well, the temperature by its way tends to be equalized; the focus is extended by time, due to the very effective heat-exchanger – the blood-stream. The heated tumor strongly exchanges its heat with its healthy surrounding, extending the focus gradually and increasing the local blood-flow. This unwanted effect has some problematic consequences:

1. The heating focus is growing, it is not correct any more, so the healthy tissue is also heated up,
2. The distributed spots of the tumour (local metastases) can be covered only by on average, covering the area completely with the intermediate healthy parts,
3. The natural movements of the patients (i.e. due to the breathing) cannot be followed by the focus,
4. The blood-flow is increased locally, supplying the tumor with nutrients (first of all with glucose) and the higher temperature gains the local metabolic rate as well,
5. The intensive tumor-metabolism produces high level of lactic acid in the volume, which lowers the pH and forces the blood to buffer it. The blood starts to shift to alkaline and

the alkaline blood delivers more oxygen to the volume, by positive feedback mechanism,

6. The intensive blood-flow has a risk of the further disseminations and metastases,
7. The heat flow to the surroundings can damage the healthy neighbourhood,
8. Enlarging the sphere having certain temperature gradients increases the area of the injury current which supports the cell-proliferation,
9. The growing heated volume is uncontrolled, the vigilance of the process becomes complicated,
10. The incident energy might burn the skin, so surface cooling is necessary. The heat-sink of the surface decreases the incident power, but its quantity has no measurable parameters. This is the reason why only the temperature in the target will orientate the control of the treatment process,
11. The necessary temperature measurement is mostly invasive, which could cause many complications, including inflammation, bleeding, infection, dissemination of the cells, etc.
12. The microwave heating might do harm not only by its unwanted hot-spots, but also with its ability to create carcinogens in situ.

These technical challenges are definitely complex, and can make the actual hyperthermia treatment uncontrolled. This branch of problems could be the reason for some controversial results and the weak acceptance of the conventional hyperthermia among medical experts.

2. Malignant diseases – To heat or not to heat?

The popular terms *"heat-dose"*, *"temperature-gain"*, *"thermal dose"*, *"energy-intake"*, *"energy-dose"* may have different definitions in various individuals who use them. Our first task is to clarify the differences between these (in popular literature many times used as synonyms) terms.

Nevertheless, the temperature is not heat, not even energy. Temperature, in this sense, is a hypothetical value of the average energy. Particles have various energies and it could happen no any individual particle has such definite energy as the average (the temperature) indicates.The temperature is an average; we can define it only on a large number of participating units (particles). The average energy of the various particles at normal human body temperature (ideal thermodynamic model) is ~ 2.5 kJ/mol. This relatively large energy is embedded and blocked in the actual system. (It is so large, that if it could be liberated within one second, the obtained power would be 2.5 kW/mol.) This average thermal energy limits the internal bonds and interactions, because any lower energy bond will be destroyed by this thermal background. This internal energy could make abrupt changes by such chemical reactions, by which activation energy is smaller (or equal) than the actual thermal average energy. The weakest bonds in life are the hydrogen-bridges, having 18 kJ/mol in ice [89] and ranging 3-30 kJ/mol in various compounds in living objects [90].

Pumping heat into a system can increase its temperature. The result of heating is not a definite temperature. The resulting temperature always greatly depends on how the heat is consumed in the system, and how the system transfers this energy to its environment.

Pumping the same energy into identical volumes, but having different surfaces, the temperature increase will be definitely different, because the volume is differently cooled down by the environmental conditions. Furthermore, the heat can make structural or other rearrangement in the material, it could be transformed into work without temperature increase of the system. For example: melting the ice absorbs energy without temperature increase, still it is completely transformed into liquid. The heat, which is pumped in to the system at this phase transition does not increase the temperature; its energy is used completely to change the structure of the material from solid to liquid.

Other clear example is the Sun radiation to the Earth. A huge part of the energy of the Sun's radiation is converted to the meteorology (like wind or rain), their mechanical effects (like waves in the ocean, like distortion of the rocks). The Sun's energy is the solely energy-source of the life processes, and this energy of the Sun makes our oil reserves, allowing us to use this energy for various applications in our everyday life. So the simple electromagnetic radiation (the spectrum of the Sun) is converted to the various kinds of energies in the Earth. Only a fraction of the radiation is realized as heat and rising temperature.

Other simple example is the human energy-intake: a female adult eats ~1600 kcal/day. When she takes more energy a day, it will not change her body temperature at all. However, when she gets this energy from radiation, she will starve, despite of the fact that she gets more energy than she could take from nutrients.

When there are so serious differences between the heat and temperature, why do we confuse them? The main reason is: we fix our attention to simple situations when we heat such materials which distribute the energy immediately all over the system, making thermal equilibrium without internal work (reactions, dilatation, etc.) in the system. In such cases, of course, all the heat energy increases the internal energy of the system, and so it is distributed in it, and proportionally increases its temperature.

When we fix our attention to such systems, like heating water in its liquid form, the applied heat and temperature are strictly proportional in a certain interval (when the water is definitely liquid). However, we have a problem even in this simple system. When a phase-transition occurs, we lose this proportionality completely. At the/a study of hyperthermia in living systems, we have to well distinguish the overall energy, the heat energy and the temperature (which is not energy) from each other.

"The use of thermodynamics in biology has a long history rich in confusion." [91]. The main complication is the fact that life cannot be studied isolated from its environment, and so the energetically open system could lead to numerous uncertainties, leading sometimes to mystification as well.

2.1. The heating paradigm

The idea of the local heating effect to burn-out the energy sources of the malignancy has dominated the hyperthermia applications from the time of Hippocrates. Its operation measured by modern methods [92], shows definite decrease of ATP and increase of lactic acid in tumors after hyperthermia treatment. The ATP depletion makes a heavy ionic-imbalance in cells [93]. Furthermore, the increased temperature can slow down or even arrest DNA replication, [94], [95].

Higher tissue temperature stimulates the immune system [94] with observed increase in natural killer cell activity [96]. Moreover, the elevated temperature distributes tumor-specific antigens on the surface of various tumor cells [97] and assists in their secretion into the extracellular fluid [98], triggering the immune reactions against the malignant cell [94].

Hyperthermia has shown significant pain-reduction during treatments [99]. This makes this method excellent to improve the quality of the patient's life and it can be applied as palliative treatment when the curative solution does not work.

Multiple effects can be counted by homogeneous heating the living organisms completely or locally. One of the decisional factors is the vasodilatation. The induced vasodilation increases:

- Blood flow
- Capillary filtration
- Capillary pressure
- Oxygen perfusion

These induce the following actions:

- Increases fibroblastic activity and capillary growth,
- Increases the oxygenation in the volume,
- Increases drug-delivery in the volume, when the drug is administered systemically,
- Increases the nutrition concentration in the volume,
- Increases the metabolic activity in the volume (higher quantity of nutrition, oxygen and higher local temperature),
- Increases the field-dependent effects, (membrane excitation, activation of signal pathways, etc.),
- Increases the effects on the blood-structure in the volume,
- Increases the micro vascular perfusion (circulation), nutrients, and phagocytes.

The chemo-drugs are delivered to the tumor by the blood-stream. Higher local temperature increases the microcirculation in the heated volume, [100], [101], [102], [103], [104], [105], [106], [107], [108], [109]; and with this it enhances the efficacy of the conventional chemo-therapies [110]. The synergy between heat-treatment and many of the chemotherapies is well-established [111], [112].

Further support is that the hot drug is more reactive [113], providing excellent possibility to synergy, which is even more effective when we consider the accelerated drug metabolism and gained pharmacokinetic parameters. The thermo-chemotherapy results in a better therapeutic effect and it increases the target specificity as well as it reduces the systemic side effects [114], [115]. In some cases the low-dose chemotherapy could be used [116], [117] with the hyperthermia promotion, it is also applied in low-dose metronomic chemo-regulation,

[118]. Furthermore, hyperthermia acts in G0 phase of cell-division which makes the action of conventional therapies possible on these cells too.

For radiotherapies, the increased microcirculation sensitizes the effect of ionizing radiation [119]. The primarily applied heat can enhance the effect of ionizing radiation because of the higher oxygen concentration in the area. Furthermore, the most efficient action of hyperthermia is in S-phase [120], which well completes the weak effect of radiotherapy in this phase of the cell-cycle. The heat-induced decrease of the DNA-dependent protein-kinase (DNA-PK), [121] is also a radio-sensitizer. Sensitizing the classical ionizing-radiation by hyperthermia has been well-known [122], [123] for a long time, and different review articles have summarized this knowledge [124], [125], [126], [127]. The advantage of combining heat-treatment with the classical ionizing-radiation is unambiguous, [128], [129], [84], the synergy between the methods is well known [130], [122] and successfully applied [131], [132], [106].

Hyperthermia has also been found to have pronounced advantages for surgical interventions. Through hyperthermia induced inhibition of angiogenesis and heat entrapment, the outline of the tumor often becomes pronounced and the size of the tumor often shrinks, making previously dangerous operations possible [133]. The feasibility of the preoperative application for locally advanced rectal cancer is well shown in a Phase II clinical trial [134]. Postoperative application of hyperthermia has also been thought to prevent relapses and metastatic processes [132]. Intraoperative radiofrequency ablation [135] and local hyperthermia [136] have also been used to improve surgical outcomes.

The combination of hyperthermia with gene-therapy also looks very promising, as shown by the successful combination of hyperthermia with HSP-promoter mediated gene therapy in cases of patients with advanced breast cancer [137]. Hyperthermia improved the results of the HSP-promoter gene therapy by inducing local HSP production and by enhancing the local rate of release from liposome [138]; it was also helpful in the double suicide gene transfer into prostate carcinoma cells [139]. It was proven that this combination therapy was highly selective for mammary carcinoma cells. Also the heat-induced gene expression could be an excellent tool in the targeted cancer gene therapy [140].

Combination with hormone therapies is also a vivid method, applied for prostate [141]; and in melanoma treatment [112]. Enzyme-therapy [142], photodynamic therapy [143], gene therapy [144], immune- [145] and other supportive-therapies [146] are used in combination with hyperthermia.

- All these factors position hyperthermia to one of the most effective treatments in oncology. Since these are mostly temperature dependent effects, an accelerated race has been started for the rising temperature and providing the highest available thermal support for the conventional therapies. Most of the applied electromagnetic techniques started to gain their power over 1 kW, providing powerful radiative, capacitive and magnetic effects to increase the temperature in depth in the targeted tissue.

2.2. Targeting complications

The large heating energy heats up the healthy surrounding as well, see Figure 10. The blood-flow will be enhanced, the nutrients supply will be higher and the result is the opposite of our aim. The situation becomes even worse by continuing the high-energy heating: the high blood-flow helps the dissemination [147], [148], [149] and could gain the metastases: Figure 11. With this, we can definitely worsen the survival and the quality of life of the patient. This problem gained the official policy in many oncological departments: avoid application of hyperthermia in oncotherapies.

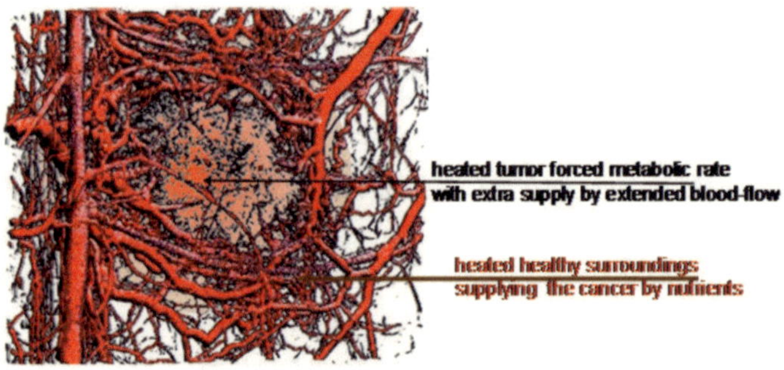

Figure 10. The real situation heats up the surroundings, the local heating does not remain locally focused

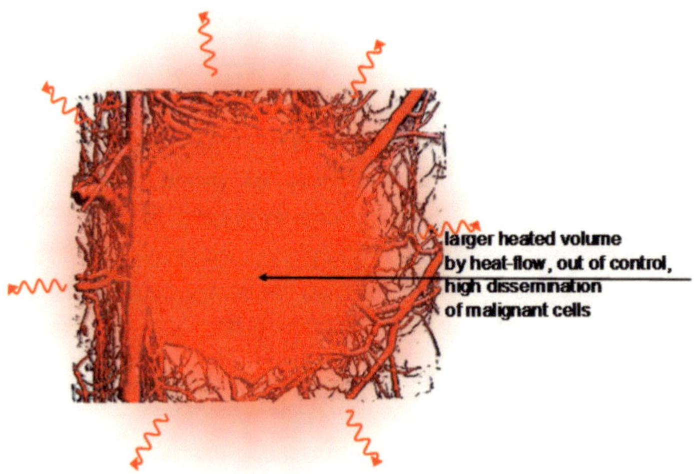

Figure 11. The large heated volume is not controlled from the focus, and makes the malignant dissemination possible by the high blood-flow in the healthy surroundings

It is plausible: the temperature spreads to the neighboring volumes independently of how precise the focus of the energy is. The energy can be focused, but the temperature seek is to be equalized and the focused energy-intake will heat up the tissue out of the focus too. This process is very rapid anyway in such good heat-conduction material as the living tissue. The cooling becomes even more emphasized, considering the physiological feedback mechanisms, which tries to reestablish the local homeostatic equilibrium by intensified blood-flow. The blood is on body temperature and this way it is an effective cooling media. This is the reason why huge energy is necessary to compensate the heat-loss of the tumor, and keeps the tumor temperature actually higher than its healthy environment.

A typical capacitive coupling solution pumps enormous energy, [150]. The rise of temperature, applying 1200 W energy after 45 min, was 4.8 °C but the reached focus differs with about 1 °C only from its untargeted neighborhood. In case of radiative applications the situation is the same. The temperature elevation in the tumor after 57 min was 4.2 °C; reached by as high power as 1300 W [151]. The overall heating obviously shows unwanted hot-spots. The elapsed time smears the relatively focused temperature. The temperature increase in the tumor was 4.2 °C on average, while in the surrounding muscle it was only 3.8 °C [151]. Is this the focus we expected? (Note, a standard speedy electric tea kettle uses 1300 W to boil a cup of water within a couple of minutes. The increase of the temperature for the ~ 0.3 liter water is ~75 ºC. We apply, in these cases, the same power reaching a temperature increase ~7 ºC during 60 minutes).

Further problems occur by a huge surface energy-density pumping high energy dose in depth. Due to the huge thermal load on the skin, more and more sophisticated methods have been/are being developed to cool the skin and to avoid its burn. A new technical race started: cooling the surface together with the increase of the incident power.

The maximal surface power density could be 1 W/cm² (10 kW/m²), for ~ 42 min, (see Figure **12.** [152]), which is a definite limit of the energy intake.

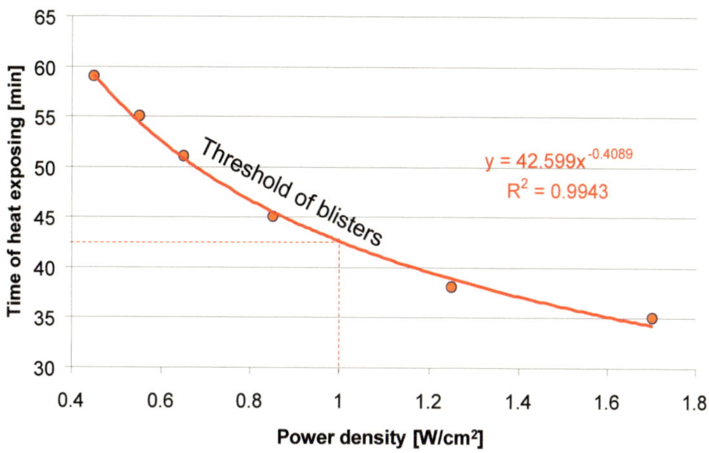

Figure 12. Threshold of surface blisters by power density through the dermal layers

In general, the injury level (threshold of blisters) depends on the full integral of the heat-flux, consequently, a longer treatment-time has lower power limit of use and for example, the 60 min treatment allows maximum 0.5 W/cm² without surface toxicity. Cooling is applied in most of the technical solutions to avoid the surface burn from overheating, see Figure 13.

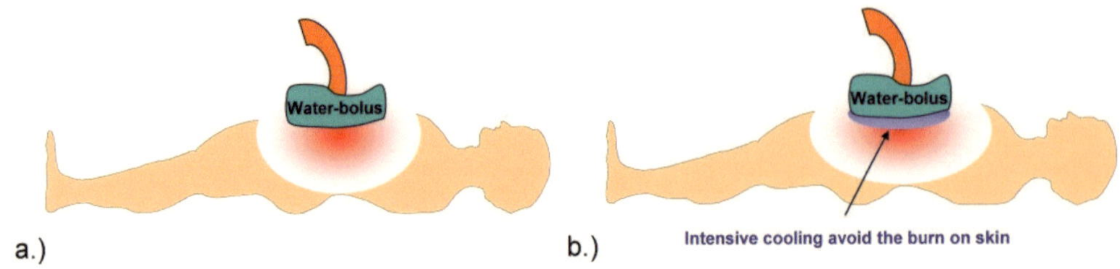

Figure 13. The incident power can overcome the threshold of blisters (a). Appropriate surface cooling is introduced to avoid this burn (b)

The surface cooling has a double effect: it cools down the surface taking away the surface energy to avoid the burn and to keep the heat-sensors (which are located in the near-surface subcutaneous area) of the body in the pleasant range of feeling.

However, the surface cooling creates serious problems too:

It makes the control of the energy intake ambiguous, no precise dose can be measured by the forwarded power. When the forwarded dose is 100 W, the cooling is 50W and the intensive cooling of the blood circulation on the surface is 30W and then maximum 20W can be absorbed in the target (see Figure 14.).

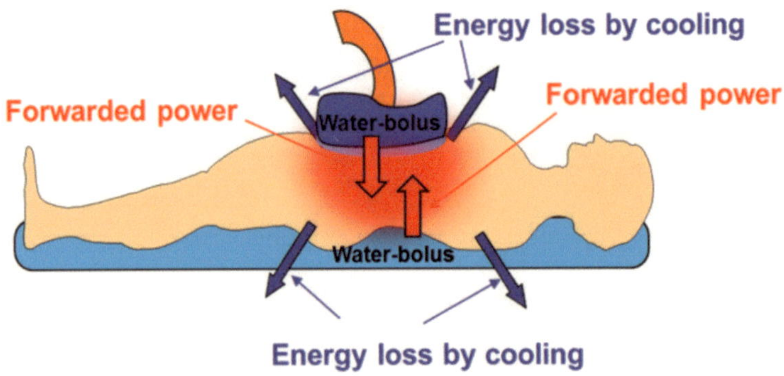

Figure 14. The forwarded power and the cooling power work oppositely. No idea about the real power pumped into the body

The high energy loss in the surface area is mainly due to the adipose layers, which are good electric- and heat-isolators [153]. Their isolation ability depends on their thickness, and it is controlled by the blood perfusion. When we cool down the surface, the homeostatic control will increase the isolating layer (see Figure 15.) by reducing the blood-flow in the area.

There is a misleading competition on the power, which is applied for local hyperthermia. The subcutane adipose tissue is an electric- and heat-flow blockade, and its conductivity decides the current transport at a fixed power transmission. The applied voltage depends on the contact area and on the applied frequency as well. The available devices for local heating range from 150W to 2000W and, in fact, the local temperature in the tumor ranges between

40-45 °C. The local maximal temperature in most cases depends more on the patient than on the incident power. At the end, the origin of the heat-flow will not exceed the 1 W/cm² on average. The higher isolation will absorb more energy, and so we need more cooling for safety and so on, see Figure 16. It is a positive feedback regulation, requesting enormous energies.

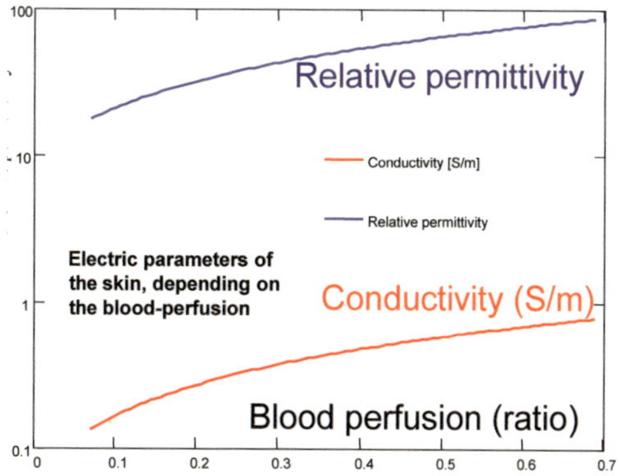

Figure 15. The blood-perfusion changes the conductivity and the relative permittivity as well

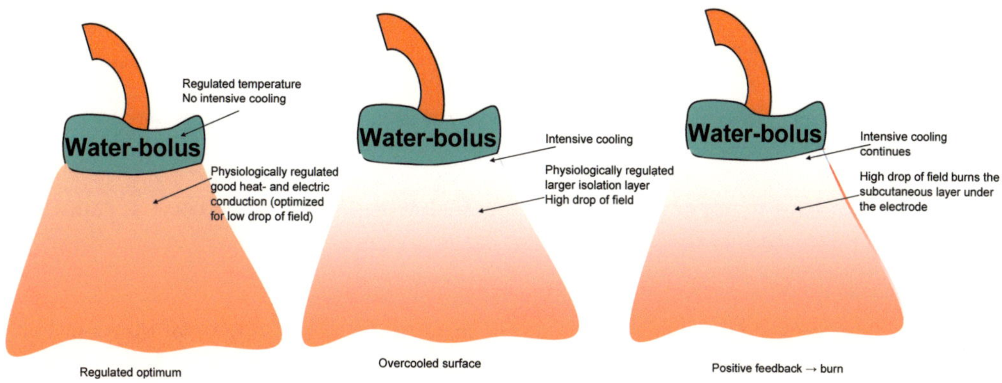

Figure 16. The physiologically regulated optimum is necessary for energy control. The large cooling grows the physiological reaction, creates a layer of isolation, which accelerates the dangerous surface overheating by positive feedback

Further complication in the control is the value of blood-flow, which is temperature dependent. The physiologic effects connected with the blood-flow are considered to be important and it is studied in details, [154], [155], [156], [157], [158].

The cooling energy is indefinite. The applied definite heating is modified with this energy-factor, making the really applied energy immeasurable. The hyperthermia dose must be the physically correct, accepted specific-energy absorption rate in J/kg, as we do it in the case of ionizing radiation too. The dosing in this case requests other, deep-inside measurement for indication of the process: the temperature as the character of the really absorbed energy. However, it is again problematic from a technical point of view: in fact, the absorbed energy distribution and the gained temperature are very different [159]. The reason is simple: provide the same energy to identical volume but the blood-flow is different in every case so it will result in different temperature. The physiology modifies the temperature! It is not possible to match the specific absorption rate (SAR) and the developed temperature.

The measurement of the power is missing, due to the fact that cooling is immeasurable and has a modifying effect on the temperature. This makes the temperature measurement in the target important, as this is the only parameter which gives us some idea about the absorbed energy, (see Figure 17.). This (generally invasive, measurement) makes it possible to have orienting value of the absorbed power in general, and sometimes it is important for safety to avoid the unwanted hot spots as well. For the successful energy dose control we have to know the energy taken away by the cooling. This underlines the importance of the control of the surface cooling triggered by the actual physiological conditions in the subcutaneous capillary bed.

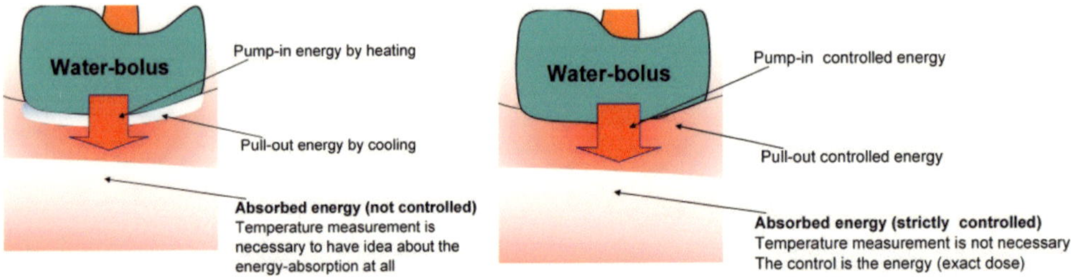

Figure 17. The control of both the energies together with the physiological parameters make oncothermia safe and effective

The full unsuccessful temperature focusing together with the intensive cooling process in conventional hyperthermia is, borrowing the words from Shakespeare, "much ado about nothing".

Dr. Storm a recognised specialist of hyperthermia formulated [78] a general opinion: "The mistakes made by the hyperthermia community may serve as lessons, not to be repeated by investigators in other novel fields of cancer treatment."

2.3. What to learn from nano-scale energy-liberation?

The general idea of microscopic heating is simple: the heating energy is not liberated in a sudden single step, but regulated and multiple small energy liberation does the same job, (see Figure 18). In our case, the forwarded energy selectively targets the most influential areas. Instead of the high, general energy pumping into the lesion, the energy is liberated at the membranes of the malignant cells.

The microscopic effects, instead of the large energy liberation, is one of the most update thinking in energy source developments.

The conventional engines in vehicles use the energy of explosion of different chemicals (e.g. petrol, diesel, kerosene). The explosion by a spark or heating over their activation energy liberates large energy in a short time, and only a small fraction of this could be applied beneficially, most of the energy is radiated, conducted or lost in various other ways. One of the largest losses is the heat-exchange by the high temperature, which somehow has to be used again (e.g. intercooler, turbo). The latest solution, however, is the set of microscopic explosions, promoting the chemical reactions individually by a membrane control (i.e. fuel cell solution) and using the energy step-by-step as a sum of the micro-reactions. The relatively low efficacy combusting engines are intended to be replaced by the fuel-cell energy-sources combined with electric motors, which are based on the membrane regulated microscopic reactions of gases. (Mostly hydrogen and oxygen gases are in use.)

In fact, life "invented" the controlled energy-liberation by micro-processes, blocking the sudden, explosion-like energy liberation, driving the processes small subsequent energy-conversion steps instead. In the living objects the energy is liberated gradually in a "ladder" of multistep processes, and this is also moderated by surface reactions.

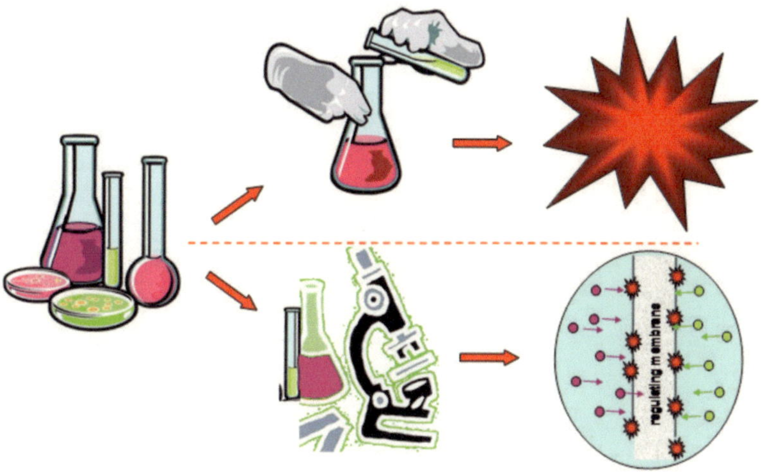

Figure 18. The difference between macro- and micro-liberation of energy. The latter is much more efficient.

The applied power and its efficacy are usually not connected. Good examples can be found in our everyday life, in systems like the standard light bulbs and the energy safe ones using a fraction of the power for the same light; or the various power-consumptions of cars, having equal performance, or the various fuel consumption of them having the same engine-power. The incandescent bulb creates light by high-temperature filament, which heats up the environment, having only 10% efficacy.

Fluorescent technology solves this task more smartly: it makes the energy-liberation selective where the effect radiates light only (see Figure 19.). Fluorescent particles turn the UV from mercury excitation to visible light. The full process has approx. 45% efficacy.

The LED technology is even more effective, because no intermediate mercury-plasma is used, direct annihilation of the electrons and electron-holes emit the light with over 90% efficacy! (see Figure 20.)

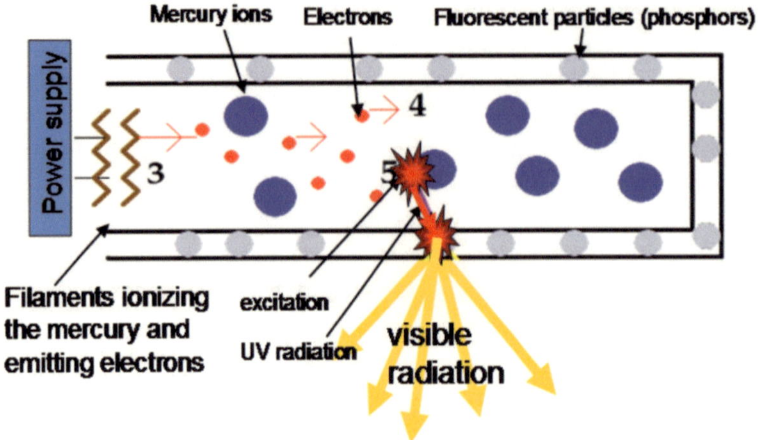

Figure 19. Fluorescent technology. The energy is liberated by micro-"explosions", excited by an UV radiation of the mercury-plasma

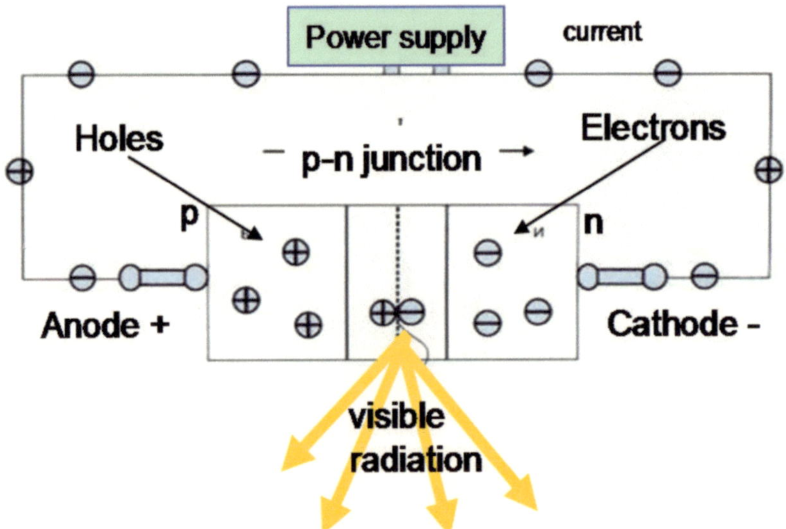

Figure 20. LED technology. The energy is liberated by micro-"explosions" by using the energy of the excited electrons

This way, the more intensive light (virtually higher temperature micro-explosions) need less energy by the block of the wasted energy to heat up the environment instead of the visible light emission: the same light-emission needs 60W, 13 W and 5 W in cases of incandescent, fluorescent or LED light-sources.

The present main-stream thinking of oncological hyperthermia is a typical loss of aims by illusions: the temperature only makes conditions that are implements and not the aim. The question "Tool or goal?" has become relevant to study the temperature alone. By a simple example of mixing the tool and the goal in our everyday life: the graduation is a tool for our professional life, however, when somebody regards the certificate of studies as a goal, its application, the aim of the study is lost.

Mixing the tool with the action creates false goal in hyperthermia application: increase the temperature alone. This "auto-suggestion" creates such a situation when magnetic resonant imaging (MRI) is applied to control the temperature during the treatment, instead of using this capable imaginary method to see what is happening in the tumor indeed.

3. Bioelectromagnetic selection – To select or not to select?

In hyperthermia applications the macroscopic heating centers on the equal (homogeneous) temperature of the entire targeted volume, irrespective of its content and the ratio of the tumor-cells in the target, (see Figure 21./a.). However, the target volume has only a small fraction of active malignant cells, and the heating process would be enough for those alone, avoiding heating (and wasting energy) to the other part of the target-volume. The micro-heating concept works differently, and heats the selected malignant cells only absorbing the energy non-equally in the target (see Figure 21/b.).

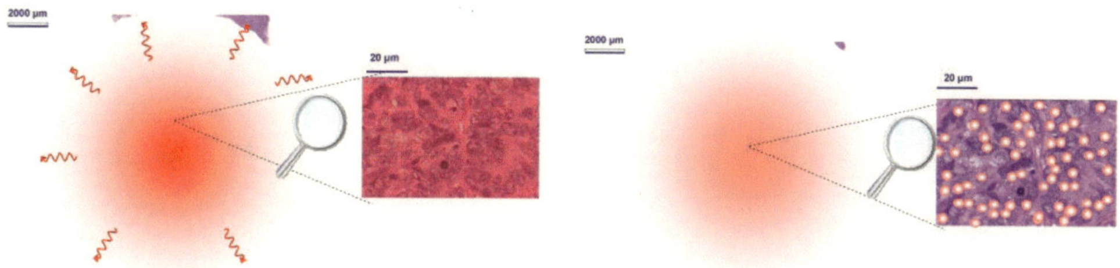

a.) b.)

Figure 21. The schematics of macroscopic and microscopic heating of tumor

In this case, the lost energy is minimal; the efficacy of the energy utilization and its control is maximal. The energy is concentrated in this case directly to the chemical reactions and does not involve the above listed losses. The energy liberated by the micro reactions is used for the desired job in full, while the explosion-like, huge energy-supply in short time cannot be used optimally, due to the intensity of the immediate offer for the available energy is too much for prompt use. This causes a large demand of waste and a low efficacy of the desired effect. The problem of the heating, however, is that it shows a false, specious effect of applications in biology. When the liberated energy is not used as active biochemical or biophysical driving-force then the waste appears as a simple growth of the temperature in the target. This deceptive illusion seems to have higher efficacy. This, of course, heats everything in the target. The excess energy is wasted in the neighborhood of the malignancy and gaining the average energy of all the parts in the target, irrespective its malignancy or its electrolyte state. This is a typical wasting of energy, using it for the actually not-necessary energizing of healthy parts. This massive heating forces the homeostatic feedback mechanisms acting against the growth of drastic temperature growths.

The oncological hyperthermia application, which uses the nano-scale heating technology (called oncothermia, [160]); the radiofrequency (RF) current flows through the chosen volume of the body (see Figure 22.), heating up the cell-membrane individually (see Figure 23.). The cell-membrane is a good isolator and so the current is most dense at the extracellular electrolyte in the immediate vicinity of the cells. Of course, when the absorbed energy is too much, the individual cellular-heating does not work, all the volume will be equally heated. This is again the declaration of the well- known rule: "the difference between the poison and the medicament is only their dose".

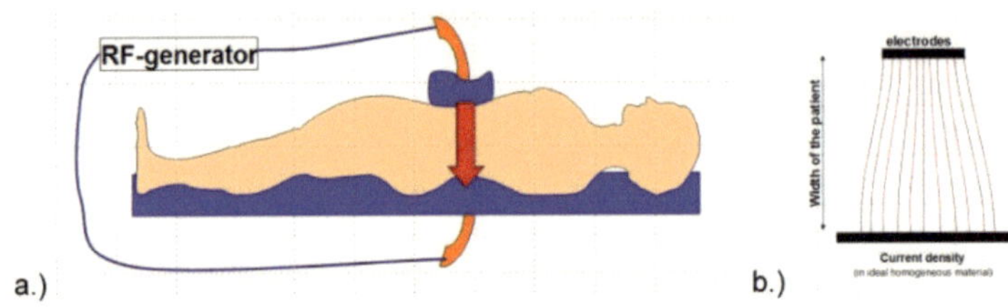

Figure 22. Both electrodes are always active, independently of its size or form. The current starts in one and ends on the other. The energy density is different, and many safety functions differ

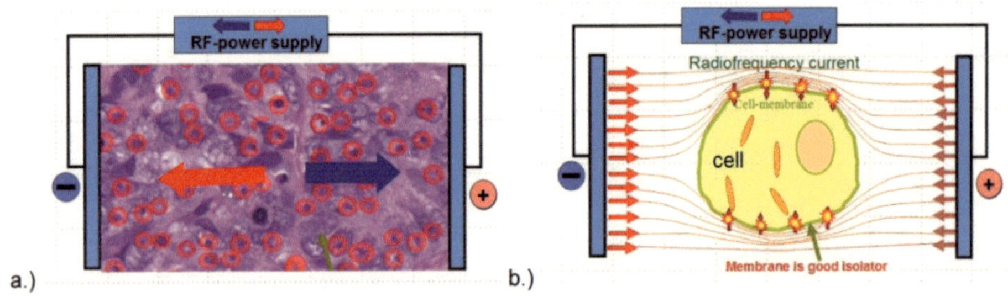

Figure 23. The selection mechanism of the optimally applied RF-current targets the cellular membrane, concentrates the energy in nano-range of the cell

Generally, a certain power interval is necessary for optimal efficacy, both the too high and the too low are non-optimal. The cars form a trivial example: the cold engine needs more fuel to be heated up for its optimal use, but it must be cooled down and kept in a definite range of temperature by a cooling system for its optimal work.

The average heating cannot produce high-efficacy. The high efficacy requests high selectivity for the accurate control of the process. The simple control of the average wastes a part of energy. This "waste" is expended energizing the particles, which are not involved in the desired process. The particles in the targeted process, which would like to have more power for the actual effect, have also the average only. Simple examples could be quoted from the everyday life again: when I would like to honor somebody's excellent work, it would be inefficient to honor everybody in average, being sure that the person whom the honor is due is also among the members of the group.

The proper selection has to choose not only the cells in general from the heated volume, but especially the malignant cells have to be selected from the target. This task could be solved using the specialties of malignant cells in comparison with their healthy counterparts.

3.1. Selection by Warburg's effect (conductivity selection)

As Otto Warburg discovered, the malignant cells behave completely differently from their healthy counterparts, [161], having mitochondrial dysfunction to produce ATP. (For this discovery a Nobel-prize was granted for him.) Warburg's work nowadays has its renaissance [162], [163]; showing the validity of the dominance of non-mitochondrial (fermentative) way of ATP production. The fermentative way of the metabolic ATP production is anyway "ancient" chemical reaction, which was characteristic at the beginning of the evolution of life, when the oxygen, the general electron acceptor was available only in a small amount in the atmosphere. It is the fermentative way to utilize the energy of glucose converting it into lactic acid (*$CH_3CHOHCOOH$*), producing only 2 ATPs in one cycle.

The metabolism in healthy cells is mainly governed by the convertible energy-source of ATP. The citrate (Krebs) cycle by mitochondria, the "energy plant" in cells, produces 36 ATPs with excellent efficacy with the help of oxygen (see Figure 24/a.). The fermentative ATP production is a low efficacy process in malignant cells, (see Figure 24/b.*)*, however, (due to its simplicity) it can occur in large amount, its overall energy-flux can be higher than obtained from the high efficacy process.

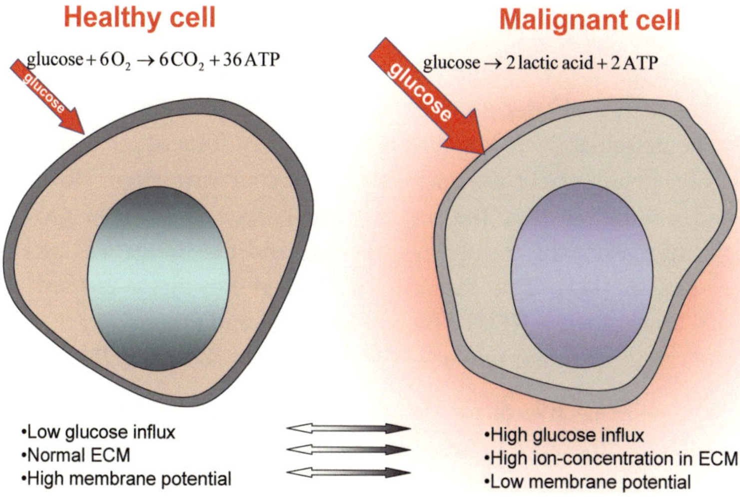

Figure 24. Differences in healthy and malignant cells

The malignant cells are in frequent and permanent cellular-division. The energy-consumption for the intensive division is higher than the energy requirement for the healthy cells in homeostasis. This is available only when the glucose intake is at least 18 times higher, because its ATP production is 18 times less than normal. This allows the cell to supply energetically all the normal processes and make the differentiation and development, the adaptation and evolution possible. This is a huge additional part of the glucose influx to the anyway high Warburg process. The higher glucose metabolism can be measured by positron emission tomography (PET) [164]. When we take the higher reproduction (proliferation) rate of malignant cells into account, (which requests more energy than for the cells in homeostasis), the final products ("waste") are produced intensively. Hence, these cells are surrounded by "waste" compounds, their extracellular electrolyte is denser in ions, and the pH in their vicinity is lower. Consequently, the higher metabolism increases the ion-transport and the ion-concentration in the area of the malignant cell, which lowers the impedance (gains the conductivity) of that volume. This irregular behavior can be measured and imaged by the Electric Impedance Tomography (EIT), [165]. One of the applications of this effect can be applied even in the prophylactics like mammography [166].

In consequence of the physical differences, the malignant cells are distinguishable by their biophysical parameters; their electric properties differ from normal. The main differences are:

- The efficacy of the ATP production in the cancerous cell is low. The large ATP demand for the proliferative energy-consumption allows less ATP for active membrane stabilization by K^+ & Na^+ transport, so the membrane potentiating weakens [167].
- The cellular membrane of cancerous cells differ electrochemically also from the normal and its charge-distribution also deviates [168].
- The membrane of the cancerous cell differs in its lipid and sterol content from their healthy counterpart [169].
- The membrane-permeability is changed by the above differences. In consequence of these, the efflux of the K+, Mg++ and Ca++ ions increase, while the efflux of Na+ decreases together with the water-transport from the cell. Therefore, the cell swallows, and its membrane potential decreases further [170]. (The efflux of K+ regulates the pH of the cell, takes the protons out from the cytosol). The concentration of Na+ increases in the cytosol, and parallel to this, the negative ion-concentration also grows on the glycocalix shell, decreasing the membrane potential and the tumor will be negatively polarized on average, [171]. This fact was well used for direct current treatment (electro-chemical cancer therapy (ECT)) by Nordenstrom and others.
- The conductivity (σ) of the tumor tissue will be higher than normal, [172].

The conductance (as a self-selective factor choosing optimal current path, see Figure 25.) ranges from 20% to 4000% difference between the healthy and malignant tissues. The data sporadically fluctuate, but generally the tumor has lower impedance than its healthy counterpart does! This is exactly what is used in the oncothermia technique.

There are numerous proofs of the conductive selection.

- In a simple theoretical investigation [173] an elliptical "tumor" is introduced into an otherwise homogeneous body. Making use of the appropriate Green's function, the changes in conductivity between the tumor and the surrounding region can be determined.
- A precise diagnostics has been established by careful calculation of electric impedance of human thorax as well [174], and the 3-D electrical impedance tomography is intensively studied, [165].

- The increase of the current density in the tumor can be visualized by the RF-CDI (radiofrequency current density image), which is a definite, MRI-conducted measurement of the real processes, [175], [176], [177], [178].

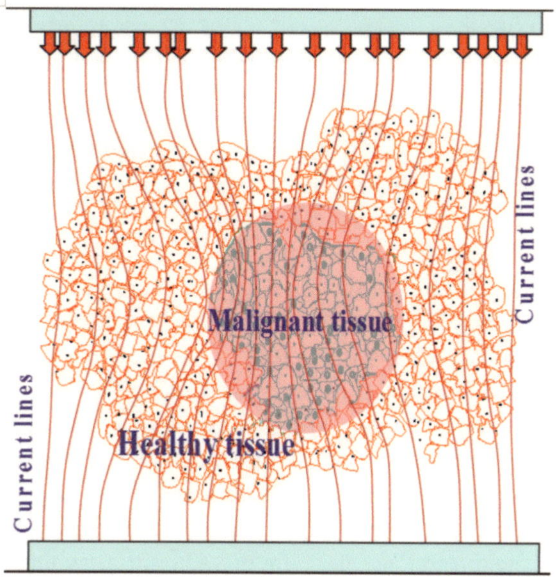

Figure 25. Effective and automatic focusing of oncothermia is a strong selective factor of the tumor and the malignant cells

Together with these effects, further add-ons are expected by oncothermia: the intensive heat transfer on the cellular membrane intensifies the ionic-transports [179], which (in positive feedback) changes the ionic motility and conductivity. In addition, the gain of the blood perfusion by the increasing temperature (below 39 °C) will lower the impedance (increase the conductance) [92], [180] which is an additional positive feedback selectivity at the beginning of the treatment. In the advanced cases, the blood-perfusion is increased by the neo-angio-genesis [181]. This extra perfusion (generally till T=39 °C) lowers the impedance (increases the conductivity), which is again a selectivity factor.

The positive feedback of growing temperature effectively increases the conductivity, [182]. The measured gain of the selectivity is 2% in °C, [183], which is in the range of 36→43 °C, that is 14% increase.

3.2. Selection by Szent-Gyorgyi's effect (dielectric selection)

The living material is not an ordered solid. Contrary to the crystals [184], it is hard to introduce the co-operation. The living matter is in aqueous solution, which is mostly well ordered, nearly crystalline (semi-crystalline, [185]) in the living state. This relative order formed the "dilute salted water" into the system having entirely different mechanical, chemical, physical, etc. behaviors from the normal aqueous solutions. Indeed, the important role in the living systems of the so-called ordered water was pointed out in the middle of the sixties, and later it was proven, [186]. At first the ordered water was suggested as much as 50% of the total amount of the water in the living bodies [187]. The systematic investigations showed more ordered water [188], [189] than it was expected before. Probably the ordered water bound to the membrane is oriented (ordered) by the membrane potential, which probably decreases the order of the connected water. Consequently, it increases the electric permeability of the water [190], and so decreases the cell-to-cell adhesion and causing cell-division and proliferation [190].

According to the Warburg's effect the metabolism gradually favors the fermentation in malignancy. The end-products of both the metabolic processes are ions in the aqua-based electrolyte. The oxidative cycle products dissociate like $6CO_2+6H_2O \rightarrow 12H^+ + 6CO_3^{2-}$ while the lactate produced by fermentation dissociates: $2CH_3CHOHCOOH \rightarrow 2CH_3CHOHCOO^- + 2H^+$. Assuming the equal proton production (by more intensive fermentation energy-flux) the main difference is in the negative ions. The complex lactate-ion concentration grows rapidly and increases its osmotic pressure. Keep the pressure normal, the dissolvent (the monomer water) has to be increased as well, seeking to solvent by non-ordered water. Indeed, it is measured in various malignancies that the water is changed to be disordered, [191], [192], [193], so in these cases the ordered water concentration in cancerous cells is smaller than in their healthy counterpart. Consequently, the hydrogen ionic transmitter becomes weak, the removal of the hydrogen ions becomes less active. This decreases the intracellular pH and the proton gradient in mitochondria, which directly worsens the efficacy of ATP production. To compensate the lowered proton-gradient, the membrane potential of mitochondria grows. This lowers the permeability of the membrane, decreases the mitochondrial permeability transition (MPT), which have a crucial role in apoptosis, [194], [195]. (The high mitochondrial membrane potential and low K-channel expression were observed in cancerous processes, [196].). These processes lead to apoptosis resistance, and for the cell energizing the ATP production of the host cell (fermentation) becomes supported. The free-ion concentration increases in the cytoplasm, and so the HSP chaperone stress proteins start to be produced. This process needs more ATP as well as it is anti-apoptotic agent, so the process could lead to the complete block of apoptosis. Rearranging (disordering) the water structure needs energy [197]. It is similar to the way the ice is melted with latent heat from zero centigrade solid to liquid with unchanged temperature conditions. This drastic change (phase transition) modifies the physical properties (like the dielectric constant) of the material without changing the composition (only the microscopic ordering) of the medium itself.

The decisional role of the two metabolic pathways (the oxidative and the fermentative) was studied by Szent-Gyorgyi [190], having an etiology approach and using additional formulation. His interpretation describes the cellular states by two different stages. The alpha-state of the cell is the fermentative status, (see Figure 26.).

This was general in the early development of life, when free oxygen was not available. The aggressive electron acceptor was not present [198]. In this stage, only simple, primitive life forms could exist. The main task was to maintain life with their unlimited multiplication. This state was only reproduction oriented, to develop complex structures and complicated work-division was not possible. All the living objects in alpha state are autonomic, they compete with each other and cooperative communication does not exist between them. With the later presence of free oxygen beta-state of life was developed. The oxygen made it possible to exchange higher value of electric charges, the unsaturated protein allowed more complex interactions and started the diversity of life. The cells, in this state, are cooperative, the task from the only multiplication became more complex, including the optimal energy-consumption, the diversity for optimal adjustment to life. This is the phase, which integrated the mitochondria for oxidative ATP production, and so produced the energy in high efficacy.

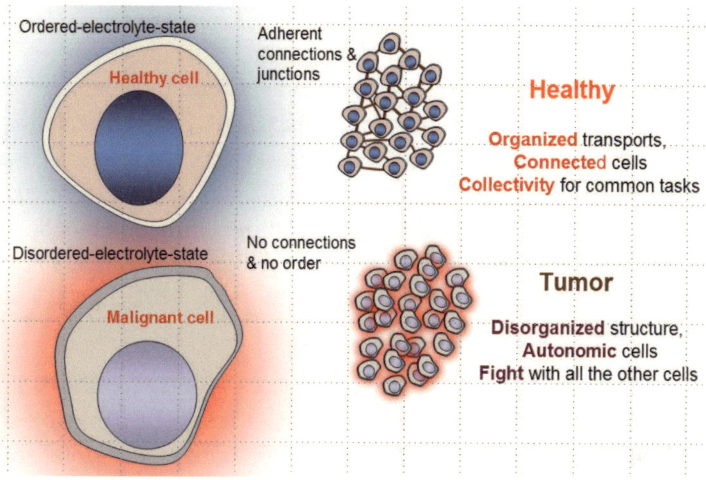

Figure 26. The dielectric (order) differences between healthy and malignant cell-environments

The historical development of the life from alpha- to beta-stages has been generalized [190], introducing the same states for the actual stage of the cells in developed complex living systems. (Further on Greek letters α and β will be used to denote those states.)

The highly organized living objects are mainly built up from cells in β-state. Their cell-division becomes controlled. This control is mandatory, because the division needs autonomic actions, the cooperative intercellular forces slack, a part of the structure has to be dissolved and rearranged, so the cell in division state is again in non-differentiate state, similar to the α one.

The α state is the basic status of life. In this status the highest available entropy is accompanied by the lowest available free-energy. All complex living systems could easily be transformed into this basic state when it becomes instable. Then by the simple physical constrains (seek to low free energy and to high entropy) the cells try (at least partly) realize the α-state again. Once more, the system (or a part of it) contains cells with high autonomy and proliferation-rate. By simple comparison of Szent-Gyorgyi's states and Warburg's metabolic pathways are common: the α- and β-states correspond with the fermentative and oxidative metabolism, respectively. In other words, α-state prefers the host cell ATP production (anaerobic) but when the perfect mitochondria function works, that is β-state.

These states are mixed (the cell works in both metabolic activities) and it is only a question of quantity in their category. In normal homeostasis the β-state characteristics is about 70%. The actual balance fixes the actual status. The balance could be formulated by the cell status of co-operability ($\alpha \leftrightarrow \beta$); or formulated by metabolic ways (*fermentation* ↔ *oxidation*) or could be formulated with the acting parts of metabolism: (*host-cell* ↔ *mitochondrion*). The meaning of all the formulations is equal: the actual energetic state is described. Note the interesting relation between the energy flux and co-operability. The high energy-flux makes the cells less cooperative and more primitive, while the low energy-flux makes the cells not only cooperative but also sophisticated, highly effective in energy production and in environmental adaptation as well. (It also has interesting similarity with the organizing of societies [199], but it is outside our present topic.)

Differences of the metabolic processes of vertebrates and invertebrates are (terrestrial, pelagic and benthic) well mirrored in the scaling exponent, [200]. The benthic invertebrates (n=215) have the lowest average scaling exponent (p_{mean}=0.63, [near to ⅔], CI_{mean}=0.18), which metabolizes basically on anaerobic way, [201], while all studied animals (n=496) have (p_{mean}=0.74, [near to ¾], CI_{mean}=0.18), [200]. The scaling of the metabolic activity is also different in mitochondrial or non-mitochondrial metabolism. The mitochondrial metabolism is always aerobic, its scaling exponent is nearly p=¾, [202], [243], while the non-mitochondrial respiration scaling is near to ⅔ [203].

One question arises immediately: what mechanism makes control on the balance of β-and α-states in the highly developed living objects? The electromagnetic behavior of electrolytes in living systems might give us the answer [204]. The cooperative cells mostly run on oxidative metabolism, and their division is controlled by the cells in their neighborhood. There are two basic reasons for normal cellular division, and it could be a regular division keeping the homeostasis of the given tissue, replacing the elder cells with young daughter cells, or it could be a forced, constrained division (like by wound-healing, reparations, embryonic development, constrained tissue-specific cell-production, etc.). The questions are: which process starts the division and which finishes it?

It is easy to start the division. The cell-division certainly requires extra energy, much larger than it is in normal conditions. This could be a mechanism described above: the changing concentration of one or more components needs more dissolvent, which is provided by the order-disorder transition of the intracellular aqueous electrolyte as well as the osmotic water-flow through the cellular membrane. The concentration misbalance can be created by outside stimuli (like injury currents) or by inside enrichment of a component due to aging or to metabolic misbalance. The order-disorder water transition does not only change the hydrogen-ion diffusion, but it also changes the dielectric constant of the medium [204]. The more disordered liquid increases the dielectric constant (in other words, the ability of electric isolation increased). This is directly connected with the promoted charge-division and the suppressed polymerization activity in subcellular level, creating positive feedback to the fermentation processes. The balance is broken, and turned to the phase where the α-state is dominant. It is not necessarily a malignant transition. This happens with any regular cell division as well. This is the "motherhood" of the cell, making it possible to "deliver" the daughter cells. The "individualism" of the mother-cell is explainable with the extreme high energy demand of the division process. When the daughter cells appear, they must accept the previous order. Their "infancy" is normal, as the "babyhood" is normal after the deliveries. The "babyhood" period has to be limited in time, and the newly born cell has to find its normal collective function. Consequently, the process might go wrong, if after finishing the division, the daughter cells do not find the way of the co-operability and the β-state again. When it is not the case, the cells are blocked in the α-state, their proliferation becomes uncontrolled. This unfortunate case, however, is not a simple process originated from one single defect. It is a disturbance of a complex controlling mechanism [190], which well correlates anyway with the single "renegade cell" concept [205], showing a long process to produce "a renegade cell" as the ancestor of the billion-cell group called cancer. According to the epidemiological research, for a complex damage to occur and for the cancer to develop at least five different mutations have to be coincidently present to be malignant. [206].

Again we are back to the main question: what is the mechanism to re-establish the β-state after the division of the cell. We think, that the down-regulation of the energy-flux has the same active elements as the up-regulation had at the start of the division. The clue is again the order-disorder transformation in the aqueous solution. As we told, at the beginning of the division, a huge energy has to be ready to supply the process, a large number of proteins and other cellular elements (lipids, enzymes, etc.) have to be produced, and all need ATP desperately. In α-sate the conditions are ready for that. When the division is over, two new daughter cells appear, the energy-consumption drastically drops to the normal level of the two cells. The doubled cytoplasm and all the cellular elements had enough dissolvent capacity even in the ordered water case. The hydrogen-bridge proton bifurcation can be reorganized, there are no opposite environmental driving forces. The sudden doubling of the cellular elments cools down the liquid to solid. It goes through the same phase transition (disorder-order transition) as it was (only the opposite direction) when the division started. This again (like in the liquid phase transitions) lowers the free energy, and in all (together with the environment, where the extra heat is radiated) increases the entropy. Note, the entropy apparently decreases (information build up) in the local cellular level, the overall conditions have to be considered for the full picture.

As we showed, the metabolic pathways could drastically modify the development of the cell, and it could be the primary source of the malignant deviations. The balance of the oxidative and fermentative metabolism tunes the cellular ability to behave collectively or constrict autonomy, being individual. These conditions of course well depend on the energy (and signaling) exchange of the cell with its actual environment. The intracellular transport properties also have to be different at changing metabolic pathway. The intensive energy flux of the fermentative metabolism increases the liberated heat in the cell, and so the temperature gradient between the extra- and intracellular compartments. The growing temperature difference could reach a critical threshold, when the heat flow turns from conductive to convective [207]. (This phenomenon works like the well-known Benard instability, [208].) The convective way promotes the ionic flows through the cellular membrane increasing the glucose permeability and so supports the fermentation way of metabolism together with the changes of the intracellular circulations, [209], [210]. This complex change could down-regulate the mitochondrial oxidative metabolism.

At the divisional processes the intracellular flows and all pathway activities are probably higher both at regular and at malignant cell-division. Possibly the order-disorder transition of the aqueous solution also has a role in the changes [211].

However, finishing the division, the daughter cells are separated, a higher surface suddenly appears and the separated volumes limit the intracellular flows and change the order of structure as well. It decreases the gradient through the membrane. This regulates the heat-flow through the cellular membrane and changes the energy-exchange from convective to the conductive one again [207]. The conductive heat-exchange does not support the intensive diffusion of the large-molecule glucose, so the oxidative way becomes necessary and regular. The two daughter cells have less than half energy-consumption (each) than it was requested by the mother cell. It is because the mother cell was large (doubled its volume) and was intensively producing various elements to complete the daughter cells. Instead of the division conditions where the high energy-request gained the energy-demand and preferred the high-energy flux fermentative metabolism, the normal homeostatic conditions will dominate again.

The significantly larger permittivity and conductivity in tumor-tissue in vitro is explained on this basis, [212]. Both the conductivity and dielectric differences between the healthy- and tumor-tissues at the applied 13.56 MHz frequency in most cases of the malignancies are over 15% [213], [172]. It is clinically proven, that the cancerous and healthy tissues of the hepatic tumors are significantly different [214]. Also the VX-2 carcinoma can be measured [215]: rabbit-liver at low frequency in vivo had a conductivity 6-7.5 times higher, permittivity 2-5 times lower than in the healthy parts (impedance difference is about 600%), while for 10 MHz region it is 200%. With impedance tomography we can make a distinction between the living and necrotic malignancy as well, [214]; both the conductivity and permittivity are higher in the malignant liver, but the frequency dependence of necrotic tissue differs.

The dielectric properties are also distinguishable by the water content of the malignant tissue, which is higher than that of their healthy counterpart. The proliferating cells control their cell-volume by their water content, in the malignant growth [216], and this effect increases the conductivity and generally the dielectric properties in the given tissue.

The high dielectric constant allows the additional selection (focusing): the higher dielectric constant absorbs more from the RF-energy, (see Figure 27.).

3.3. Selection by order-disorder effect (fractal physiology selection)

The non-equilibrium phenomena is well formulated in the description of the Avrami-equation [217], pioneered by Kolmogorov [218], by Johnson & Mehl [219] and by others, [220], [221]. The description could serve as a mathematical model for different biological processes, [222], [223]. Experimental data which were collected by Cope [224], [225], and by others [226], [227], show a definite universality to describe the real processes.

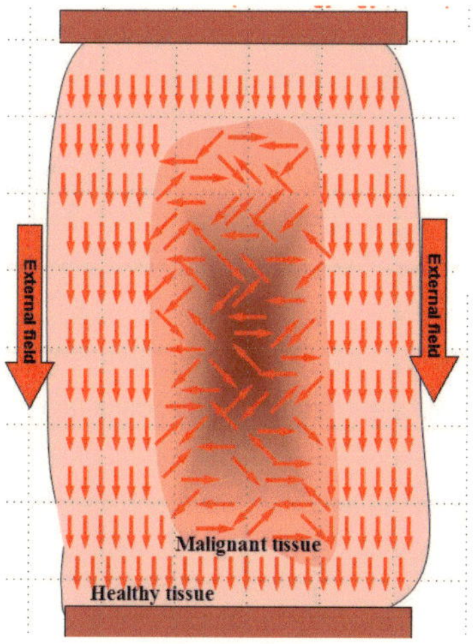

Figure 27. The disordered state could absorb more form the applied electric field energy than the ordered one

The modern physiology is an essentially interdisciplinary subject, combining the knowledge of various fields, like the electronic structure approach of solid-state physics (e.g. Szent-Gyorgyi, [228], [229]), the superconductivity (e.g. Cope, [230]), the electromagnetism (e.g. Liboff, [231], [232]), the thermodynamics (e.g. Schrodinger, [233], Katchalsky & Curran [234]), etc. Various modern approaches were developed in the last decades based on this complexity, like self-organization ([235], [236],), fractal physiology ([237], [238], [239], [240]), and the bioscaling ([241], [242], [243]).

The healthy cells work collectively, their energy-consumption as well as their life-cycles and the availability of resources are controlled collectively by the various forms of the self-organizing, [244], [245]. The healthy cells are organized this way, their standard cycles, reactions and structures are complexly regulated in both internal and external areas. The healthy cells have special "social" signals [246] commonly regulate and control their life. They are specialized for work-division in the organism and their life-cycle is determined by the collective "decisions".

What makes the difference in the absorption? It is the missing collective order in malignancy. The cancerous cells behave non-collectively; they are autonomic. They are "individual fighters", having no common control over them, only the available nutrients regulate their life. The order, which characterizes the healthy tissue is lost in their malignant version, the cellular communications are missing [247].

The malignancy has a special fractal structure, which can be identified by impedance measurements on Erlich solid tumors [248]. This structure (due to its definite percolative self-similarity) is a better conductor [249] than the non-fractal healthy tissue.

The living matter has a highly self-organized hierarchical structure. It is in non-equilibrium and its processes are non-stationer, [250]. The subsystems of living organisms are multiple, connected with various physical, chemical and physiological processes and the interacting signals change in a wide range. The simplest biological systems show various processes on different time-scales in vivo, which are connected by bio-scaling [241]. There are no two identical living objects exist, the living matter is variable, changeable and mutable, [240]. It differs from the lifeless [251]. While the thermal and quantum fluctuations in lifeless are negligible by the size of the system; the living object has a high number of homologue phase-states randomly transformed and altered into each other, they mutate by the time, which is unchanged among identical environmental conditions. In contrast, the permanent and immanent change makes the living object possible for adaptation, for mutation and for natural selection. This dynamism appears in the change of the confirmation state of proteins optimizing the enzymatic reactions of life. Due to these fluctuations, the living matter is "noisierand" because of its self-similar [252] and self-organized [244] behavior, its power-spectrum shows pink-noise (1/f noise), [238], [239].

The highest deficiency of information (highest entropy) is achieved by the noise, which has Gaussian distribution [253] (Gaussian noise). Because the effective power-density of pink-noise is constant in all characteristic scales, the Gaussian pink-noise then has maximal entropy in all the scales. The living system has special fractal dynamism, [254], in consequence of its self-similar stochastic behavior, it fluctuates by the pink-noise, [255]. The maximal entropy of Gaussian pink-noise allows an important conclusion: the noise of the living state has maximal entropy (stable dynamic equilibrium) in all of the characteristic scales.

The cell motility probed by noise analysis of thickness shear mode resonators [256]. The noise analysis of the electric currents has become a new tool in the field, [240]. Absorption and fluctuations of giant liposomes were studied by electrochemical impedance measurements, [257].

Oncothermia uses these new approaches to fit in the best curative performance. This new approach (the fractal physiology) is applied for oncothermia. The carrier electric field delivers the time-fractal structure to the tissues enhancing considerable the selection between the connected healthy cellular community and the individual autonomy of the malignant proliferation.

The disordered structure of malignancy is a good absorbent. To show it again by a simple example: when somebody's hair is in order, the comb slides through the over-combed hair. However, when the same hair is disordered, combing is able even to cut out the hair by their energy-absorption mechanisms. In malignancy the disorder makes the same energy-absorption process, (see Figure 28.).

The order-disorder selection method is similar to the process when the light goes through the windows-glass (see Figure 29.). When the glass is transparent to that specific set of colors (visible light, definite interval of frequencies) its absorption is almost zero, all energy goes through it. However, when it has any bubbles, grains, precipitations etc. those irregularities will absorb more from the energy, their transparency is locally low, their energy absorption is high, they are heated up locally. It is a self-selection depending on the material and the frequency (color) which we apply in the given example.

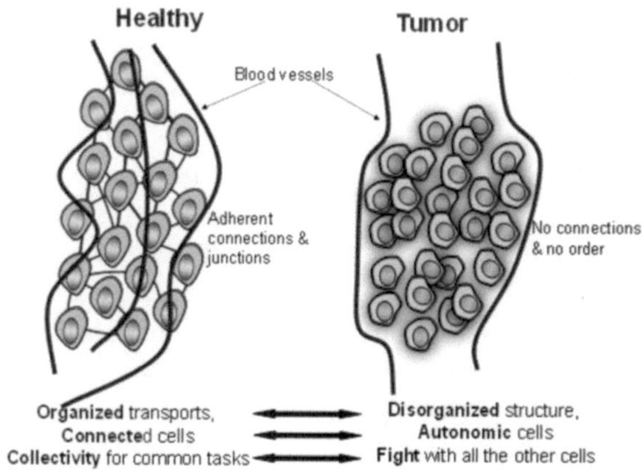

Figure 28. The malignant absorption selects by the disorder of the cancer, having no transparency for the well-chosen modulated RF carrier frequency (It is a patented method and know-how of oncothermia.)

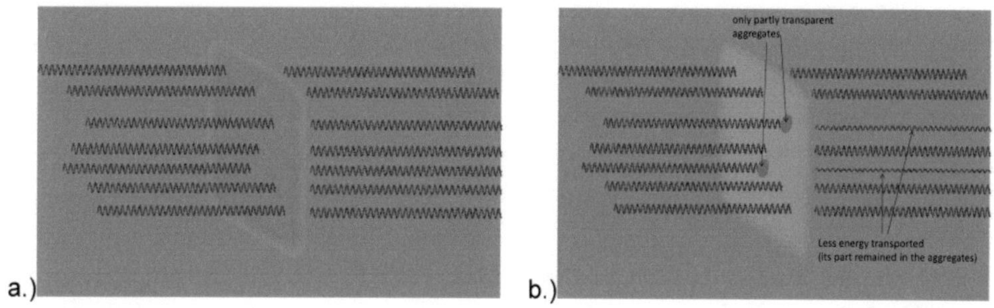

Figure 29. The transparency of the glass. In full transparent case all the energy goes over the glass (a), but when the glass has aggregates, those absorb a part of energy (b), and they will be hotter than their environment

This is the effect, which is used by oncothermia with some modulation. The carrier frequency delivers the information (modulation frequencies), for which the cancer cells are much less "transparent" than their healthy counterparts are. Malignant cells are heated up by the selectively absorbed energy.

3.4. Effect of electric field on malignancies

The physiology is an interdisciplinary subject. It uses numerous principles and discoveries. Its electronic structure approach derived from solid state physics (e.g. Szent-Gyorgyi, [228], [229]), the superconductivity approach (e.g. Cope, [258]), the electromagnetic resonances (e.g. Liboff, [259], [232]), the thermodynamics of life (e.g. Schrodinger, [233], Katchalsky & Curran [234]), etc. are all parts of the physiology, and make it really complex like the phenomena of the life itself is.

The important category of the hyperthermia was generated by electric fields [260], [198],which is even a hot topic in science presently[261], [262]. The electric conductive heating started in the late 19th century is called "galvanocautery" [263]. The method was further developed by D'Arsonval, introducing the impedance (alternating current [*AC*], later higher frequencies, even spark-generated currents) calling it *"Arsonvalization"*, [264], and later a more modernized method was the *"fulguration"* [265]. The Arsonvalization method had fantastic popularity at the turn of the 19th-20th centuries, developing three different branches: the interstitial hyperthermia, including the galvanic heat-stimulation (*electro-chemical-cancer-treatment*), the ablation techniques and the capacitive coupling. The first capacitive coupled device on conductive basis was the *"Universal Thermoflux"*. It was launched on to the market by such a giant of the electric industry in that time as Siemens, which was later further developed, and the new device by the name *"Radiotherm"* was launched on the market in the early 1930s. The first start of the new capacitive-coupling technologies was in 1976 by LeVeen [266] and has been widely applied since then [267], [268], [74]. Many hyperthermia devices use capacitive coupling since its treatment is easy.

An electric field application without an increase in temperature (using less than 5W power) has also been found effective against cancer [269], [270], [271], [272], [273], [274], by using galvanic (DC) current applications. The control of these treatments is the tissue-resistance and the quality parameter is the applied charge load, [275], [276]. Numerous devices were developed and applied widely, but the expected breakthrough result was missing. An entirely new line was started with Professors Rudolf Pekar, [277], [278], [279], Bjorn Nordenstrom [273], [274] and Xin You Ling [280], [281], [282]; and continued by others [283], [284], [285], [286], [287], [288], [289]. Remarkable results were produced by this method; and the biological mechanisms involved in electromagnetic field are intensively investigated [290], [72], and the effect of electric field is studied on various side of its complex behavior, [261], [262]. Recently, the effect of electric field has been used for special therapies in oncology, [291], [292], [293], [294].

A sophisticated study was performed to study the synergy of temperature and modulated electric field [295]. The model was HT-29 human colorectal carcinoma cell-line being xenografted to nude mice (BALB (nu/nu)). For comparison we performed low temperature oncothermia experiment, where the bolus of the upper-electrode was cooled down. The intensive cooling kept the tumor near the physiological temperature (38 °C) while the oncothermia field was identical with the heating conditions of 42 °C. The result is surprisingly interesting (see Figure 30). The effect of electric field made nano-range heating only, the overall temperature had a minor role in the cell-killing mechanism.

3.5. Other selection factors

There are numerous selection effects existing to distinguish the malignant cells. Here we comprehensively list some of them.

The missing cell-junctions and the characteristic isolation of the malignant cells from each other [247], [296] create a free extracellular pathway between the cells, definitely increasing the conductivity of the extracellular electrolyte. Furthermore, the decrease of the epithelial barrier function (tight-junction permeability changes) can be measured by electric impedance measurement, [297].

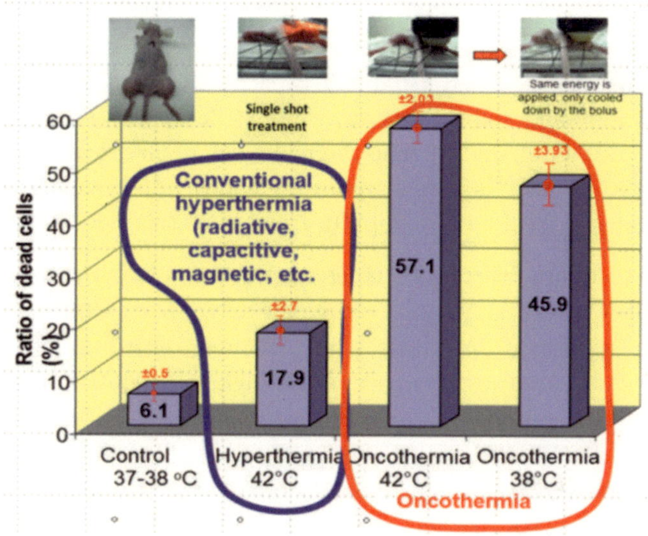

Figure 30. Oncothermia was 3 times more effective than hyperthermia on the identically high (42 °C) temperature. However, cooling down the tumor during the treatment, the death-rate decreased only slightly, exceeding more than 2 times the classic hyperthermia on high temperature

The special membrane effect (rectification on membranes, [298]), is also a factor of the cellular selectivity of cancer by RF electric field. The impedance measurement is useful for the control of other treatment modalities. It adequately measures the distortion, made by irradiation [299], and the drug-effect can also be controlled, [300]. Such usual practice, like following the wound healing, is also objectively traceable [301]. Bioimpedance vector pattern can distinguish cancer patients without disease versus locally advanced or disseminated diseases [302].

The impedance measures selectively, differentiates between the cancerous and healthy tissue, and is able to distinguish the extra- and intra-cellular electrolyte. Selective impedance measurements are provided clinically as well. Many comparative studies have been provided for malignant tissues, however, the results are not identical; the measurements very much depend on the conditions. (This is a trivial consequence of many factors, which we listed above.) However, all the studies measured lower impedance in the tumor than in their healthy counterpart in all of the tissue and staging of the tumor, in vitro and in vivo as well.

Hyperthermia increases biochemical reaction rates [303] and therefore the metabolic rate as well. The metabolic heat production of tumor depends on the doubling time of its volume [304]. The high metabolic rate keeps the temperature for tumor tissues higher than its neighborhood, [305]. This works as selection factor for heating of tumor tissue. Therefore, in case of 6 °C increase the amount of growth will be 1.8-times higher [306] than its healthy counterpart.

It has been long known that hyperthermia can cause the softening or melting of the lipid bilayer [307], [308], [155], it can change lipid-protein interactions [309], and it can denature proteins [310]. All of these events can arrest the cell-cycle of the tumor.

Heat-treatment cause structural alteration in transmembrane proteins, causing a change in the active membrane transport and membrane capacity [311] leading to substantial changes in potassium, calcium, and sodium ion gradients [312], membrane potential [313], [314], cellular function [315], [316], and causing thermal block of electrically excitable cells [317], [303]. The thermo tolerable cells have significantly higher (~15%) membrane potential than the naïve cells [314], and the difference rapidly grows by the elapsed time at 45°C.

In chemo-thermo-therapies the role of chaperone proteins is important. Chaperones (stress- or heat-shock-proteins) are highly conserved proteins, which are vital in almost every living cell and on their surfaces during their whole lifetime, regardless of their stage in the evolution, [318]. Any kind of change in the dynamic equilibrium of the cell life (environmental stresses, various pathogen processes, diseases, etc.) activates their synthesis [319]. Excretion of the chaperones is the 'stress-answer' of the cells to accommodate themselves to the new challenges. As a consequence of the stressful 'life' of malignant cells, the molecular chaperones are present in all cancerous cells [320], [321], [322] to adapt the actual stress to help tumor-cell survival. Moreover, the shock-proteins are induced by every oncological treatment-method, which are devoted to eliminate the malignancy: after conventional hyperthermia [323], after chemotherapy [324], after radiotherapy [325] or even after photo-therapy [326] intensive HSP synthesis was shown. By the stress adaptation the induction or over-expression of the stress proteins generally provide effective protection of the cell against apoptosis [327], but their extracellular expression acts oppositely: it makes a signal to the immune system on the defect of the actual cell [328]. Furthermore, induction of various HSPs (HSP27, HSP70, and HSP90) was observed in numerous metastases and the HSP90 homologue, GRP94 may act as a mediator of metastasis generation. HSP generally degrades the effect of the hyperthermia therapy because it may increase the tumor cell survival, and its massive induction may generate the tumor thermo-tolerance and in parallel drug- and radio-tolerance. Heat treatment can also lead to multi-drug resistance [329].

Non-temperature dependent effects (mainly field stresses) can also produce chaperone-synthesis [330]. The HSP manifestation in the biopsies might give a good clinical indication for the treatment response [331].

On the other hand, the chaperone HSP70 assists to freeze the actual dynamic equilibrium (the "status-quo") and so tries to re-establish the cellular communication in the extra-cellular electrolyte [328]. It is shown that their expression on the cell-membrane gains the apoptotic signals and enhances the immune reactions, [328]. HSP participates in the activation of the p53 tumor-suppresser [332] and has been associated with the tumor-suppresser retinoblastoma protein [333].

Recently, numerous scientific theories have also concentrated on the significance of thermally induced non-thermal effects, such as heat-shock protein (HSP) production [334],

[335]. Development of the thermo-tolerance is one of the suppressors of hyperthermia efficacy [323]. From the point of view of the thermo-tolerance, one of the most prominent chaperone proteins is the HSP72. The concentration of this HSP is 5-10 times lower in the healthy cells than in the malignant ones, and both grow by the heat-treatment [336]. However, responding to the heat treatment, their concentration in healthy cells is: multiplied by 8 or 10, while during the same heat treatment the HSP72 multiplication creates only 1.2-1.5 times higher concentration in malignant cells, [323].

4. Cellular effects – To kill or not to kill?

Like Nobel-laureate A. Szent-Gyorgyi formulated: from the point of view of life, it is not interesting how the monkey goes through the forest, but it is essential how the forest goes through the monkey [as nutrition]. In hyperthermia we have to have the same change of paradigm: it is not important how the incident energy increases the temperature, but that is essential how the incident energy changes the structure and the chemical bonds in the targeted tissue.

4.1. Apoptotic cell killing

The above described mechanism targets the membrane of the malignant cells, and excites numerous pathways essential for the cellular fate, (see Figure 31.). The excitations have serious consequences on membrane:

- Induces apoptotic signal
- Forms membrane-HSP
- Makes the membrane more transparent
- Forms higher motility of membrane domains
- Rebinds the E-cadherin adherent connections
- Damages the cell-membrane
- Rectificates, demodulates the modulated signal (stochastic effects are involved)

The effects in the cytoplasm are also remarkable. The transmembrane temperature gradient

- Dilutes the cytoplasm
- Develops higher intracellular pressure
- Activates apoptotic pathways
- Activates death receptors
- Suppresses the proliferation
- Arrests the DNA replication

These effects were shown in multiple, different experiments. The basic repeated phenomena are the time-delay of the action, selection and tumor destruction of oncothermia became trivial hours after the treatment (see Figure 32., [337]). The numerous apoptotic bodies show the character of the process.

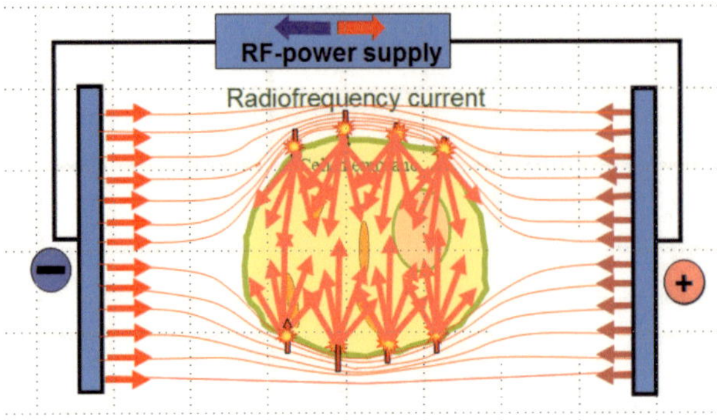

Figure 31. Numerous pathways are excited

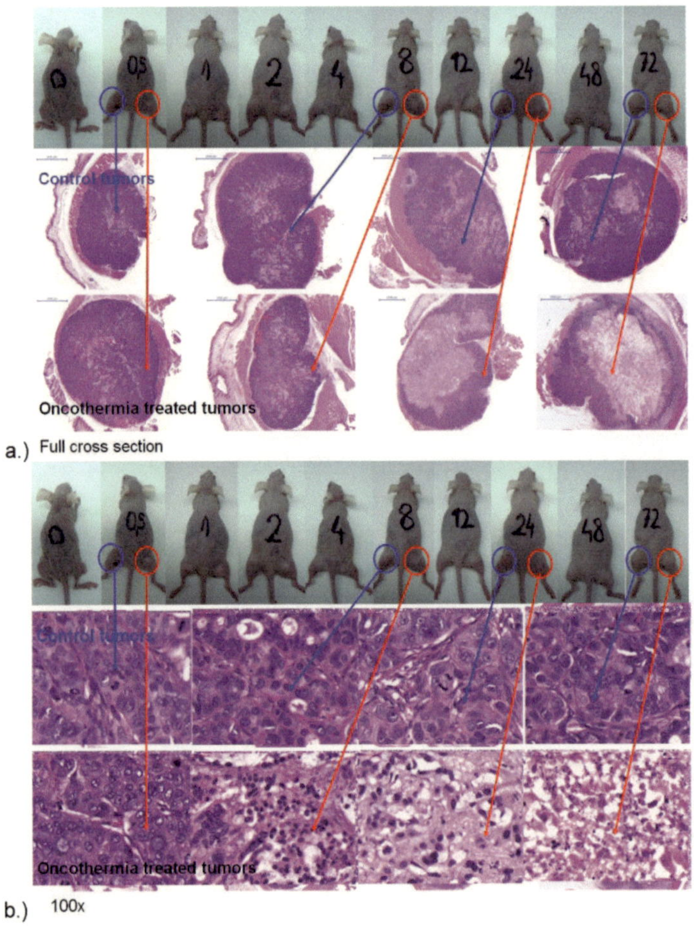

Figure 32. Morphological observations show extended cell-destruction in the large volume of the tumor (field effect is active, temperature doesn't change, self-focusing). The destruction has a time-delay, hours are requested for the natural processes to be well- activated to fight. The numbers indicated on the mice are the hours after the single shot of 30 min oncothermia treatment, (HE Staining). (a) full cross section of the tumor, (b) magnification of the tissue by 100x

The time delay indicates the long-duration processes, which were identified as programmed cell-death (apoptosis), by various investigations: macro- and micro-morphology, enhanced activity of p53 tumor-suppressor, cleaved caspase 3 involvement, Tunel reaction, DNA fragmentation (laddering), etc. (see Figure 33., [337]). The rebuilt external apoptotic pathways are shown by reestablished E-cadherin connections, by enreachment of beta-catenin and its relocalization into the nuclei, by connexin induction, by activation of death-toll receptors, like FADD, FAS, DR-5, etc.

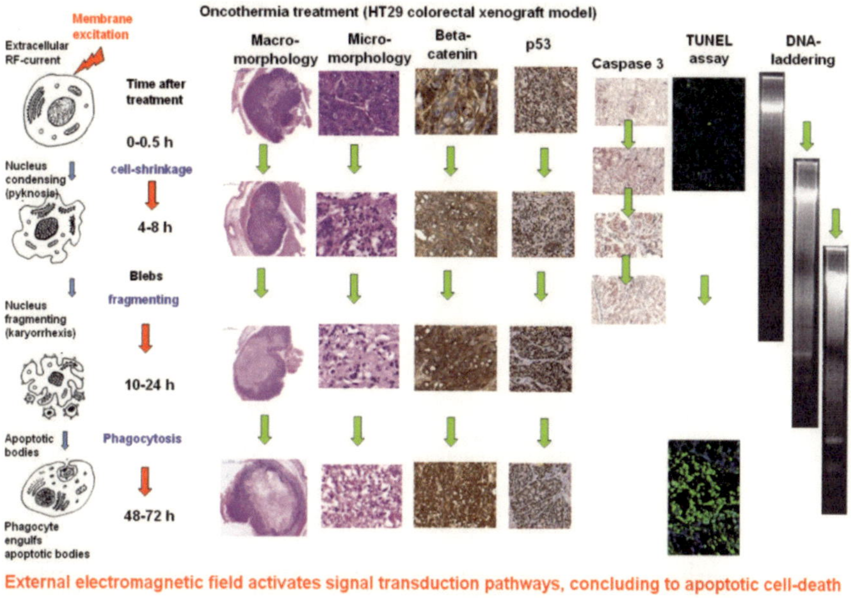

Figure 33. External electromagnetic field activates signal transduction pathways, concluding to apoptotic cell-death. (Oncothermia treatment (HT29 colorectal xenograft model)

This apoptotic process is non-toxic (no inflammatory reactions afterwards) and promotes the immune reactions (works parallel with these).

The cellular selection is proven by various experiments. One of these is the definite selection of malignant cells in co-cultures, [338]. The effect on healthy human keratinocytes (HCK) co-cultured with human fibroblasts (see Figure 34.) was marginal, and was regenerated by the time. The co-culture with immortalized (but not malignant) HaCaT keratinocytes is affected slightly, but the malignant A431 cell-line was selected from the co-culture (see Figure 35.).

The time-delay and the relocalization of the beat-catenin to the cell-nuclei is shown in vitro (HepG2 cell-line) and in vivo (HT29 xenograft) shown in Figure 36. [339].

The time delay is shown in the Tunel reactions (see Figure 37.), indicating the late apoptotic phases dominantly after 24 h of the single shot treatment.

An interesting measurement was provided by Ki67 proliferation marker, measured in the living tumor part after the single-shot treatment of oncothermia, (see Figure 37, [340]). The surviving, living malignant cells in the treated tumor had definitely and significantly suppressed Ki67 marker compared to its untreated counterpart in all the time-scale investigated.

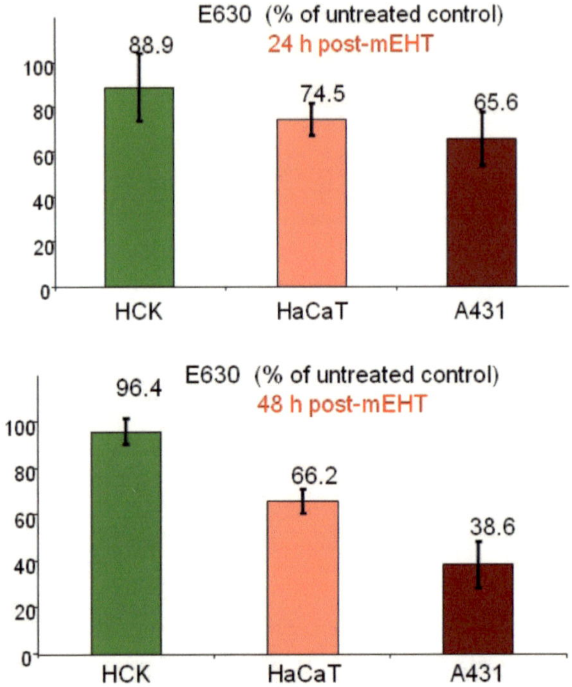

Figure 34. Co-culture with normal human skin fibroblasts as a model of a squamous carcinoma growing within connective tissue cells (100.000/ml) were exposed to oncothermia. Samples were incubated for 24 h at 37°C, fixed and stained with crystal violet. Cellular metabolic activity was measured using the MTT assay (standard colorimetric test) and quantitated at 630 nm. (Data represent the mean value ± S.E.M. of 4-6 separate experiments assayed in triplicate, but some experiments were repeated up to 12 times to obtain reliable data.)

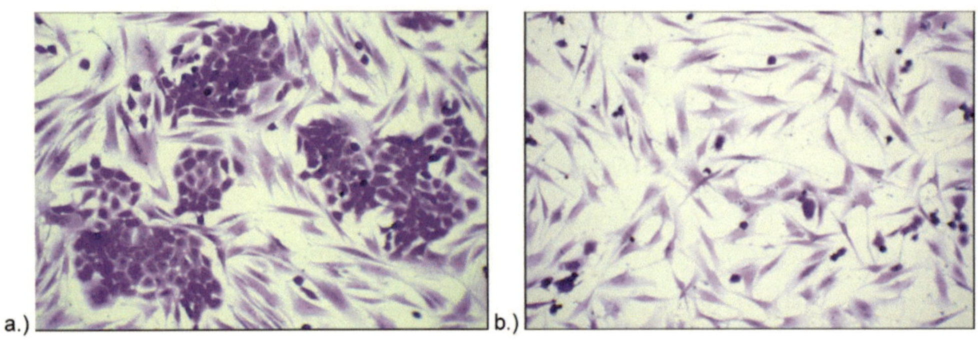

Figure 35. The selection of the malignant cells is effective in the co-culture of the malignant A431 human keratinocytes and healthy human fibroblasts. [a – before oncothermia, b – after oncothermia]. The healthy cells remain intact, while the malignant cells are damaged and cleared. (Experiment is described in Figure 34.)

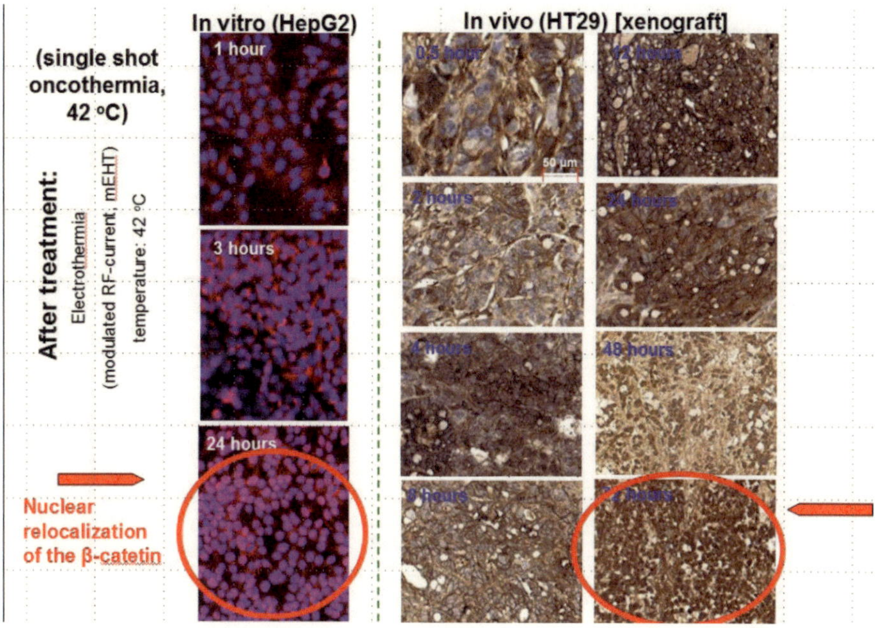

Figure 36. The beta-catenin relocalization into the nuclei

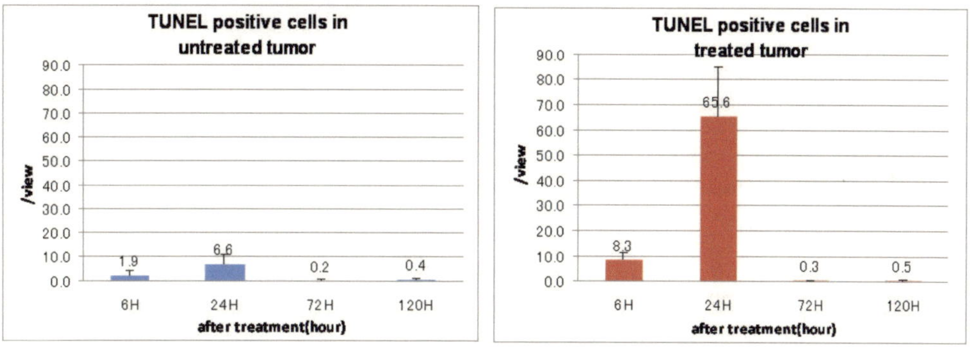

Figure 37. TUNEL assay: enzymatically label the DNA fragments resulted by apoptotic process

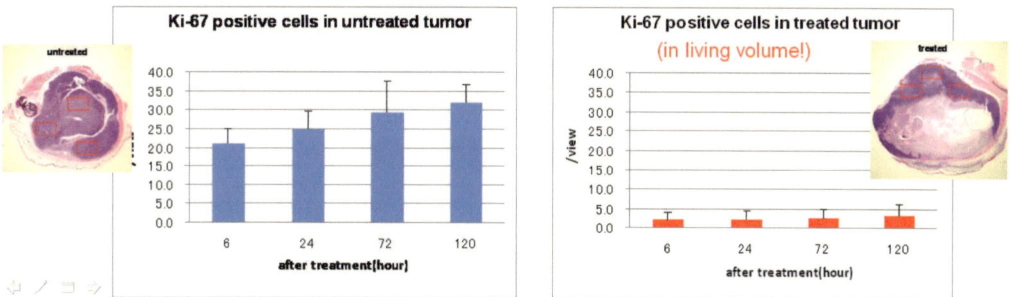

Figure 38. Colon26 (murine colorectal cancer) cell line derived allograft (CID mice), single shot. (Ki-67: proliferation marker protein, expressed in the nuclear membrane only in the dividing cells.)

The cleaved Caspase-3 (as important part of the apoptotic pathway) was activated (see Figure 39., [341]), as well as the death toll receptors became overexpressed (see Figure 40., [341]).

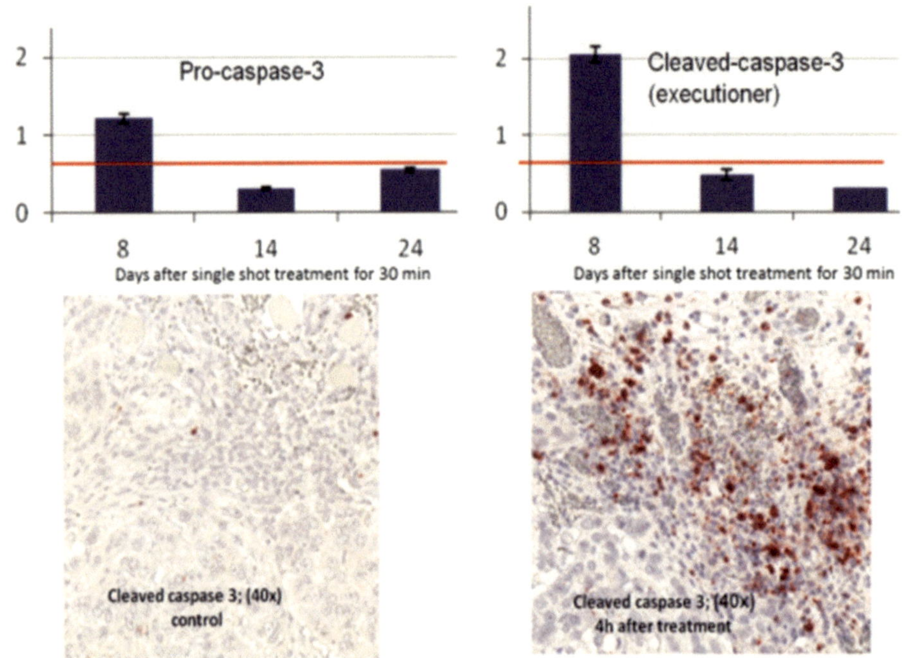

Figure 39. HT29 human colorectal carcinoma cell-line xenograft model in nude mice. Caspases, or cysteine-aspartic proteases or cysteine-dependent aspartate-directed proteases are a family of cysteine proteases that play essential roles in apoptosis (programmed cell death), necrosis, and inflammation (the red line is for the reference value) [Reference: untreated control]

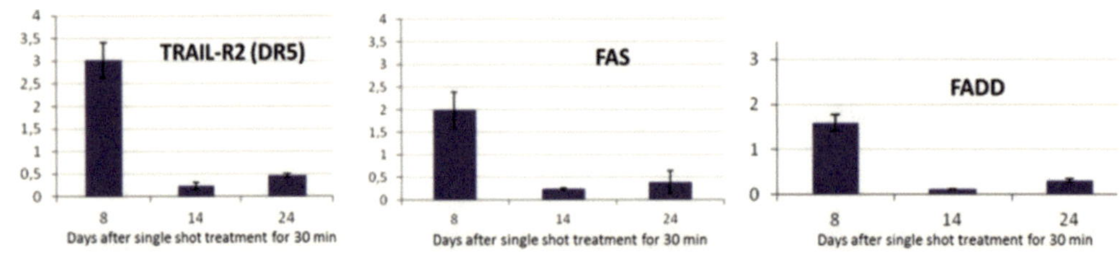

Figure 40. HT29 human colorectal carcinoma cell-line xenograft model in nude mice. Death receptor activity (the red line is for the reference value) [Reference: untreated control]

4.2. Suppressing the dissemination of malignant cells

Oncothermia is different from this point of view as well. It blocks the dissemination, avoids their motility due to the lazy connections with the tumor. Oncothermia makes it by the reestablishing the cellular connections (see Figure 41. [337]), which is also great success to save life. The built up connections can force not only the sticking together, but make bridges between the cells for information exchange to limit the individuality and the competitive behavior of the malignant cells.

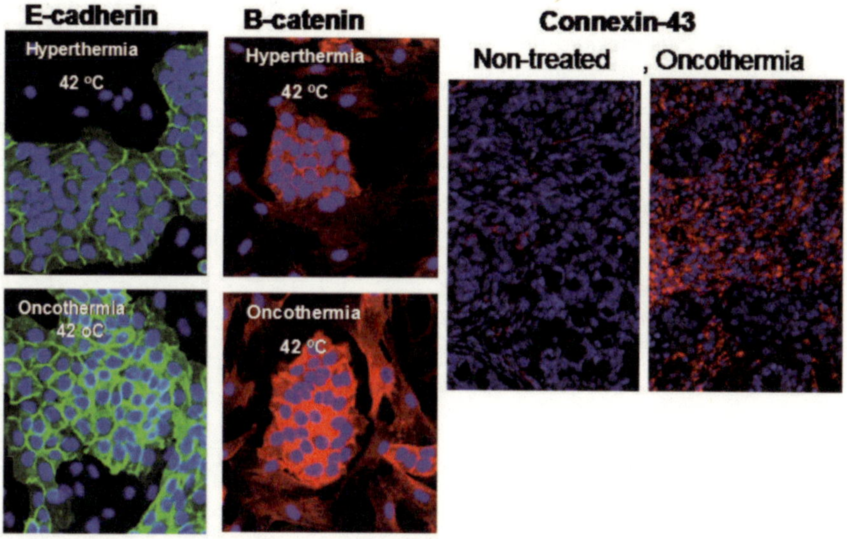

Figure 41. Oncothermia can reestablish the adherent cell connections (E-cadherin and β-catenin) as well as the gap-junctions (Connexin-43). These could reestablish the cellular communication and can stop the dissemination of tumor cells

This "gluing mechanism" is not only important for the external apoptotic signal, but makes the malignant cells less mobile, their motility is reduced and the dissemination risk is decreased.

4.3. Action on far distant metastases

The main danger of malignancies is the metastases, attacking the organs which are crucial for life. When the tumor grows somewhere without endangering the important systems like the respiratory system, central nervous system, cardiovascular system, etc., it is not life-threatening. These tumors are local (benign or early malignant), their elimination is possible. The real life-threatening danger is the malignancy, when the cells are disseminated from the tumor-lesion by the various transport systems (lymph, blood), or their effect becomes systemic by one of the general mechanisms of the organism.

The heavy life-threatening effect of metastases has been observed on statistical basis on colorectal adenocarcinoma collecting data for 15 years [342]. The long- term (10 years) survival was around 90% when no metastases were present, 60% in case of regional metastases and only 15% when distant metastases were developed in the patient. The blood-transported cells can be blocked easily by the brain, lung, kidney, liver, etc., causing fatality. The challenge of the treatments is to recognize the tumor early, to avoid the metastases, and/or to block the dissemination as much as possible.

In veterinarian clinical trial of dogs having osteosarcomas without evidences of metastases, the local radiation combined complementary with whole body hyperthermia was studied. The result was surprisingly bad [343], [344]: the combined treatment was not effective on the primer tumor, but rapid and massive metastases were developed in far distance organs including the lung. This blocked the research in this direction, the veterinarian application of the hyperthermia even in combined therapies was not plasticized in veterinary field.

One of the interesting, and so far not completely understood process, is the systemic effect of the local treatments called abscopal (out of the target) or bystander effect [345]. This phenomenon shows a systemic effect only by local treating, see Figure 42. The effect was shown in mice experiments [346], see Figure 43, and also in human, see Figure 44., [347].

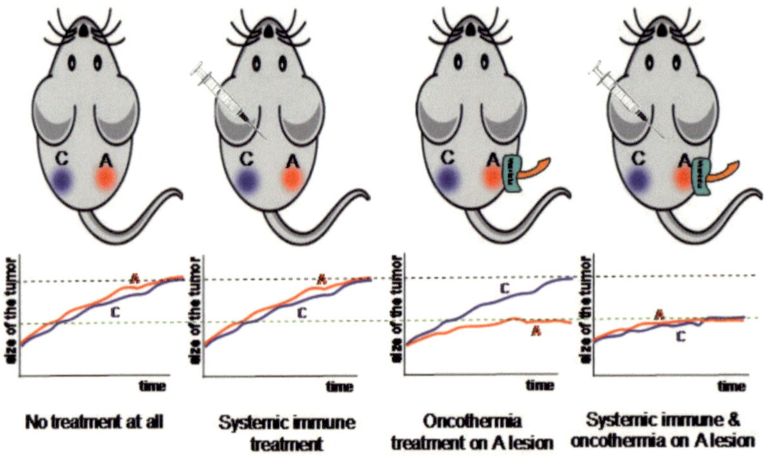

Figure 42. The mice have two distant tumors in left and right femoral region. The growths of the tumors are equal. When we treat the mice systemically with immune supporters, no change can be seen. When we treat the A tumor locally with oncothermia, that tumor does not grow so quickly as the reference C. However, when we apply the systemic immune therapy and the local oncothermia for the only A-lesion, surprisingly, the C lesion is also suppressed

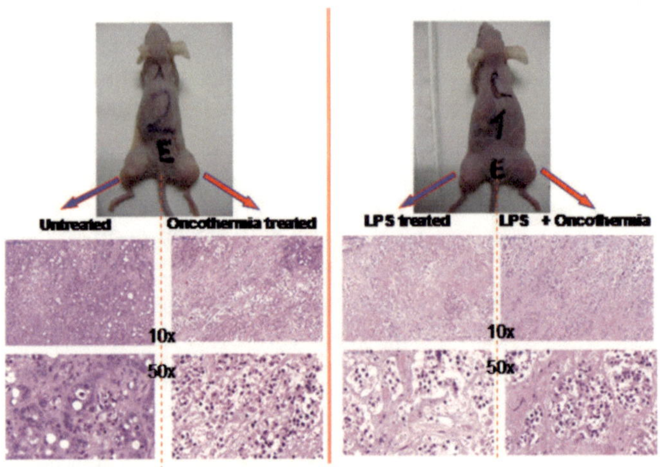

Figure 43. E. coli LPS sc. to the dorsal region of the animal 24 h before the oncothermia treatment. 100ug LPS in 100uL Salsol solution. 30 min oncothermia with pink noise AM modulation (41-42°C tumor core temperature) Sampling: animals were sacrificed 72 h after the treatment

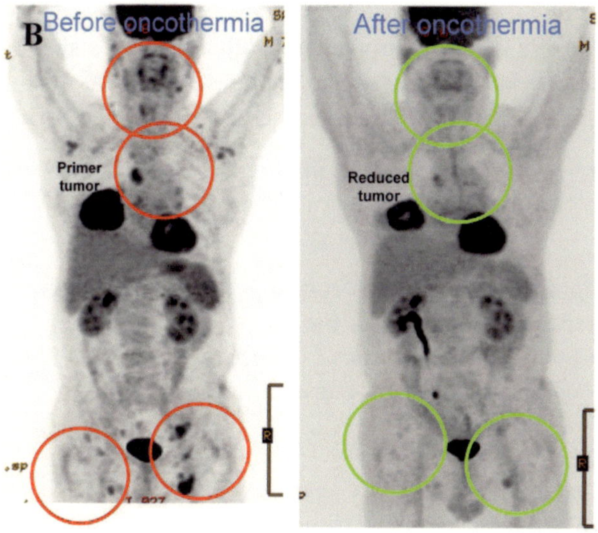

Figure 44. Investigator: Prof. Dr. Seong Min Yoon, Institute: Division of Hematology-Oncology, Department of Internal Medicine, Samsung Changwon Hospital, Sungkyunkwan University, S.Korea Patient: SAsc, 72 y, male, Primer-tumor: Non-small cell lung cancer; Size: 9.5 cm right middle lobe, Metastases: in sentinel and distant lymph-nodes, Tumor-classification: cT2 cN2 M0, stage IIIB, Treatment: trimodal protocol: 28x1.7 Gy; support: 250 microgram Leukine and Oncothermia 6x; Only the primer tumor was locally treated

4.4. Some clinical results

Oncothermia has a long-time history with large number of documented case reports and clinical trials [160]. During more than 20 years 43 studies were performed involving more than 2000 patients altogether from 14 clinics in 4 countries (see Table 1.) Details of the clinical effects are summarized in the publications as well as in the specialized monograph [160].

The clinical trials of oncothermia are dominantly retrospective. To develop randomized clinical trials is a challenge for patients. Patients do not agree to be in the control-arm at any case. In most of the cases they are registered for oncothermia because the other methods (conventional gold standards) failed. In these cases progression could occur anyway due to drug-resistance, organ-overload (kidney, liver, etc.), tumor-relapses, psycho-resistance, etc.

The advanced cases at the conditions described above emphasize not only the complexity of the individual situation of patients, but also underlines the fact that oncothermia is applied as the facility of the "no other is possible" many time hopeless cases providing over 3rd line treatment approach. This high-line treatment process is in general palliation (the first goal is to provide acceptable quality of life), which is an important factor for oncothermia as well. However oncothermia even in these advanced situations has curative value, and makes curative therapy in 3rd-line or over. The professional literature clearly shows the rare facility of the evidence-based clinical trials for these high-line treatments. Other evidences have to be shown when randomized controlled trials are not possible, [348]. The challenges of evaluation appear forcefully in case of patients with advanced stages having inoperable (or partly resected) tumors, having relapsed malignancies, patients who are resistant on the gold-standard treatments, etc. Oncothermia is facing to this challenge as well.

We have to make special attention evaluating of the clinical results performed by oncothermia. The complications make definite challenges to objective evaluation. The main challenges are:

- Oncothermia is applied in higher (usually third and subsequent) treatment-lines, boosting or resensitizing the effect of the conventional therapies. Oncothermia is mostly applied in cases when the conventional therapies fall. In most of the cases oncothermia therapy is applied when the patient has/is
  - Inoperable lesion
  - Radio-resistant
  - Chemo-resistant (refractory)
  - Improper blood-counts
  - Liver-failure
  - Kidney failure
  - Psycho-resistance

  In most of the cases the complex combination of the above problems occurs. Due to these conditions, oncothermia is applied in higher line of the therapies. This sequence of the treatments is mostly determined by the individual decisions of the physicians [349], usually without having help from any evidence based statistical approvals.
- Usually it is applied in palliative care; many patients are in terminal phase. This patient care has very limited statistical evidence based trials; the medical decision-making processes are usually well tailored to the individual patients [350], [351].
- Only few controlled randomized clinical trials are available for oncothermia. The results have to be concluded from observational studies and from the historical and data-base comparisons. USA- and EU-databases (SEER [352], Eurocare [353]) are mostly used. Due to the not solved problem between the hypothesis check confidence of evidence based medicine and the observational studies [354], [355], this data-comparison is acceptable. Make the result as objective as they could be, we compared the collected results of the same localizations and the same protocols from various clinics. The common significant difference from the databases can be accepted as evidence.
- In the case of long-survivals, we have to consider, that oncothermia is taken only in a small fraction of the overall survival. The patients are treated by oncothermia in their definite late stages, after prognosis "no curative help" by continuing the gold-standards alone. In consequence, the long overall survival generally is not the result of the oncothermia, but the selection of the patients in their end. Oncothermia effect in these cases can be negligible, irrespective of its real efficacy. The chance to measure the efficacy is the first year survival rate (%), when the patients with the most aggressive kind of the given cancer do not survive the following year after the diagnosis. If they start the oncothermia in the first year, the survival-rate result can be an objective sign of the efficacy.

- Special cases are treated on Intend-to-Treat population. This makes the patient selection not objective enough, but the dominantly metastatic patient's spectrum compensates for this lack of selection. In this case, we have an automatic selection of advanced (many times terminal) cases.
- The generally low quality of life (QoL) in combination of supportive therapies weaken the measurability of oncothermia alone. However, due to the fact that oncothermia is not proposed as monotherapy, the combination objectively measures the benefit, if the supportive therapies alone would not be successful at all.
- The patients are treated with oncothermia in their very advanced, metastatic states. The local oncothermia treatment, of course, concentrates on definite localizations, (primary or metastatic) which again lowers the full measurability of the oncothermia in the development of the cancer. This is the main reason why oncothermia measures first of all the overall survival rates, which are good objective parameters of the treatment efficacy in general.
- The quality of life (QoL) of the patients is an important characteristic of such a method as oncothermia. In a generally controlled and randomized study a trial effect exists [356], which is not the case in oncothermia applications. However, it could be negative outcome, that in a strict competitive market the opinions are not independent and objective [357] and of course the conflict of interest could make considerable bias [358], [359].

On the above bias structure the characteristics of the clinical studies could be described as – Single arm, open label, observational for intention-to-treat (ITT) population, dominantly for the patients in late/advanced stages, where the conventional methods have failed. Mostly the survival rate was the studied endpoint. The inclusion criteria were the inoperable and in progression after chemo- and/or radio-therapy. Exclusions were only the well-known, above described contraindications of oncothermia.

The oncothermia challenge is its use when the conventional treatments are unsuccessful. In consequence, its effect could be active only in a small (last) fraction of the overall survival. When patients have long overall survival by the conventional treatments alone, oncothermia is applied only in the last stage of the disease so objectively the life-elongation by oncothermia can not be observed.

To make an objective evaluation, we have special considerations how to get the evidences from the available information pool and find the objective evidences. It is a complex challenge, having four basic approaches. These methods highlight the objective information and their parallel results make the obtained data evidence-based. The five legs are:

1. **Fast course case comparison.** Use the survival of the rapid, fast course cases (most advanced, drastically quickly developing cases) in comparison with large databases. (Only the survival is considered as relevant parameter, the clinical outcomes (responses) are not studied as evidences.)
2. **Comparison of clinics.** Compare the obtained data of the independent clinics, using the same protocol for the same cohort.
3. **Quality of life comparison.** Collect the data about the quality of life and the adverse effects limiting the application of oncothermia.

4. **Create a quasi-control arm**. Patients having no benefit from oncothermia could form a quasi-arm for control. The "no benefit" category could be defined when the patient survival is short from the time of the first oncothermia treatment.
5. **Parametric evaluation.** Use the available latest statistical knowledge to find the relevant parameters of the survivals and use the best fit of the parametric distribution for evaluation.

Study	Number of patients	1st year survival (%)	Median overall survival (m)	Resposnding patients/ratio (%)	Median overall survival of responding patients (m)	Median overall survival of non-responding patients (m)	Reference
Brain gliomas	27	86.2	23.6	43	66.2	18.2	[360], [361]
Brain-glioma study Phase II, Retrospective	140	71.7					[362], [363]
Astrocytoma	40		25.8	80	40.2	20.2	
Glioblastoma	92		16	73	21.9	13.1	
Diffuse astrocytoma	8		52.9				
Glioma (WHO IV) Study, Phase II, prospective, two arms	45		15				[160], [364]
Passive arm	36	40	11				
Active arm	9	65	14.5	43	66.2	18.2	
Recurrent glioblastoma study, Phase II, retrospective,	19	68.0	21.8	59	32.6	12.4	[365]
Glioma study, Phase II, retrospective	36	60.0					[366]
Astrocytoma	9		106				
Glioblastoma	27		20				
Glioma study, Phase II, retrospective	179						[367]
Astrocytoma	53	100	103				
Glioblastoma	126	76	16				
Advanced, relapsed brain gliomas, Phase II, retrospective	12		10	25			[368]
Brain glioma WHO III-IV, Phase I, safety prospective	15						[369], [370], [371], [372]
Head and neck study, Phase II. retrospective	64	92.2	26.1				[160], [373]
Bone-metastases, monotherapy, Phase II, retrospective	6	100	40.1				[160], [373]

Study	Number of patients	1st year survival (%)	Median overall survival (m)	Responsnding patients/ratio (%)	Median overall survival of responding patients (m)	Median overall survival of non-responding patients (m)	Reference
Refractory bone-metastases study, Phase II, retrospective	11			90.9			[374]
Breast cancers	103	97.1	52.1	45	274.8	10.9	[160] , [373]
Colorectal cancer ()	218	84.9	28.5				[160] , [373]
Sigma	12			34.1			
Rectum	92			57.1	58	21	
Colon	114			44.2	109.8	23.2	
Colon cancer study, , Phase II, prospective, three arms, randomized	154						[375] [376]
Clifford TCM	53			75			
Monotherapy	50			81			
Combined therapy	51			91			
Esophagus study, Phase II, retrospective	12	41.7	28.5	35	29.4	8.5	[160], [377]
Rectum cancer study, Inoperable→operable, Phase II, retrospective	7			71			[378]
Kidney cancer study, Phase II, retrospective	39	84.6	35.9	48	78.4	33.7	[160], [373]
Liver metastases from various origin, Phase II, retrospective	25		20.5				[379]
Liver metastases from various origin, Comparative study, Phase II, retrospective	28						[374]
With radiotherapy	16			81			
With chemotherapy	8			38			
Monotherapy	4			25			
Liver metastasis form colorectal origin, Phase II, retrospective	80	86.0	24.1				[380]
Passive arm		53	11				
Active arm	80	91	24.1				
With chemotherapy	30	80	21.5				
Monotherapy	50	92	24.4				
Liver metastasis form colorectal origin, Phase II, retrospective	15		23	80			[381]

Study	Number of patients	1st year survival (%)	Median overall survival (m)	Resposnding patients/ratio (%)	Median overall survival of responding patients (m)	Median overall survival of non-responding patients (m)	Reference
Liver metastasis form colorectal origin, Phase II, retrospective	22		28				[382]
Rectal cancer, non-operable, , Phase II, retrospective	65			96			[383]
Liver metastasis	29			86			
Metastatic brain tumors study, Phase II, retrospective	15	90.0	46.2	73	48.2	16.1	[368]
Non-small cell lung cancer meta-analysis	311						[384]
Passive arm	53	26.5	14				
Active arm	258	67.0	15.8	21	53.4	18.1	
Non-advanced (WHO<III)	77		11	17			
Advanced (WHO≥III)	140		14.7	88			
Lung carcinoma study, Phase II, retrospective	61	67.2	16.4				[385], [160]
Pancreas tumor study, Phase II, retrospective	26	46.2	11.6				[386]
Liver metastasis form colorectal origin, Phase II, retrospective	30		22				[387]
Pancreas tumor study, Phase II, retrospective	107						[385]
Passive arm	34		6.5				
Active arm	73	52.1	9.93	58	25.5	8.4	
Pancreas tumor study, Phase II, retrospective	30	31.0		41	34.4	5.6	[388], [389]
Pancreas tumor study, Phase II, retrospective	42	52.4	12.3				[390]
Pancreas tumor study, Phase II, retrospective	13	40.0	11.9				[391]
Pelvic gynecological cancer studies, Phase II, retrospective	74						[392]
Cervix	38	86.8	27.6	25	63.5	20.9	
Ovary	27	100	37.8	67	132.7	19.4	
Uterus	9	100	61.5	62	68.5	32.0	
Prostate cancer study, Phase II, retrospective	18	88.9	38.8	72	53.4	7.6	[377]

Study	Number of patients	1st year survival (%)	Median overall survival (m)	Resposnding patients/ratio (%)	Median overall survival of responding patients (m)	Median overall survival of non-responding patients (m)	Reference
Esophagus study, Phase II, retrospective	7		6.8	100			[378]
Soft tissue sarcoma study, Phase II, retrospective	16	100	35.9	31	115.3	31.3	[160]
Stomach cancer study, Phase II, retrospective	68	58.9	14.4				[160]
Urinary bladder cancer study, Phase II, retrospective	18	85.0	36.5	73	42.0	22.6	[160]

Table 1. Summary of the studies made by oncothermia treatment

We show, as spectacular examples, two important categories in comparison with the literature: the sensitive extra-cranial (non-invasive) brain glioma treatments and the treatments of the aggressive pancreas tumors.

4.4.1. Comparison of brain studies

Some more open-label, single arm, monocentric, retrospective and intention-to-treat frame oncothermia studies were published at professional conferences, [393], [394], [395], [396], [397] as well.

The comparison of the median survivals for anaplastic astrocytoma and for glioblastoma multiform obtained by different clinics shows good correlations. Their glioblastoma multiform (WHO IV) results are ranging from 14-25.2 months median survival (weighted mean is 19.1 months), while the literature ([352], [398], [399], [400]), uses only 10.5 months weighted mean.

According to the RTOG classifications [401], we divided the patients into two groups: age under- and over-50 years. By this division in cases of glioblastoma oncothermia has 14.4 and 19 months for over and under 50 years of ages, [397]; while RTOG has 9.7 and 13.7 months, [401]; respectively. The method shows successful applications in pediatric cases as well, [402].

The results are pretty coherently above the statistical values of the large databases SEER [352] and the gold-standard radiotherapy (RT) and RT+PCV [398]. The results of oncothermia show advantages in comparison with the publications on Temozolomide [399], [400], too.

The first-year survival rates compared to SEER [352] and EUROCARE [353] databases as well as to the recent chemotherapy of Temozolomide also show significant advantages (more than 25% increase) of oncothermia.

No serious side effects were observed [403]. Patients tolerated the treatments well during the whole treatment period. Most of the patients were well relaxed, some even fell asleep during the treatment. Patients reported better quality of life, but this information was not objectively measured.

The results well indicate the feasibility and the benefit of the oncothermia showing a valid treatment potential and safe application. Oncothermia is a potential way to escape from the present impasse situation and could treat brain gliomas successfully. Question of Editorial of JAMA "Where to go from here?" [404] could be answered with the help of the oncothermia way.

4.4.2. Comparison of pancreas efficacy studies I. & II

For clear evidence of the results, let us compare the first year survivals and the median survivals obtained in various clinics in comparison to the historical control and the large databases. The weighted average of five clinics of the first year survival percentages and the median survival times are 47.5 % and 12.4 months for oncothermia, while the references (large databases SEER and EUROCARE) show 15.6 % and 7.3 months, respectively.

5. Future – To join or not to join?

Oncothermia formulated a new paradigm: [72], and made it clear "What is against the acceptance of hyperthermia?" [83]. The problem is the misleading aim of getting uncontrollable temperature as dose and ignoring the physiological reaction of the patients.

The philosophy of oncothermia simply follows the line of Hypocrates: "Nil Nocere" ("Do not harm"). Of course this has to be understood as "be natural as much as possible". Oncothermia supports the natural processes of living organisms, applying the normal physiological and biophysical reactions of the body, using these to fight against the malignancy on standard way. The basic problem of the malignancy is that the immune system and all the protective mechanisms of the organism do not fight against this lesion, do not recognize the danger, they handle it as a normal tissue, supply and try to solve the irregularities, if it was a wound. By the appropriate selective mechanism, oncothermia is able to "discover" these irregularities, showing their differences from the normal tissue and activate the standard protective, defense mechanisms in the body to fight.

5.1. Natural treatment paradigm

The natural therapy must help the body's internal corrective actions to reestablish the healthy state. In normal healthy state the body is in homeostasis, which is controlled by numerous negative feedback loops, making the actual state definitely "constant" despite its energetically open status, (see Figure 45.). The disease breaks up the relative equilibrium, and the body tries to reestablish the homeostasis. For this enhanced negative feedback control is enforced (see Figure 46.). Recognizing the disease, we act with our medical knowledge, and in many cases, we work against the natural homeostasis, the constrained action induces new homeostatic negative feedback. The body starts to fight against our constraints together with the disease (see Figure 47.). This controversial situation happens with classical hyperthermia, when the constrained massive temperature change is physiologically down-regulated (or at least the physiology works against it by the systemic [like blood-flow] and local [like HSP] reactions). Oncothermia disclaims the old approach, introducing a new paradigm: with the application of micro-heating, it induces considerably less physiological feedback to work against the action, and with the application of the electric field it uses such effect, for which the body has no physiological answer. With this new paradigm, oncothermia helps the natural feedback mechanisms to reestablish the healthy state (see Figure 48.).

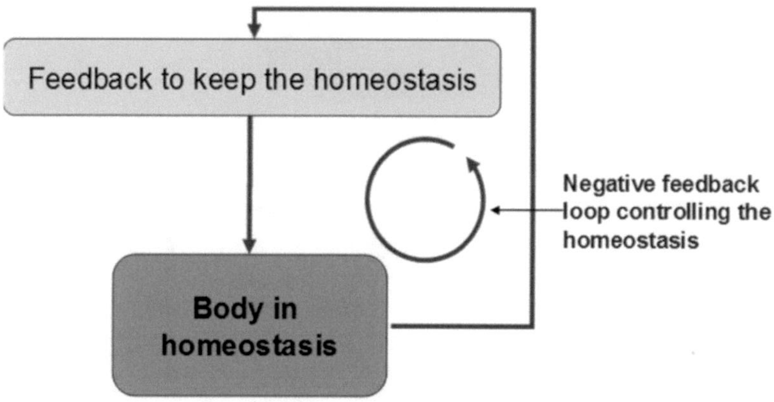

Figure 45. The natural healthy state is stabilized by the negative feedback loops of physiology

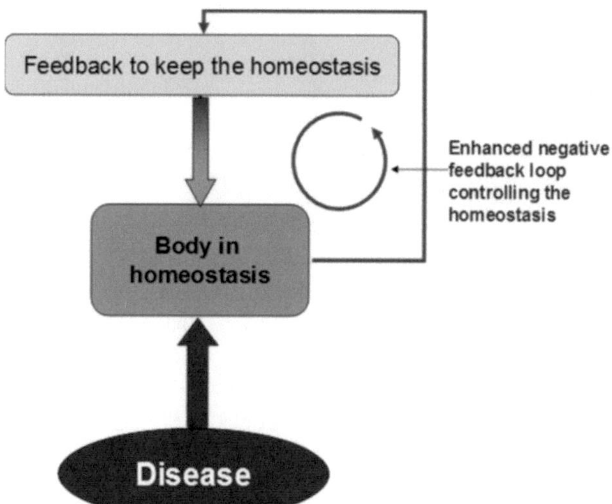

Figure 46. The disease breaks the homeostasis, so the physiology tries to compensate and correct the damage

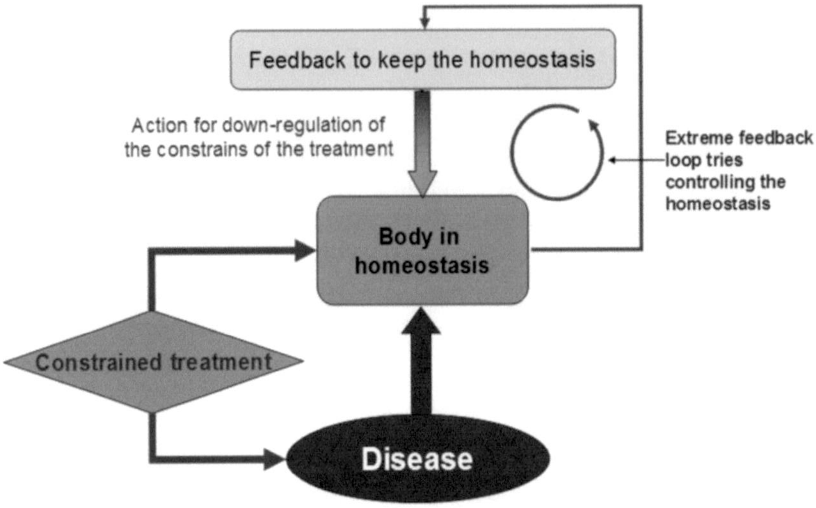

Figure 47. The classical hyperthermia introduces a new constrained effect which induces even more physiological feedback, forcing the body for the "double front" fight

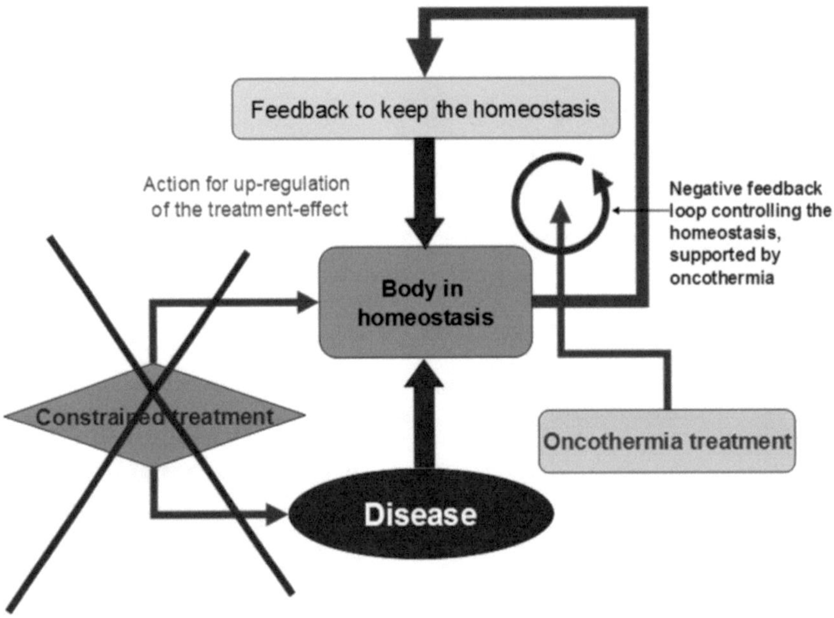

Figure 48. Oncothermia acts differently. It helps the natural feedback loops for natural corrections

Oncothermia blocks the physiological positive feedbacks, reestablishes the homeostasis to the level, which the actual conditions allow. The blocks are effective:

- The growth of cancer itself has a positive feedback loop. The rate of proliferation depends on the actual mass of the tumor, so the tumor mass gradually grows. Selective blocking of malignant autonomy could eliminate the positive feedback loop of malignancy.

- The lowering of the pH of the tumor is also a positive feedback loop. By the blocking of the high metabolic rate, the pH-loop is eliminated as well.
- The injury current loop also has positive feedback. This is broken by the flow of the electric current density.
- The neoangiogenesis is also a positive feedback, supporting the tumor by its accelerated nutrition demand. The electric current prefers the new vessels for conduction, blocking their actions.
- The growing temperature decreases the impedance (increases the conductance by the mobility of the ions) in the tumor. This positive feedback loop is used till the temperature does not increase too much. The step-up heating uses this effect and controls this loop.
- The growing temperature blocks the blood-flow in the tumor, which traps the heat in the center of the tumor. The heat-trap makes necrosis in the center of the tumor, which is anyway very acidic, and in most cases it is necrotized naturally. In artificial focusing, this necrotized volume remains the main target, however it does not need more energy. The real danger of the tumor is the vividly living outer "shell" which is responsible for metastases and for the volume-occupying rapid growth as well. The oncothermia current flows through this "shell" irrespective of how large the necrotic center is, and makes the oncothermia effective. It is shown, that after oncothermia the proliferation activity is drastically suppressed even in the possible remaining tumor tissue, which of course was massively targeted by the RF current.

5.2. Epilogue

Hyperthermia is an ancient treatment. It was the very first one in oncology, but it could not find its established place among the "gold standards" of the oncotherapies. The controversial results were originated from the paradigm to constrain the temperature growth in the process. The constrained forces made physiological contra-reactions keep the homeostasis, which unfortunately contains the malignant tissue as well. The actions have to be selective, and have to be gentle enough to work together with the natural processes, and not against them.

Oncothermia selects the malignant cells and acts differently from the physiological homeostatic reactions (heat-flow on the membrane supported by the electric field effects). It is natural, it is not against the homeostasis and physiology does not work against the action. The main task is to direct the physiology in the standard way, and act on such normal line. The positive feedback loops (the avalanche effects), which may destroy the normal homeostatic equilibrium have to be stopped.

Oncothermia follows the update demands of the modern oncology:

- It is a personalized therapy,
- It is non- toxic,
- It elongates the survival time of the patients,
- It completes the curative actions with increased quality of life
- It has good cost/benefit ratio

The introduced new paradigm by oncothermia solved the classical challenges:

- Challenge (1): "The biology is with us while the physics is against us" (Overgard J., [405]).
- *Oncothermia solution:* "The biophysics is with us"
- Challenge (2): "The biology and the physics are with us while the physiology is against us" (Osinsky S., [88]).
- *Oncothermia solution:* "The fractal physiology is with us"
- Challenge (3): "Reference point is needed!" (Fatehi D. van der Zee J., et. al. [406]).
- *Oncothermia solution:* "Back to the gold standards, use the energy instead of temperature"

The task for the future is challenging, and we are expecting professionals to repeat our results and come with us to fight in the war against cancer [407].

Author details

Andras Szasz, Nora Iluri and Oliver Szasz
Department of Biotechnics, St.Istvan University, Hungary

6. References

[1] Fischler M.P., Reinhart W.H. (1997). "Fever: friend or enemy?". Schweiz Med Wochenschr 127 (20): 864–70
[2] Christian Raetz and Chris Whitfield (2002) Lipopolysaccharide Endotoxins Annu. Rev. Biochem. 71:635-700
[3] Rosenberg H, Davis M, James D, Pollock N, Stowell K (2007). "Malignant hyperthermia". Orphanet J Rare Dis 2: 21.
[4] Su F, Nguyen ND, Wang Z, Cai Y, Rogiers P, Vincent JL (2005). "Fever control in septic shock: beneficial or harmful?". Shock (Augusta, Ga.) 23 (6): 516–20
[5] Milligan AJ (1984) Whole-Body Hyperthermia Induction Techniques. Cancer Res 44:4869s-4872s
[6] Galvagno SM (2003) Emergency Pathophysiology: Clinical Applications for Prehospital Care. Teton New Media, Jackson, USA, Ch.30, p.361
[7] Smith E (2002) Egyptian Surgical Papyrus dated around 3000 B.C. (cited by: van der Zee J: Heating the patient: a promising approach? Ann. Oncol. 13:1173-1184
[8] Bruch W (1866) Verhandlungen ärztlicher Gesellschafter. Berl Klin Wschr. 3:245-246
[9] Schamberg J, Tseng H (1927) Experiments on the therapeutic value of hot baths with special reference to the treatment of syphilis, and some physiologic observations. Am J of Syphilis XI:337-397
[10] Seegenschmiedt MH, Vernon CCA (1995) Historical Perspective on Hyperthermia in Oncology. Seegenschmiedt MH, Fessenden P, Vernon CC (eds): Thermoradiotherapy and thermochemotherapy Vol 1, Springer/Verlag Berlin Heidelberg

[11] Medieval literature – 1. Medieval Turkish Surgical manuscript from Charaf ed-Din, 1465 (Paris, Bibliotheque Nationale), 2. Armamentarium chirurgicum of Johann Schultes, Amsterdam 1672 (Paris, Bibliotheque de Faculte Medicine), cited by: Seegenschmiedt MH, Vernon CC:A Historical Perspective on Hyperthermia in Oncology, In: Seegenschmiedt MH, Fessenden P, Vernon CC (eds): Thermoradiotherapy and thermochemotherapy Vol 1, Springer/Verlag Berlin Heidelberg 1995
[12] Busch W (1866) Uber den Einfluss welche heftigere Erysipeln zuweilig auf organisierte Neubildungenausuben. Vrh. Naturhist. Preuss Rhein Westphal 23:28-30
[13] Coley WB (1893) The treatment of malignant tumors by repeated inoculations of erysipelas with a report of ten original cases. Am J Med Sci 105:487-511
[14] Westermark F (1898) Uber die Behandlung des ulcerierenden Cervixcarcinoms mittels konstanter Warme, Zentralbl. Gynaekol. 22:1335-1337
[15] Westermark N (1927) The effect of heat on rat tumors. Skand. Arch. Physiol. 52:257-322
[16] Overgaard K (1934) Uber Warmeterapie bosartiger Tumoren. Acta Radiol. [Ther.] (Stockholm) 15:89-99
[17] Muller C (1912) Therapeutische Erfahrungen an 100 mit kombination von Rontgenstrahlen un Hochfrequenz, resp. Diathermie behandeleten bosartigen Neubildungen, Munchener Medizinische Wochenschrift 28:1546-1549
[18] Adam J (1923) Carcinoma of right tonsil and soft palate treated by diathermy. Journ. of laryngol. a. otol. No. 4
[19] Barney (1969) Efficiency of the high frequenz current on tumors of the bladder. Boston med. a. surg. journ. No. 1.
[20] Bordier (1924) Puissance de la diathermie dans le cancer. Paris Medical, No. 10.
[21] Bruni (1921) La cura dei tumori benigni della vesicae con la diathermia. Rif med. Vol. 37.
[22] Corbus Budd (1921) Presentation of a case of prickle celled carcinoma of the penis treated by diathermy and radium. Urol. and. cut. rev. p. 204.
[23] Czerny (1911) Therapie des Krebses. Münch. med. Wochenschr. Nr. 58.
[24] Czerny (1910) Methoden der Krebsbehandlung. Münch. med. Wochenschr. Nr. 17.
[25] Davies Colley (1922) Periostal sarcoma of the temporal bone treated by diathermy. Proc. of the Royal. Soc. of Med. Vol. 15.
[26] Grenouville et Lacaille (1921)Behandlung der Blasentumoren mittels Diathermie. Journ. D'urol. p. 316.
[27] Gould u. Pearce (1913) The Treatment of inoperable cancers. The Lancet
[28] Johnson (1922) Diathermy in the treatment of malignant growths. Americ. Journ. of Electrotherapeut A. Radiol. Nr. 11.
[29] Müller Chr (1913) Die Krebskrankheit und ihre Behandlung mit Röntgenstrahlen und hochfrequenter Elektrizität Resp. Diathermie. Strahlentherapie. Bd. 2., H. 1.
[30] Müller Chr (1913) Die Röntgenbehandlung der malignen Tumoren und ihre Kombinationen. Strahlentherapie. Bd. 3.
[31] Novak (1922) The treatment of malignant tumors of the pharynx and larynx by diathermy Illinois Med. Journ. Vol. 41.

[32]Patterson (1923) Diathermy for malignant diseases of the month, pharynx and nose. With notes on seventeen successful cases. Brit. Med. Journ. p. 56
[33]Renner (1914) Behandlung der Blasentumoren mit Hochfrequenzströmen. Berl. Klin. Wochenschr. Nr. 37.
[34] Schmidt L. u. Kollischer (1916) Diathermy in malignant tumours of the bladder. Surg. Gynecol. A. Obstetr, V. 23.
[35] Stephan (1912) Histologische Untersuchungen über die Wirkung der Thermopenetration auf normale Gewebe und Carcinom. Beitr. z. klin. Chirurg. Bd. 77. H. 2.
[36] Steward (1922) Diathermy in the treatment of malignant disease. Practit. V. 108.
[37] Syne (1923) Surgical diathermy in the treatment of malignant disease of the troat. Glasgow. Med. Journ. No. 4.
[38] Syne (1923) Cases of malignant disease of the pharynx treated by surgical diathermy. Journ. of Laryngol. A. Otol. No. 4.
[39] Telemann (1911) Hochfrequenzströme in der Medizin. Dtsch. med. Wochenschr. Nr. 18.
[40] Theilhaber (1912) Behandlung der Carcinomkranken nach der Operation. 6. Internat. Kongr. f. Geburtsh. u. Gynäk. in Berlin
[41] Theilhaber (1913) Operationslose Behandlung des Carcinoms. Berl. klin. Wochenschr. Nr. 8.
[42] Theilhaber (1913) Die Verhütung der Rezidive nach Krebsbehandlung. Krebskongr. in Brüssel
[43] Theilhaber (1918) Die Behandlung der Krebskranken nach Entfernung der Geschwülste. Jahreskurse f. ärztl. Fortbild
[44] Theilhaber (1919) Die akute Entzündung als Heilmittel. Wien. Klin. Wochenschr. Nr. 29.
[45] Theilhaber (1919) Der Einfluss der Diathermiebehandlung auf das Carcinomgewebe. Münch. med. Wochenschr. Nr. 44.
[46] Theilhaber (1923) Der Einfluss der cellulären Immunität auf die Heilung der Carcinome, (insbesondere der Mamma und des Uterus). Arch. f. Gynäkol. S. 237.
[47] Werner: Die Rolle der Strahlentherapie bei der Behandlung maligner Tumoren. Strahlentherapie. Bd. 1. H. 1. u. 2.
[48] Werner u. Caan (1911) Elektro und Radiochirurgie im Dienste der Behandlung maligner Tumoren. Münch. med. Wochenschr. Nr. 23.
[49] Wyeth (1923) Die Diathermie bei der Behandlung maligner Tumoren. Americ. Journ. of. Electrotherapeut. a Radiol. No. 5.
[50] Kluger MJ (1991) Fever: Role of Pyrogens and Cryogens. Physiological Reviews 71:93-127
[51] Devrient W (1950) Überwärmungsbäder. A.Marcus&E.Weber's Verlag Berlin
[52] Hoff F (1957) Fieber, Unspezifische Abwehrvorgänge, Unspezifische Therapie. Georg Thieme Stuttgart
[53] Lampert H (1948) Überwärmung als Heilmittel. Hippokrates Stuttgart
[54] Schmidt KL (1987) Hyperthermie und Fieber. Hippokrates Stuttgart

[55] Heckel M (1990) Ganzkörperhyperthermie und Fiebertherapie – Grundlagen und Praxis. Hippokrates Stuttgart

[56] Heckel M (1992) Fiebertherapie und Ganzkörper-HT, Bessere Verträglichkeit und Effizienz durch thermoregulatorisch ausgewogene, kombinierte Anwendung beider Verfahren. ThermoMed 14-19

[57] Vaupel P, Kruger W (1992) Warmetherapie mit wassergefilterter Infrarot-A-Strahlung, Grundlagen und Anwendungsmoglichkeiten. Hippocrates, Verlag Stuttgart

[58] Hildebrandt B, Drager J, Kerner T et al (2004) Whole-body hyperthermia in the scope of von Ardenne's systemic cancer multistep therapy (sCMT) combined with chemotherapy in patients with metastatic colorectal cancer: a phase I/II study. Int. J. Hyperthermia, 20:317-333

[59] Ardenne A. Von, Wehner H (2005) Extreme Whole-Body Hyperthermia with Water-Filtered Infrared-A Radiation. Eurekah Bioscience Collection, Oncology, Landes Bioscience

[60] Wust P, Riess H, Hildebrandt B (2000) Feasibility and analysis of thermal parameters for the whole-body hyperthermia system IRATHERM 2000. Int. J. Hyperthermia 4:325-339

[61] Kraybill W, Olenki T (1998) A phase I study of fever-range whole body hyperthermia (FR-WBH) in patients with advanced solid tumors: correlation with mouse models, Int. J. Hyperthermia, 2002, Vol. 18, No. 3, 253-266 and Burd R, Dziedzic ST: Tumor Cell Apoptosis, Lymphocyte Recruitment and Tumor Vascular Changes Are Induced by Low Temperature, Long Duration (Fever-Like) Whole Body Hyperthermia, Journal of Cellular physiology 177:137-147

[62] Toyota, Strebel, Stephens, Matsuda, Bull (1997) Long Duration - Mild Whole Body Hyperthermia with Cisplatin: Tumour Response and Kinetics of Apoptosis and Necrosis in a Metastatic at Mammary Adenocarcinoma, Int. J. Hyperthermia, 13:497-506

[63] Sakaguchi Y, Makino M, Kaneko T et al (1994) Therapeutic Efficacy of Long Duration – Low Temperature Whole Body Hyperthermia When Combined with Tumor Necrosis Factor and Carboplatin in Rats. Cancer Research 54:2223-2227

[64] Ostberg R (2000) Use of mild, whole body hyperthermia in cancer therapy. Immunological Invest. 29:139-142

[65] Appenheimer MM, Chen Q, Girard RA, Wang WC, Evans SS (2005) Impact of Fever-Range Thermal Stress on Lymphocyte-Endothelial Adhesion and Lymphocyte Trafficking. Immunological Inestigations, 34:295-323

[66] Shah A, Unger E, Bain MD et al (2002) Cytokine and adhesion molecule expression in primary human endothelial cells stimulated with fever-range hyperthermia. Int. J. Hyperthermia, 18:534-551

[67] Ostberg JR, Gellin C, Patel R, Repasky EA (2001) Regulatory Potential of Fever-Range Whole Body Hyperthermia on Langerhans Cells and Lymphocytes in an Antigen-Dependant Cellular Immune Response. The Journal of Immunology; 167:2666-2670

[68] Burd R, Dziedzic TS, Xu Y et al (1998) Tumor Cell Apoptosis, Lymphocyte Recruitment and Tumor Vascular Changes Are Induced by Low Temperature, Long Duration (Fever-Like) Whole Body Hyperthermia. J. Cellular physiology, 177:137-147

[69] Dahl O, Dalene R, Schem BC, Mella O (1999) Status of clinical hyperthermia. Acta Oncol. 38(7):863-873

[70] Senior K (2001) Hyperthermia and hypoxia for cancer-cell destruction. Lancet Oncology, 2:524-525

[71] Wust P, Hildebrandt B, Sreenivasa G, Rau B et al (2002) Hyperthermia in combined treatment of cancer. Lancet 3:487-497

[72] Szasz A, Szasz O, Szasz N (2001) Electrohyperthermia: a new paradigm in cancer therapy. Wissenschaft & Forschung, Deutsche Zeitschrift für Onkologie, 33:91-99

[73] Szasz A, Szasz N, Szasz O (2003) Hyperthermie in der Onkologie mit einem historischen Uberblick. Wissenschaft & Forschung, Deutsche Zeitschrift für Onkologie; 35:140-154

[74] Abe M, Hiraoka M, Takahashi M et al (1986) Multi-institutional studies on hyperthermia using an 8-MHz radiofrequency capacitive heating device (Thermotron RF-8) in combination with radiation for cancer therapy. Cancer. 58:1589-1595

[75] Pacing Clin Electrophysiol. 2000 Jan;23(1):8-17. Tissue temperatures and lesion size during irrigated tip catheter radiofrequency ablation: an in vitro comparison of temperature-controlled irrigated tip ablation, power-controlled irrigated tip ablation, and standard temperature-controlled ablation. Petersen HH, Chen X, Pietersen A, Svendsen JH, Haunsø S., http://www.ncbi.nlm.nih.gov/pubmed/10666748

[76] Percutaneous cryoablation techniques and clinical applications, Servet Tatlı, Murat Acar, Kemal Tuncalı, Paul R. Morrison, Stuart Silverman
http://www.dirjournal.org/pdf/DIREPUB_1922_online.pdf

[77] Hornbach NB (1987) Is the community radiation oncologist ready for clinical hyperthermia? RadioGraphics 7:139-141

[78] Storm FK (1993) What happened to hyperthermia and what is its current status in cancer treatment? J Surg Oncol 53:141-143

[79] Brizel DM (1998) Where there's smoke, is there fire? Int J Hyperthermia 14:593-594

[80] Sneed PK, Dewhirst MW, Samulski T et al (1998) Should interstitial thermometry be used for deep hyperthermia? Int. J. Radiat. Oncol Biol. Phys. 40:1205-1212

[81] Oleson JR (1989) If we can't define the quality, can we assure it? Int. J. Radiat. Oncol Biol. Phys 16:879

[82] Nielsen OS, Horsman M, Overgaard J (2001) A future of hyperthermia in cancer treatment? (Editorial Comment), European Journal of Cancer, 37:1587-1589

[83] Szasz A (2006) What is against the acceptance of hyperthermia? Die Naturheilkunde Forum-Medizine 83:3-7

[84] Oleson JR (1991) Progress in hyperthermia? Int. J. Radiat. Oncol Biol. Phys 20:1147-1164

[85] Oleson JR (1993) Prostate cancer: hot, but hot enough? Int. J. Radiat. Oncol Biol. Phys. 26: 369-370

[86] van der Zee J (2002) Heating the patient: a promising approach? Annals of Oncology 13:1173-1184

[87] Smythe WR, Mansfield PF (2003) Hyperthermia: has its time come? Ann Surg Oncol 10:210-212

[88] Osinsky S, Ganul V, Protsyk V et al (2004) Local and regional hyperthermia in combined treatment of malignant tumors: 20 years experience in Ukraine, The Kadota Fund International Forum 2004, Awaji Japan, June 15-18

[89] Markovitch, O., Agmon, N.: Structure and energetics of the hydronium hydration shells. J. Phys. Chem. A. 111(12), 2253–2256 (2007)

[90] Jeffrey GA (1997) An Introduction to Hydrogen Bonding (Topics in Physical Chemistry). Oxford University Press, USA

[91] Morowitz HJ (1992) Beginnings of Cellular Life: Metabolism Recapitulates Biogenesis. Yale University Press, p 69

[92] Vaupel PW, Kelleher DK (1996) Metabolic status and reaction to heat of normal and tumor tissue, In: Seegenschmiedt MH., Fessenden P., Vernon CC. (Eds.) Thermo-radiotherapy and Thermo-chemotherapy, Vol. 1. Biology, physiology and physics, Springer Verlag, Berlin Heidelberg, pp. 157-176

[93] Kabakov AE, Gabai VL (1997) Heat Shock Proteins and cytoprotection: ATP-deprived mammalian cells. (Series: Molecular Biology Intelligence Unit), Springer Verlag, New York, Berlin, Heidelberg

[94] Keszler G, Csapo Z, Spasokoutskaja T et al (2000) Hyperthermy increase the phosporylation of deoxycytidine in the membrane phospholipid precursors and decrease its incorporation into DNA. Adv Exper Med Biol 486:333-337

[95] Dikomey E, Franzke J (1992) Effect of heat on induction and repair of DNA strand breaks in X-irradiated CHO cells. Int J Radiat Biol 61(2):221-233

[96] Shen, R.N., Lu, L., Young, P., et, al.: Influence of elevated temperature on natural killer cell activity, lymphokine-activated killer cell activity and lecitin-dependent cytotoxicity of human umbilical cord blood and adult blood cells. Int. J. Radiat. Oncol. Biol. Phys. 29, 821-26 (1994)

[97] Srivastava PK, DeLeo AB, Old LJ (1986) Tumor Rejection Antigens of Chemically Induced Tumors of Inbred Mice. Proc Natl Acad Sci USA 38(10):3407-3411

[98] Csermely P, Schnaider T, Soti C et al (1998) The 90 kDa Molecular Chaperone Family: Structure, Function and Clinical Applications A Comprehensive Review. Pharmacol Ther 79(2):129-168

[99] Gonzalez-Gonzalez, D.: Thermo-radiotherapy for tumors of the lower gastro-instenstinal tract. In: M.H. Seegenschmiedt, M.H., Fessenden, P., Vernon, C.C. (eds.) Thermo-radiotherapy and Thermo-chemiotherapy. Biology, physiology and physics, Vol. 1, pp. 105-119, Springer Verlag, Berlin, Heidelberg (1996)

[100] Reinhold HS (1987) Tumor microcirculation, In:Field SB and Franconi C (Eds): Physics and Technology of hyperthermia, NATO ASI Series, Series E: Applied Sciences, No. 127, Martinus Nijhoff Publishers, Dordrecht/Bosto/Lanchester, pp.448-457

[101] Reinhold HS (1987) Effects of hyperthermia on tumor microcirculation, In:Field SB and Franconi C (Eds): Physics and Technology of hyperthermia. NATO ASI Series, Series E: Applied Sciences, No. 127, Martinus Nijhoff Publishers, Dordrecht/Bosto/Lanchester, pp.458-469

[102] Tanaka Y (2001) Thermal responses of microcirculation and modification of tumor blood flow in treating the tumors, In: Kosaka M, Sugahara T, Schmidt KL, Simon E (Eds.): Thermotherapy for Neoplasia, Inflammation, and Pain. Springer Verlag Tokyo, pp. 407-419

[103] Reinhold HS, Blachiewicz, Berg-Blok (1978) Decrease in tumor microcirculation during hyperthermia, In: Streffer C, vanBeuningen D, Dietzel F, Röttinger E, Robinson JE, Scherer E, Seeber S, Trott K-R (Eds): Cancer Therapy by hyperthermia and radiation. Urban & Schwarzenberg, Baltimore-Munich, pp.231-232

[104] Dudar TE, Jain RK (1984) Differential response of normal and tumor microcirculation to hyperthermia. Cancer Research, 44:605-612

[105] Hudlicka O, Tyler KR (1984) The effect of long-term high-frequency stimulation on capillary density and fibre types in rabbit fast muscles. J. Physiol. 353:435-445

[106] Endrich B, Hammersen F (1986) Morphologic and hemodynamic alterations in capillaries during hyperthermia, In: Anghileri LJ, Robert J. (Eds.): Hyperthermia in Cancer Treatment. CRC Press, Inc. Boca Raton Florida, US, Vol II. pp. 17-47, (Ch. 2)

[107] Zant G. van (1986) Effects of hyperthermia on hematopoietic tissues, In: Anghileri LJ, Robert J. (Eds.): Hyperthermia in Cancer Treatment. CRC Press, Inc. Boca Raton Florida, US, Vol II. Pp. 59-73, (Ch. 4)

[108] Hales JRS, Hirata K (1986) Aspects of circulatory responses in animals pertinent to the use of hyperthermia in cancer treatment, In: Anghileri LJ, Robert J. (Eds.): Hyperthermia in Cancer Treatment. CRC Press, Inc. Boca Raton Florida, US, Vol II. Pp. 49-58, (Ch. 3)

[109] Ingram DL, Mount LE (1975) Man and animals in hot environments, Topics in environmental physiology and medicine. Springer Verlag, Berlin, Heidelberg, New York,

[110] Urano M (1994) Thermochemotherapy: from in vitro and in vivo experiments to potential clinical application, In: Urano & Douple (eds.) Hyperthermia in Oncology 4:169-204

[111] Ohno T, Sakagami T, Shiomi M et al (1993) Hyperthermai therapy for deep-regional cancer: thermochemotherapy, a combination of hyperthermia with chemotherapy. In: Matsuda T (ed) Cancer treatment by hyperthermia, radiation and drugs, Taylor&Francis, London-Washington DC, pp 303-316

[112] Piantelli M, Tatone D, Castrilli G et al (2001) Quercetin and tamoxifen sensitize human melanoma cells to hyperthermia. Melanoma Research 11:469-476

[113] Pilling MJ, Seakins PW (1995) Reaction kinetics. Oxford Science Publications, Oxford University Press, Oxford

[114] Wiedermann GJ, Feyerabend T, Mentzel M et al (1994) Thermochemotherapie: grunde fur die kombinationsbehandlung mit hyperthermia und chemotherapie. Focus Mul 11:44-50

[115] Issels RD, Abdel-Rahman S, Salat C et al (1998) Neoadjuvant chemotherapy combined with regional hyperthermia (RHT) followed by surgery and radiation in primary recurrent high-risk soft tissue sarcomas (HR STS) of adults (updated report), J. Cancer Res. Clin. Oncol. 124:R105

[116] LeVeen HH, Rajagopalan PR, Vujic I et al (1984) Radiofrequency thermotherapy, local chemotherapy, and arterial Occlusion in the treatment of non-resectable cancer. Am Surg 50(2):61-65

[117] Okamura K, Nakashima K, Fukushima Y et al Hyperthermia with low dose chemotherapy for advanced non-small-cell lung cancer. http://www.isshin.or.jp/okamura/awaji2004/awaji1.html

[118] Franchi F, Grassi P, Ferro D et al (2007) Antiangiogenic metronomic chemotherapy and hyperthermia in the palliation of advanced cancer. European Journal of Cancer Care 16(3):258-262

[119] Streffer C, (1995) Molecular and cellular mechanism of hyperthermia In: Seegenschmiedt MH., Fessenden P., Vernon CC. (Eds.) Thermo-radiotherapy and Thermo-chemotherapy, Vol. 1. Biology, physiology and physics, Springer Verlag, Berlin Heidelberg, pp. 47-74

[120] Roti JL, Laszlo A (1988) The effects of hyperthermia on cellular macromolecules. In: Urano M, Douple E (eds) Hyperthermia and Oncology Vol 1, Thermal effects on cells and tissues, VSP Utrecht, The Netherlands, pp 13-56

[121] Okumura Y, Ihara M, Shimasaki T, Takeshita S, Okaichi K (2001) Heat inactivation of DNA-dependent protein kinase: possible mechanism of hyperthermic radio-sensitization, in: Thermotherapy for Neoplasia, Inflammation, and Pain, (Kosaka M, Sugahara T, Schmidt KL, Simon E (Eds.)), Springer Verlag Tokyo pp. 420-423

[122] Urano M, Douple E. (eds) (1992) Hyperthermia and Oncology: Volume .2. Biology of thermal potentiation of radiotherapy. VSP BV Utrecht The Netherlands, VSP BV Utrecht, The Netherlands

[123] Perez CA, Brady LW, Halperin EC et al (2004) Principles and Practice of Radiation Oncology. 4th edition, Lippincott Williams and Wilkins, Philadelphia

[124] Molls M (1992) Hyperthermia – the actual role in radiation oncology and future prospects. Strahlenterapie und Oncologie 168:183-190

[125] Seegenschmiedt MH, Feldmann HJ, Wust P (1995) Hyperthermia – its actual role is radiation oncology. Strahlentherapie und Oncologie 171:560-572

[126] Emami B, Scott C, Perez CA et al (1996) Phase III study of interstitial thermoradiotherapy compared with interstitial radiotherapy alone in the treatment of recurrent or persistent human tumors: a prospectively controlled randomized study by radiation therapy oncology group. Int J Rad Oncol Biol Phys 34(5):1097-1104

[127] Wust P, Rau B, Gemmler M et al (1995) Radio-thermotherapy in multimodal surgical treatment concepts. Onkologie 18(2):110-121

[128] Hentschel M, Wust P, (2000), Hyperthermia: bald eine entablierte Therapie? MTA Spectrum, 12:623-628

[129] Hager ED, Birkenmeier J, Popa C, (2006), Hyperthermie in der Onkologie: Eine viel versprechende neue Methode? Deutsche Zeitschrift fur Onkologie, 38:100-107

[130] Hehr T, Wust P, Bamberg M et al (2003) Current and potential role of thermoradiotherapy for solid tumors. Onkologie 26(3):295-302

[131] van der Zee J, Gonzalez Gonzalez D, van Rhoon GC et al (2000) Comparison of radiotherapy alone with radiotherapy plus hyperthermia in locally advanced pelvic tumors: a prospective, randomised, multicentre trial. Dutch Deep Hyperthermia Group. Lancet 355(9210):1119-1125

[132] Kodama K, Doi O, Higashyama M et al (1993) Long-term results of postoperative intrathoracic chemo-thermotherapy for lung cancer with pleural dissemination. Cancer 72(2):426-431

[133] Masunaga S, Hiraoka M, Akuta K et al (1990) Non-Randomized Trials of Thermoradiotherapy versus Radiotherapy for Preoperative Treatment of Invasive Urinary Bladder Cancer. J Jpn Soc Ther Radiol Oncol 2: 313-320

[134] Rau B, Wust P, Hohenberger P et al (1998) Preoperative Hyperthermia Combined with Radiochemotherapy in Locally Advanced Rectal Cancer – A Phase II Clinical Trial. Annals of Surgery 227(3):380-389

[135] Pearson AS, Izzo F, Fleming RYD et al (1999) Intraoperative radiofrequency ablation of cryoablation for hepatic malignances. Amer J Surg 178(6):592-598

[136] Kouloulias VE, Kouvaris JR, Nikita KS et al (2002) Intraoperative hyperthermia in conjunction with multi-schedule chemotherapy (pre- intra- and post operative), by-pass surgery, and post-operative radiotherapy for the management of unresectable pancreatic adenocarcinoma. Int.J Hyperthermia 18:233-252

[137] Ohtsuru A, Braiden V, Cao Y (2001) Cancer Gene Therapy in Conjunction with Hyperthermia Under the Control of Heat-Inducible Promoter. In: Kosaka M, Sugahara T, Schmidt KL (eds) Thermotherapy for Neoplasia, Inflammation, and Pain, Springer Verlag .Tokyo, pp 464-470

[138] Gaber MH, Wu NZ, Hong K et al (1996) Thermosensitive liposomes: extravasation and relase of contents in tumor microvascular networks. Int J Radiat Oncol Biol Phys 36(5):1177-1187

[139] Balckburn LV, Galoforo SS, Corry PM et al (1998) Adenoviral-mediated transfer of heat-inducible double suicide gene into prostate carcinoma cells. Cancer Res 58(7):1358-1362

[140] Huang Q, Hu JK, Zhang L et al (2000) Heat-induced gene expression as a novel targeted cancer gene therapy strategy. Cancer Res 60(13):3435-3439

[141] Yerushalmi A, Shani A, Fishelovitz Y et al (1986) Local microwave hyperthermia in the treatment of carcinoma of the prostate. Oncology 43(5):299-305

[142] Oleson JR. Calderwood SK. Coughlin CT. Dewhirst MW. Gerweck LE. Gibbs FA. Kapp DS. (1988), Biological and Clinical Aspects of Hyperthermia in Cancer Therapy. Am. J. Clin. Oncology 11:368-380

[143] Henderson BW, Waldow SM, Potter WR, Dougherty TJ. (1985) Interaction of Photodynamic Therapy and Hyperthermia: Tumor Response and Cell Survival Studies after Treatment of Mice in Vivo. Cancer Research 45:6071-6077

[144] Lohr F. Hu K, Huang Q. Zhang L. Samulski T. Dewhirst M. Li C. (2000) Enhancement of radiotherapy by hyperthermia-regulated gene therapy International Journal of Radiation OncologyBiologyPhysics, 48:1513-1518

[145] Skitzki JJ. Repasky EA. Evans SS. (2009) Hyperthermia as an immunotherapy strategy for cancer, Current Opinion in Investigational Drugs 10:550-558

[146] Vertrees RA. Jordan JM. Zwischenberger JB (2007) Hyperhtermia and Chemotherapy: The Science. In: Current Clinical Oncology, Intraperitoneal Cancer Therapy, Hlem CW. Edwards RP. (Eds.) Humana Press, Totowa NJ, USA

[147] Oliveira RS, Bevilacqua FRG, Chammas R (1997) Hyperthermia increases the metastatic potential of murine melanoma. Braz J Med Biol Res, 30:941-945

[148] Shah SA, Jain RK, Finney PL (1983) Enhanced metastasis formation by combined hyperthermia and hyperglycemia in rats bearing Walker 256 carcinosarcoma. Cancer Lett. 19(3):317-23

[149] Nathanson SD, Nelson L, Anaya P, Havstad S, Hetzel FW (1991) Development of lymph node and pulmonary metastases after local irradiation and hyperthermia of footpad melanomas, Clinical and Experimental Metastasis 9:377-392

[150] Brochure of Thermotron RF-8. (Yamamoto Vinita, Osaka, Japan)

[151] Gellermann J, Wlodarczyk W, Hildebrandt B, Ganter H, Nicolau A, Rau B, Tilly W, Fähling H, Nadobny J, Felix R, Wust P, (2005) Noninvasive Magnetic Resonance Thermography of Recurrent Rectal Carcinoma in a 1.5 Tesla Hybrid System Cancer Res 65:5872-5880

[152] Stoll AM (1967) Heat transfer in Biotechnology, in: Advances in heat Transfer, (Eds.: Hartnett JP, Irvine TF.) 4:65-139, Academic Press Inc. New York, London

[153] Cooper TE, Trezek GJ (1971) Correlation of thermal properties of some human tissue with water content. Aerospace Med. 42:24-27

[154] Ardenne M. von, Reitnauer PG (1977) Krebs-Mehrschritt-Therapie und Mikrozirkulation. Krebsgeschehen 9:134-149

[155] Streffer C (1990) Biological basis of thermotherapy, In: Gautherie M (Ed.): Methods of hyperthermia control, Clinical Thermology. Springer Verlag, Berlin, Heidelberg, New York, London, Paris, Tokyo, Hong Kong

[156] Law MP (1988) The response of normal tissues to hyperthermia, In: Urano M, Douple E. (Eds.) Hyperthermia and Oncology: Vol.1. Thermal effects on cells and tissues. VSP BV Utrecht The Netherlands, pp. 121-159

[157] Prescott DM (1996) Manipulation of physiological parameters during hyperthermia, In: Seegenschmiedt MH., Fessenden P., Vernon CC. (Eds.) Thermo-radiotherapy and Thermo-chemotherapy, Vol. 1. Biology, physiology and physics. Springer Verlag, Berlin Heidelberg, pp. 177-189

[158] Muftuler TL, Hamamura MJ, Birgul O, Nalcioglu O (2006) In Vivo MRI Electrical Impedance, Tomography (MREIT) of Tumors. Technology in Cancer Research and Treatment, 5(4):381-387

[159] van der Zee J, (2005) Presentation on Conference in Mumbai India (http://www.google.com/#sclient=psy&hl=en&site=&source=hp&q=%22van+der+Zee%22+Mumbai+ext:ppt&btnG=Google+Search&aq=&aqi=&aql=&oq=&pbx=1&bav=on.2,or.r_gc.r_pw.&fp=e7df6ea8d325b7b2, accessed Apr. 2011)

[160] Szasz A, Szasz N, Szasz O (2010) Oncothermia – Principles and Practices, Springer Verlag, Heidelberg

[161] Warburg O (1966) Oxygen, The Creator of Differentiation, Biochemical Energetics, Academic Press, New York, 1966; (Warburg O: The Prime Cause and Prevention of Cancer, Revised lecture at the meeting of the Nobel-Laureates on June 30, 1966 at Lindau, Lake Constance, Germany)

[162] Garber K (2004) Energy boost: The Warburg effect returns in a new theory of cancer. Journ. Nat. Canc. Inst. USA 96:1805-1806

[163] Hsu PP, Sabatini DM (2008) Cancer metabolism: Warburg and Beyond. Cell 134(5):703-707

[164] Oehr P, Biersack HJ, Coleman RE (Eds) (2004) PET and PET-CT in Oncology. Springer Verlag, Berlin-Heidelberg

[165] Babaeizadeh S (2007) 3-D Electrical Impedance Tomography of piecewise contant domains with known internal boundaries. IEEE Trans. Biomed. Eng. 54:2-10

[166] TransCan TS (2000) Transcan Medical Ltd. Migdal Ha'Emek, Israel, distributed by Siemens AG, Germany,

[167] Marino AA, Iliev IG, Schwalke MA, Gonzalez E, Marler KC, Flanagan CA (1994) Association between cell membrane potential and breast cancer. Tumour Biol, 15:82-89

[168] Cure JC (1995) Ont he electrical charateristics of cacer. II> International Congress of Electrochemical Treatment of Cancer. Jupiter, Florida

[169] Revici E (1961) Research in Pathophysiology as Basis Guided Chemotherapy, with Special Application to Cancer. Princeton, NJ> D. Van Nostrand Compani

[170] Seeger PG, Wolz S (1990) Succesful Biological Contol of Cancer. Neuwieder Verlagsgesellschaft Gmbh

[171] Cure JC. (1991) Cancer an electrical phenomenon. Resonant 1(1)

[172] Foster KR, Schepps JL (1981) Dielectric properties of tumor and normal tissues at radio through microwave frequencies. J. Microwave Power 16:107-119

[173] Peirce A (Tutor): IAM-CSC-PIMS senior undergraduate math modeling workshop, The Institute of Applied Mathematics (IAM), The University of British Columbia

[174] Metherall P (1998) Three-dimensional electrical impedance tomography of the human thorax. PhD thesis, University of Sheffield

[175] Mikac U, Demsar F, Beravs K, Sersa I (2001) Magnetic Resonance Imaging of alternating electric currents. Magnetic Resonance Imaging 19:845-856

[176] Joy M, Scott G, Henkelman M (1989) In vivo detection of applied electric currents by magnetic resonance imaging. Magnetic Resonance Imaging, 7:49-54

[177] Seersa I, Beravs K, Dodd NJF et al (1997) Electric current Imaging of Mice tumors. MRM 37:404-409

[178] Scott GC, Joy MLG, Armstrong RL, Henkelman RM (1995) Electromagnetic considerations for RF current density imaging. IEEE Trans. Med. Imaging 14:515-524

[179] Szasz A, Vincze Gy, Szasz O, Szasz N (2003) An energy analysis of extracellular hyperthermia. Magneto- and electro-biology, 22:103-115

[180] Pence DM, Song CW (1986) Effect of heat on blood-flow, In: Anghileri LJ, Robert J. (Eds.): Hyperthermia in Cancer Treatment, Vol. II. CRC Press, Inc. Boca Raton Florida, US, pp.1-17

[181] Häfner H-M, Bräuer K, Eichner M et al (2005) Analysis of Cutaneous Blood Flow in Melanocytic Skin Lesions. J. vascular Res. 42:38-46

[182] McRae DA, Esrick MA, Mueller SC (1997) Non-invasive, in-vivo electrical impedance of EMT-6 tumors during hyperthermia: correlation with morphology and tumour-growth delay. Int. J. Hyperthermia, 13:1-20

[183] Esrick MA, McRae DA (1994) The effect of hyperthermia induced tissue conductivity changes on electrical impedance temperature mapping. Phys. Med. Biol. 39:133-144

[184] Mott NF, Jones H (1958) The theory of the properties of metals and alloys. Dover Publ Inc, New York

[185] Cope FW (1969) Nuclear magnetic resonance evidence using D2O for structured water in muscle and brain. Biophys J 9(3):303-319

[186] Damadian R (1971) Tumor detection by nuclear magnetic resonance. Science 171(3976):1151-1153

[187] Cope, F.W.: A review of the applications of solid state physics concepts to biological systems. J. Biol. Phys. 3(1), 1-41 (1975)

[188] Hazlewood CF, Nichols BL, Chamberlain NF (1969) Evidence for the existence of a minimum of two phases of ordered water in skeletal muscle. Nature 222(195):747–750

[189] Hazlewood CF, Chang DC, Medina D et al (1972) Distinction between the Preneoplastic and Neoplastic State of Murine Mammary Glands. Proc Natl Acad Sci USA 69(6):1478-1480

[190] Szentgyorgyi, A.: The living state and cancer. Physiological Chemistry and Physics 12, 99-110 (1980)

[191] Gniadecka M, Nielsen OF, Wulf HC (2003) Water content and structure in malignant and benign skin tumors. Journal of Molecular Structure 661-662:405-410

[192] Beall PT et al (1979) Water-relaxation times of normal, preneoplastic, and malignant primary cell cultures of mouse mammary gland. In: 23rd Annual Meeting of the Biophysical Society, Atlanta, Georgia, USA, 26-28 February 1979

[193] Chung, S.H., Cerussi, A.E., Klifa, C., et. al.: In vivo water state measurements in breast cancer using broadband diffuse optical spectroscopy. Phys. Med. Biol. 53, 6713-6727 (2008)

[194] Fiskum G (2000) Mitochondrial participation in ischemic and traumatic neural cell death. Journal of Neurotrauma 17(10):843–855

[195] Ichas F, Mazat JP (1998) From calcium signaling to cell death: two conformations for the mitochondrial permeability transition pore. Switching from low- to high-conductance state. Biochimica et Biophysica Acta 1366:33–50

[196] Bonnet S, Archer SL, Allalunis-Turner J et al (2007) A Mitochondria-K+ Channel Axis Is Suppressed in Cancer and Its Normalization Promotes Apoptosis and Inhibits Cancer Growth. Cancer Cell 11(1):37–51

[197] Chidanbaram, R., Ramanadham, M.: Hydrogen bonding in biological molecules-an update. Physica B 174(1-4), 300-305 (1991)

[198] Szentgyorgyi A (1960) Introduction to a Submolecular Biology. Academic Press, New York, London

[199] Akerlof GA, Shiller RJ (2009) Animal spirits. Princeton University Press, Princeton and Oxford

[200] Moses ME, Hou C, Woodruff WH et al (2008) Revisiting a model of oncogenic growth: estimating model parameters from theory and data. Am Nat 171(5):632-645

[201] Pamatmat MM (2005) Measuring aerobic and anaerobic metabolism of benthic infauna under natural conditions. Journal of Experimental Zoology 228(3):405-413

[202] West GB, Woodruf WH, Born JH (2002) Allometric scaling of metabolic rate from molecules and mitochondria to cells and mammals. Proc Natl Acad Sci U S A 99(1):2473–2478

[203] Lane N (2006) Mitochondria: Key to Complexity. In: Martin W (ed) Origins of Mitochondria and Hydrogenosomes, Chapter 2, Springer, Heidelberg, Germany

[204] Szentgyorgyi A (1998) Electronic Biology and Cancer. Marcel Dekkerm New York

[205] Weinberg RA (1998) One renegade cell. Basic Books, A Member of the Perseus Books Group, New York

[206] Cairns J (1975) The Cancer Problem. Scientific American 233(5):64-72, 77-78

[207] Kurakin, A.: Scale-free flow of life: on the biology, economics, and physics of the cell. Theor. Biol. Med. Model. 6:6 (2009)

[208] Getling AV, Rayleigh-Benard C (1998) Structures and Dynamics. World Scientific, Singapore

[209] Hochachka PW (1999) The metabolic implications of intracellular circulation. Proc Natl Acad Sci USA 96(22):12233-12239

[210] Coulson RA (1986) Metabolic rate and the flow theory: a study in chemical engineering. Comp Biochem Physiol A Comp Physiol 84(2):217-229

[211] Szentgyorgyi A (1968) Bioelectronics, A Study on Cellular Regulations, Defense and Cancer. Acad. Press, New York, London

[212] Blad B, Baldetorp B (1996) Impedance spectra of tumour tissue in comparison with normal tissue; a possible clinical application for electric impedance tomography. Physiol. Meas. 17Suppl.4A:A105-15

[213] Stoy RD, Foster KR, Schwan HP (1982) Dielectric properties of mammalian tissues form 0.1 to 100 MHz: a summary of recent data, Phys.Med.Biol. 27:501-513

[214] Haemmerich D, Staelin ST, Tsai JZ et al (2003) In vivo electrical conductivity of hepatic tumors. Physiol. Meas. 24:251-260

[215] Smith SR, Foster KR, Wolf GL (1986) Dielectric properties of VX-2 carcinoma versus normal liver tissue. IEEE Trans. Biomed. Eng. BME-33:522-524

[216] Dubois J-M, Rouzaire-Dubois B (2004) The influence of cell-volume changes on tumor cell proliferation. Eur. Biophys. J, 33:227-232

[217] Avrami MA.: Kinetics of phase change Parts: I. J. Chem. Phys. 7, 1103 (1939); Avrami. M.A.: Kinetics of phase change Parts: II. J. Chem. Phys. 8, 212 (1940); Avrami, M.A.: Kinetics of phase change Parts: III. J. Chem. Phys. 9, 1103 (1941)

[218] Kolmogorov NN (1937) On the statistical theory of the crystallization of metals. Bull Acad Sci UssR Math Ser 1:355-359

[219] Joshnson WA, Mehl PA (1939) Reaction kinetics in processes of nucleation and growth. Trans Amer Inst Mining (Metal) Engrs 135:416

[220] Augis JA, Bennett JE (1978) Calculation of the Avrami parameters fer heterogeneous solid state reactions using a modification of the Kissinger method. J Therm Anal 13:285-291

[221] Levine LE, Narayan KL, Kelton KF (1997) Finite size corrections for the Johnson-Mehl-Avrami-Kolmogorov equation. J Mater Res 12(1):124-131

[222] Cope FW (1977) Detection of phase transitions and cooperative interactions by Avrami analysis of sigmoid biological time curves for muscle, nerve, growth, firefly, and infrared phosphorescence, of green leaves, melanin and cytochrome C. Physiol. Chem. Phys. 9(4-5):443-459

[223] Cope FW (1977) Solid State physical replacement of Hodgkin-Huxley theory. Phase transformation kinetics of axonal potassium conductance. Physiol. Chem. Phys. 9(2):155-160

[224] Cope FW (1977) The kinetics of biological phase transitions manifested by sigmoid time curves: a review of approaches. Physiol. Chem. Phys. 8(6):519-527

[225] Cope FW (1980) Avrami analysis of electrical switching in hydrated melanin suggest dependence on a phase transition. Physiol. Chem. Phys. 12:537-538

[226] Suckjoon J, Bechhoefer J (2005) Nucleation and growth in one dimension. II. Application to DNA replication kinetics. Phys. Rev. E. 71(1), 011909

[227] Haiyang Z (2005) Reconstructing DNA replication kinetics from small DNA fragments. Simon Fraser University, China

[228] Szent-gyorgyi A. (1941) Towards a new biochemistry? Science 93(2426):609-611

[229] Szent-gyorgyi A (1946) Internal photo-electric effect and band spectra in proteins. Nature 157:875-875

[230] Cope FW (1971) Evidence from activation energies for superconductive tunneling in biological systems at physiological temperatures. Physiol Chemistry & Physics 3:403-410

[231] Liboff AR (1985) Geomagnetic cyclotron resonance in living cells. J. Biol. Phys. 13(4):99-102

[232] Liboff AR (2003) Ion Cyclotron Resonance in Biological Systems: Experimental Evidence. In: Stavroulakis P (ed) Biological Effects of Electromagnetic Fields, Springer Verlag, Berlin-Heidelberg, pp 6-113

[233] Schrodinger E (1967) What is life? Cambridge University Press, Cambridge, United Kingdom
[234] Katchalsky A, Curran PF (1967) Non-equilibrium thermodynamics in biophysics. Harward University Press, Cambridge, MA, USA
[235] Haken H (1987) Self-Organization and Information. Phys. Script. 35(3):247-254
[236] Sornette D (2000) Chaos, Fractals, Self-Organization and Disorder: Concepts and Tools. Springer Verlag, Berlin-Los Angeles
[237] Deering W, West BJ (1992) Fractal physiology. IEEE Engineering in Medicine and Biology 11(2):40-46
[238] West BJ (1990) Fractal Physiology and Chaos in Medicine. World Scientific, Singapore, London
[239] Bassingthwaighte JB, Leibovitch LS, West BJ (1994) Fractal Physiology. Oxford Univ. Press, New York, Oxford
[240] Musha T, Sawada Y (eds.) (1994) Physics of the living state. IOS Press, Amsterdam
[241] Brown JH, West GB (eds) (2000) Scaling in Biology. Oxford University Press, Oxford
[242] Brown JH, West GB, Enquis BJ (2005) Yes, West, Brown and Enquist's model of allometric scaling is both mathematically correct and biologically relevant. Functional Ecology 19(4):735 –738
[243] West GB, Brown JH (2005) The origin of allometric scaling laws in biology from genomes to ecosystems: towards a quantitative unifying theory of biological structure and organization. Journal of Experimental Biology 208:1575-1592
[244] Camazine S, Deneubourg JL, Franks NR et al (2003) Self-organization in biological systems. Princeton Studies in Complexity, Princeton Univ. Press, Princeton, Oxford
[245] Bak P, Tang C, Wieserfeld K (1988) Self-organized criticality. Phys. Rev. A. 38:364-373
[246] Raff MC (1992) Social controls on cell survival and death. Nature 356(6368):397-400
[247] Loewenstein WR, Kanno Y (1967) Intercellular communication and tissue growth. The Journal of Cell Biology 33(2):225-234
[248] Dissado LA (1990) A fractal interpretation of the dielectric response of animal tissues. Phys. Med. Biol. 35:1487-1503
[249] El-Lakkani A (2001) Dielectric response of some biological tissues. Bioelectromagnetics 22:272-279
[250] Walleczek J (ed) (2000) Self-organized biological dynamics & nonlinear control. Cambridge Univ. Press, Cambridge
[251] Marjan MI, Szasz A (2000) Self-organizing processes in non-crystalline materials: from lifeless to living objects. OncoTherm Kft., Budapest
[252] West GB, Brown JH, Enquist BJ (1999) The Four Dimension of Life: Fractal Geometry and Allometric Scaling of Organisms. Science 284:4
[253] Hegyi G, Vincze G, Szasz A (2007) Axial-vector interaction with bio-systems. Electr. Biol. Med. 26:107-118
[254] Goldberger AL, Amaral LAN, Hausdorff JM, Ivanov PCh, Peng C-K: Fractal dynamics in physiology: Alterations with disease and aging, PNAS Colloquium,

99:2466-2472, Suppl.1., presented in Arthur M.Sackler Colloquium of NAS, March 23-24, 2001, Irvine, CA, USA

[255] Szendro P, Vincze G, Szasz A (2001) Bio-response on white-noise excitation. Electro- and Magnetobiology, 20:215-229

[256] Sapper A, Wegener J, Janshoff A (2006) "Cell motility probed by noise analysis of thickness shear mode resonators." Anal Chem. 15;78(14):5184-5191

[257] Sapper A, Reiss B, Janshoff A, Wegener J (2006) "Adsorption and fluctuations of giant liposomes studied by electrochemical impedance measurements." Langmuir. 22(2):676-680

[258] Cope, F.W.: Evidence from activation energies for superconductive tunneling in biological systems at physiological temperatures. Physiol Chemistry & Physics 3, 403-410 (1971)

[259] Liboff, A.R.: Geomagnetic cyclotron resonance in living cells. J. Biol. Phys. 13(4), 99-102 (1985)

[260] Schwan HP (1982) Nonthermal cellular effects of electromagnetic fields: AC-field induced ponderomotoric forces. Br. J. Cancer 45:220

[261] McCaig CD, Rajnicek AM, Song B, Zhao M (2005) Controlling cell behaviour electrically: current views and future potential. Physiol. Rev. 85:943-978

[262] Szasz N (2003) Electric field regulation of chondrocyte proliferation, biosynthesis and cellular signalling. PhD theses, MIT, Cambridge, USA

[263] Granmt D, (1904) The Galvano-Cautery in the Treatment of Intra-Laryngeal Growths. The Journal of Laryngology Rhinology and Ontology, 19 : 294-297

[264] Short History of Bioelectrics, http://www.pulsedpower.eu/bioelectrics/bio_02_main.html

[265] Kratzer GL, Onsanit T. (2007) Fulguration of selected cancers of the rectum: Report of 27 cases. Diseases of Colon and Rectum, 15:431-435

[266] LeVeen HH, Wapnick S, Piccone V et al (1976) Tumor eradication by radiofrequency therapy. JAMA 235(20):2198-2200

[267] Short JG, Turner PF (1980) Physical Hyperthermia and Cancer Therapy. Proc. IEEE 68:133-142

[268] Storm FK, Morton DL, Kaiser LR (1982) Clinical radiofrequency hyperthermia: a review. Natl Cancer Inst Monogr 61:343-50

[269] Watson BW (1991) Reappraisal: The treatment of tumors with direct electric current. Med. Sci. Res., 19:103-105

[270] Samuelsson L, Jonsson L, Stahl E (1983) Percutaneous treatment of pulmonary tumors by electrolysis. Radiologie 23:284-287

[271] Miklavcic D, Sersa G, Kryzanowski M (1993) Tumor treatment by direct electric current, tumor temperature and pH, electrode materials and configuration, Bioelectr. Bioeng. 30:209-211

[272] Katzberg AA (1974) The induction of cellular orientation by low-level electrical currents. Ann. New York Acad Sci. 238:445-450

[273] Nordenstrom BWE (1983) Biologically Closed Electric Circuits: Clinical experimental and theoretical evidence for an additional circulatory system. Nordic Medical Publications, Stockholm, Sweden

[274] Nordenstrom BWE (1998) Exploring BCEC-systems, (Biologically Closed Electric Circuits), Nordic Medical Publications. Stockholm, Sweden

[275] Matsushima Y, Takahashi E, Hagiwara K et al (1994) Clinical and experimental studies of anti-tumoral effects of electrochemical therapy (ECT) alone or in combination with chemotherapy. Eur. J. Surg. S-574:59-67

[276] Chou CK, Vora N, Li JR et al (1999) Development of Electrochemical treatment at he City of Hope (USA), Electricity and Magnetism in Biology and Medicine, Ed. Bersani, Kluwer Acad. Press/Plenum Publ., pp. 927-930,

[277] Pekar R, Korpan NN (2002) Krebs - Die medizinische und die biologische Tragödie. Vienna, Munich, Berne

[278] Pekar R (1996) Die Perkutane Galvano-Therapie bei Tumoren-Schwachstrombehandlung von zugänglichen Neoplasmen und ihre vitale Hybridisation in Theorie und Praxis. Verlag W. Maudrich, Vienna, Munich, Berlin

[279] Pekar R (2002) Die perkutane Bio-Elektrotherapie bei Tumoren (The percutaneous bio electrical therapy for tumors). Verlag W. Maudrich; Vienna – Munich - Berlin

[280] Ling X-Y. (1994) Advances in the treatment of malignant tumors by Electrochemical Therapy (ECT). Eur.J.Surgery, Suppl. 574:S31-36

[281] Xin Y, Xue F, Ge B et al (1997) Electrochemical treatment of lung cancer. Bioelectromagnetics 18(1):8-13

[282] Xin Y-L (1994) Organization and Spread electrochemical therapy (ECT) in China, Eur. J. Surg. S-574:25-30, 1994, and Xin Y-L: Advances in the treatment of malignant tumors by electrochemical therapy (ECT). Eur. J. Surg. S-574:31-36

[283] Quan K (1994) Analysis of the Clinical Effectiveness of 144 Cases of Soft Tissue and Superficial Maligniant Tumors Treated with Electrochemical Therapy The European Journal of Surgery Suppl. 574:S45-49, Scandinavian University Press

[284] Song Y (1994) Electrochemical Therapy in the Treatment of Malignant Tumors on the Body Surface. The European Journal of Surgery Suppl. 574:S41-43, Scandinavian University Press

[285] Senn E (1990) Elektrotherapie. Thieme Verlag, Stuttgart

[286] Robertson GSM, Wemys-Holden SA, Dennisson AR, Hall PM, Baxter P, Maddern GJ (1998) Experimental study of electrolysis-induced hepatic necrosis, British J. Surgery, 85:1212-1216

[287] Jaroszeski MJ, Coppola D, Pottinger C et al (2001) Treatment of hepatocellular carcinoma in a rat model, using electrochemotherapy. Eur. J. Cancer, 37:422-430

[288] Holandino C, Veiga VF, Rodrigues ML et al (2001) Direct current decreases cell viability but not P-glucoprotein expression and function in human multidrug resistant leukemic cells. Bioelectromagnetics 22:470/478

[289] Susil R, Semrov D, Miklavcic D (1998) Electric field-induced transmembrane potential depends on cell density and organization, Electro- and Magnetobiology, 17:391-399

[290] Vaupel P, Hammersen F (Hrsg.) (1982) Mikrozirkulation in malignen Tumoren. Karger, Basel

[291] Kirson ED, Dbaly V, Tovary F et al (2007) Alterníting electric fields arrest cell rpliferation, in animal tumor models and human brain tumors. Proc Nat Acad Sci 104:10152-10157

[292] Barbault A, Costa FP, Bottger B, Munden RF, Bomholt F, Kuster N, Pasche B (2009) Amplitude-modulated electromagnetic fields for the treatment of cancer: Discovery of tumor specific frequencies and assessment of a novel therapeutic approach. Jornal of Experimental&Clinical Cancer Research 28:51-61

[293] Kirson ED, Dbal V, Rochlizt C, Tovarys F, Salzber M, Palti Y (2006) Treatment of locally advanced solid tumors using alternating electric fields (TTFields) – a translational study. Clinical Research 17: Phase II and III Adult Clinical Trials, Proceedings of American Association Cancer Research, 47. #5259. http://www.aacrmeetingabstracts.org/cgi/content/abstract/2006/1/1233-b

[294] National Institutes of Health US, Low Levels of Electromagnetic Fields to Treat Advanced Cancer (ADLG3) http://clinicaltrials.gov/ct2/show/NCT00805337

[295] Andocs G, Renner H, Balogh L et al (2009) Strong synergy of heat and modulated electromagnetic field in tumor cell killing, Study of HT29 xenograft tumors in a nude mice model. Strahlentherapie und Onkologie 185:120-126

[296] Loewenstein WR (1999) The touchstone of life, Molecular information, cell communication and the foundations of the life. Oxford University Press, Oxford, New York, pp 298-304

[297] Soler AP, Miller RD, Laughlin VK et al (1999) Increased tight junctional permeability is associated with the development of colon cancer. Carcinogenesis, 20:1425-1431

[298] Sabah NH (2000) Rectification in Biological Membranes. IEEE Engineering in Medicine and Biology, 19(1):106-113

[299] Osterman KS, Paulsen KD, Hoopes PJ (1999) Application of linear circuit models to impedance spectra in irradiated muscle, In: Electrical Bioimpedance Methods: Applications to Medicine and Biotechnology. Riu P, Rosell J, Bragos R, Casas O. (Eds.), Ann. New York Acad. Sci. 873:21-29

[300] Santini MT, Cametti C, Zimatore G et al (1995) A dielectric relaxation study on the effects of the antitumor drugs Lomidamineand Rhein on the membrane electrical properties of Erlich ascites tumour cells. Anticancer Res. 15:29-36

[301] Keese CR, Wegener J, Walker SR, Giaever I (2004) Electrical wound-healing assay for cells in vitro. PNAS, Proceedings Nat. Acad. Sci. USA 101:1554-1559

[302] Toso S, Piccoli A, Gusella M et al (2000) Altered tissue electric properties in lung cancer patients as detected by bioelectric impedance vector analysis. Nutrition, 16:120-124S

[303] Weiss TF (1996) Cellular Biophysics. Transport, Vol 1. MIT Press, Cambridge

[304] Gautherie M (1982) Temperature and blood-flow patterns in breast cancer during natural evolution and following radiotherapy. Biomedical Thermology, Alan R. Liss, New York, pp 21-24

[305] Head JF, Wang F, Lipari CA et al (2000) The important role of Infrared Imaging in Breast cancer. IEEE Engineering in Medicine and Biology Magazine 19(3):52-57

[306] Matay G, Zombory L (2000) Physiological effects of radiofrequency radiation and their application for medical biology. Muegyetemi Kiado, Budapest, p 80

[307] Heilbrunn LV (1923) The colloid chemistry of protoplasm. Am J Physiol 64:481-498

[308] Yatvin MB, Dennis WH (1978) Membrane lipid composition and sensitivity to killing by hyperthermia, Procaine and Radiation. In: Streffer C, vanBeuningen D, Dietzel F et al (eds) Cancer Therapy by Hyperthermia and Radiation, Urban & Schwarzenberg, Baltimore, Munich, pp 157-159

[309] Bowler, K., Duncan, C.J., Gladwell, R.T., et. al.: Cellular heat injury. Comp. Biochem. Physiol. 45A, 441-450 (1973)

[310] Belehradek J (1957) Physiological aspects of heat and cold. Annu Rev Physiol 19:59-82

[311] Wallach DFH (1978) Action of Hyperthermia and Ionizing radiation on plasma membranes In: Streffer C, vanBeuningen D, Dietzel F et al (eds) Cancer Therapy by Hyperthermia and Radiation, Urban & Schwarzenberg, Baltimore, Munich, pp 19-28

[312] Nishida T, Akagi K, Tanaka Y (1997) Correlation between cell killing effect and cell-membrane potential after heat treatment: analysis using fluorescent dye and flow cytometry. Int J Hyperthermia 13(2):227-234

[313] Weiss TF (1996) Cellular Biophysics. Electrical properties, Vol 2. MIT Press, Cambridge

[314] Ricardo R, Gonzalez-Mendez R, Hahn GM (1989) Effects of hyperthermia on the intercellular pH and membrane potential of Chinese hamster ovary cells. Int J Hyperthermia 5:69-84

[315] Mikkelsen RB, Verma SP, Wallach DFH (1978) Hyperthermia and the membrane potential of erythrocyte membranes as studied by Raman Spectroscopy. In: Streffer C, vanBeuningen D, Dietzel F et al (eds) Cancer Therapy by Hyperthermia and Radiation, Urban & Schwarzenberg, Baltimore, Munich, pp 160-162

[316] Hahn GM (1990) The heat-shock response: Effects before, during and after Gene activation. In: Gautherie M (ed) Biological Basis of Oncologic Thermotherapy, Springer verlag Berlin, pp 135-159

[317] Hodgkin, A.L., Katz, B.: The effect of temperature on the electrical activity of the giant axon of the squid. J. Physiol. 108, 37-77 (1949)

[318] Latchman DS (1999) Stress proteins. Springer Verlag, Berlin, Heidelberg

[319] Soti C, Csermely P (1998) Molecular Chaperones in the Etiology and Therapy of Cancer. Pathol Oncol Res 4(4):316-321

[320] Ferrarini M, Heltai S, Zocchi MR et al (1992) Unusual Expression and Localization of Heat Shock Proteins in Human Tumor Cells. Int J Cancer 51(4):613-619

[321] Protti MP, Heltai S, Bellone M et al (1994) Constitutive Expression of the Heat Shock Protein 72kDa in Human Melanoma Cells. Cancer Letters 85(2):211-216

[322] Gress TM, Muller-Pillasch F, Weber C et al (1994) Differenctial Expression of Heat Shock Proteins in Pancreatic Carcinoma. Cancer Res 54(2):547-551

[323] Xu M, Wright WD, Higashikubo R et al (1996) Chronic Thermotolerance with Continued Cell Proliferation. Int J Hyperthermia 12(5):645-660

[324] Pirity M, Hever-Szabo A, Venetianer A (1996) Overexpression of P-glycoprotein in Heta and/or Drug Resistant Hepatoma Variants. Cytotechnology 19(3):207-214

[325] Santin AD, Hermonat PL, Ravaggi A et al (1998) The Effects of Irradiation on the Expression of a Tumor Rejection Antigen (Heat Shock Protein GP96) in Human Cervical Cancer. Int Radiat Biol 76(6):699-704

[326] Morgan J, Whitaker JE, Oseroff AR (1998) GRP78 Induction by Calcium Ionophore Potentiates Photodynamic Therapy Using the Mitochondrial Targeting Dye Victoria Blue BO. Photocem Photobiol 67(1): 155-164

[327] Punyiczki M, Fesus L (1998) Heat Shock and Apoptosis: The Two Defense Systems of the Organisms May Have Overlapping Molecular Elements. Ann N Y Acad Sci 951:67-74

[328] Sapozhnikov AM, Ponomarev ED, Tarasenko TN et al (1999) Spontaneous apoptosis and expression of cell-surface het-shock proteins in cultured EL-4 lymphoma cells. Cell Proliferation 32(6):363-378

[329] Huot J, Roy G, Lambert H, Landry J (1992) Co-induction of HSP27 Phosphorylation and Drug Resistance in Chinese Hamster Cells. Inter J Oncology 1:31-36

[330] Goodman R, Blank M (1999) The induction of stress proteins for cytoprotection in clinical applications. First International Symposium on Nonthermal Medical/Biological Treatments Using Electromagnetic Fields and Ionized Gases, ElectroMed'99, Norfolk VA, USA, 12-14 April 1999

[331] Liu FF, Bezjak A, Levin W et al (1996) Assessment of palliation in women with recurrent breast cancer. Int J Hyperthermia 12(6):825-826

[332] Hupp TR, Meek DW, Midgley CA et al (1992) Regulation of the Specific DNA Binding Function of p53. Cell 71(5): 875-886

[333] Chen CF, Chen Y, Dai K et al (1996) A New Member of the HSP90 Family of Molecular Chaperones Interacts with the Retinoblastoma Protein During Mitosis and After Heat Shock. Mol Cell Biol 16(9):4691-4699

[334] de Pomarai D, Daniels C, David H et al (2000) Non-thermal heat-shock response to microwaves. Nature 405(6785):417-418

[335] Bukau B, Horwich AL (1998) The HSP70 and HSP60 chaperone machines. Cell 92(3):351-366

[336] Watanabe M, Suzuki K, Kodama S et al (1995) Normal human cells at confluence get heat resistance by efficient accumulation of hsp72 in nucleus. Carcinogenesis 16(10):2373-2380

[337] Andocs G, Szasz O, Szasz A (2009) Oncothermia Treatment of Cancer: From the laboratory to clinic, Electromagnetic Biology and Medicine, 28:148-165

[338] Brunner G, Klinik Hornheide, Munster Univ., Germany, Hyperthermia Symposium, Cologne, 2006

[339] Andocs G, Szasz O. Szasz A. (2009) In vitro and in vivo evidences of effects of modulated rf-conducting heating. 25th Annual Meeting of the European Society for Hyperthermic Oncology, ESHO, Verona, June 4-6.
[340] Okamoto Y, Andocs G, Kinya K. (2011) Oncothermia Research and Veterinary Application in Japan, Tottori University; Oncothermia Seminar, Toyama City, Japan
[341] Meggyeshazi N, Andocs G, Szasz A (2011) Possible immune-reactions with oncothermia. ESHO, Aarhus, Denmark, May 26-28.
[342] Konishi et al (2007) Prognosis and risk factors of metastasis in colorectal carcinoids: results of a nationwide registry over 15 years. GUT 56:863-868
[343] Lord PF, Kapp DS, Morrow D (1981) Increased Skeletal Metastases of Spontaneous Canine Osteosarcoma after Fractionated Systemic Hyperhtermia and Local X-Irradiation. Cancer Research 41:4331-4334
[344] Rice L, Urano M, Chu A, Suit HD. The influence of whole body hyperthermia on the frequency of metastasis in a murine tumor system (abstract). Proc Ann Soc Therap Radiol 21st Ann Meeting 1979:201
[345] Mole RH. Whole body irradiation-radiology or medicine? Br J Radio. 1953; 26: 234-241
[346] Saupe H (2010) Possible activation of neutrophiles by oncothermia. 1st International Oncothermia Symposium, Cologne, November 22-23
[347] Seong Min Yoon, Jung Suk Lee: (2011) Case of Abscopal effect with Metastatic Non-Small-Cell Lung Cancer , submitted to BMJ
[348] Kongsgaard UE, Werner MU (2009) Evidence-Based Medicine Works Best When There is Evidence: Challenges in Palliative Medicine When Randomized Controlled Trials are not Possible. Journal of pain and Palliative Care Pharmacotherapy 23:48-50
[349] Gardner MJ, Altman DG (1989) Statistics with Confidence, British Medical Journals Book, British Medical Journal, London
[350] Bruera E (2006) Process and content of Decision making by advanced cancer patients. J Clin Oncol 24:1029-1030
[351] Tassinari D, Montanari L, Maltoni M et al (2008) The palliative prognostic score and survival in patients with advanced solid tumors receiving chemotherapy. Supportive Care of Cancer 16:359-370
[352] Surveillance, Epidemiology, and End Results (SEER), National Cancer Institute. www.seer.cancer.gov. 2000
[353] EUROCARE-3 European Cancer Database. www.eurocare.org/profiles/index.html
[354] Benson K, Hartz AJ (2000) A comparison of observational studies and randomized, controlled trials. NEJM 342(25):1878-1886
[355] Concato J, Shah N, Horwitz RI (2000) Randomized, controlled trial, observational studies, and the hierarchy of research design. NEJM 342(25):1887-1892
[356] Pappercorn JM, Weeks JC, Cook EF et al (2004) Comparison of outcomes in cancer patients treated within and outside clinical trials: conceptual framework and unstructures review. The Lancet 363:263-270

[357] Stelfox HT, Chua G, O'Rourke K et al (1998) Conflict of interests in the debate over calcium-channel antagonists. NEJM 338(2):101-106

[358] Choudhry NK, Stelfox HT, Detsky AS (2002) Relationships between authors of clinical practice guidelines and the pharmaceutical industry. JAMA 287(5):612-617

[359] Baird P, Downie J, Thompson J (2002) Clinical trials and industry. Science 297:2211

[360] Dani A, Varkonyi A: Electro-hyperthermia treatment of malignant brain tumors, Results of hyperthermia, Seminar, St. Istvan University, Aug. 26-27., 2003. (in Hungarian)

[361] Szasz A, Dani A, Varkonyi A (2004) Az elektro-hipertermia eredményei nagyszámú beteg retrospektív kiértékelésének tükrében Magyarországon. Magyar Klinikai Onkológiai Társaság III. Kongresszusa, Budapest, Hungary, 17–20 November 2004

[362] Sahinbas H, Baier JE, Groenemeyer DHW, Boecher E, Szasz A. (2006) Retrospective clinical study for advanced brain-gliomas by adjuvant oncothermia (electro-hyperthermia) treatment. www.gimt-online.de/uploads/media/Therapieergebnisse_Giloma_Studie_01.pdf

[363] Sahinbas H, Groenemeyer D, Boecher E, Szasz A (2007) Retrospective clinical study of adjuvant electrohyperthermia treatment for advanced braingliomas, Deutsche Zeitschrift fuer Onkologie, 39:154-160

[364] Szasz A (2009) Brain glioma results by oncothermia, a review. Expanding the Frontiers of Thermal Biology, Medicine and Physics Annual Meeting of Society of Thermal Medicine, Tucson, USA, 3–7 April 2009

[365] Douwes F, Douwes O, Migeod F, Grote C, Bogovic J (2006) Hyperthermia in combination with ACNU chemotherapy in the treatment of recurrent glioblastoma. http://www.klinikst-georg.de/pdf/hyperthermia_in_combination_with_ACNU_chemotherapy_in_the_treatment_of_recurrent_glioblastoma.pdf

[366] Hager ED et al (2003) The treatment of patients with high-grade malignant gliomas with RF-hyperthermia. Proc ASCO 22:118, #47;Proc Am Soc Clin Oncol 22: 2003

[367] Hager ED et al (2008) Prospective phase II trial for recurrent high-grade malignant gliomas with capacitive coupled low radiofrequency (LRF) deep hyperthermia. ASCO, J Clin ncol, Annual Meeting Proceedings (Post-Meeting Edition) 26:2047

[368] Fiorentini G, Giovanis P, Rossi S, Dentico P, Paola R, Turrisi G, Bernardeschi P (2006) A phase II clinical study on relapsed malignant gliomas treated with electro-hyperthermia. In Vivo, 20:721–724

[369] Wismeth C et al (2006) Loco-regional hyperthermia in patients with progressive astrocytoma WHO III or glioblastoma WHO IV (RNOP-10) – a prospective single arm phase I/II study; EANO

[370] Hau P (2010) Transcranial electro-hyperthermia combined with alkylating chemotherapy in patients with relapsed high-grade gliomas: phase I clinical results. 1st International Oncothermia Symposium, 22-23 November, Cologne, Germany

[371] Wismeth C et al (2009) Transcranial electro-hyperthermia combined with alkylating chemotherapy in patients with relapsing high-grade gliomas – Phase I clinical results.

Expanding the Frontiers of Thermal Biology, Medicine and Physics Annual Meeting of Society of Thermal Medicine, Tucson, USA, 3-7 April 2009

[372] Wismeth C, Dudel C, Pascher C et al (2010) Transcranial electro-hyperthermia combined with alkylating chemotherapy in patients with relapsed high-grade gliomas – Phase I clinical results. J Neurooncol 98(3):395–405

[373] Szasz A et al (2005) Retrospective analysis of 1180 oncological patients treated by electrohyperthermia in Hungary. Jahreskongress der Deutschen Gesellschaft für Radioonkologie, DEGRO 11, Karlsruhe, 26–29 May 2005

[374] Aydin H et al (2003) Strahlen-Hyperthermie bei Lebermetastasen und bei therapieresistenten Knochenmetastasen. Hyperthermia Symposium, Cologne, Germany, 25–26. October

[375] Pang C (2012) Clinical Research on Integrative Treatment of Colon Carcinoma with Oncothermia and Clifford TCM Immune Booster. Oncothermia Journal 5:24-41

[376] Pang C (2010) Clinical Research on Integrative Treatment of Colon Carcinoma with Oncothermia and Clifford TCM Immune Booster. 1st International Oncothermia Symposium, 22-23 November, Cologne, Germany

[377] Dani A, Varkonyi A, Magyar T, Szasz A (2010) A retrospective study of 1180 cancer patients treated by oncothermia. Forum Hyperthermia accepted (pp. 1–11)

[378] Renner H. (2003) Simultane RadioThermoTherapie bzw. RadioChemoThermoTherapie, Hyperthermia Symposium, Cologne, Germany, October

[379] Szasz A (2009) Clinical studies evidences of modulated rf-conductive heating (mEHT) method. Paper presented at the 25th Annual Meeting of the European Society for Hyperthermic Oncology, ESHO, Verona, Italy, 4–6 June

[380] Hager ED et al (1999) Deep hyperthermia with radiofrequencies in patients with liver metastases from colorectal cancer. Anticancer Res 19(4C):3403–3408

[381] Panagiotou P, Sosada M, Schering S, Kirchner H (2005) Irinotecan plus Capecitabine with regional electrohyperthermia of the liver as second line therapy in patients with metastatic colorectal cancer. ESHO, Jun.8–11, Graz, Austria

[382] Ferrari VD, De Ponti S, Valcamonico F et al (2007) Deep electro-hyperthermia (EHY) with or without thermo-active agents in patients with advanced hepatic cell carcinoma: phase II study. J Clin Oncol 25:18S, 15168

[383] Vigvary Z, Mako E, Dank M (2002) Combined radiological and interventional treatment of non-operable rectal tumors and their liver metastases. Regional Radiology Conference, Maribor, Sept. 19–20, Slovenia

[384] Dani A, Varkonyi A, Magyar T, Szasz A. (2011) Clinical study for advanced non-small-cell lung cancer treated by oncothermia; Oncothermia Journal, 3:39-49

[385] Szasz A, Dani A et.al (2005) Retrospective analysis of 1180 oncological patients treated by electro-hyperthermia, DEGRO 11. Jahreskongress der Deutschen Gesellschaft für Radioonkologie, 26-29 Mai 2005, Kongresszentrum, Karlsruhe

[386] Dani A, Varkonyi A, Nyiro I, Osvath M (2003) Clinical experience of electro-hyperthermia for advanced pancreatic tumors, Conference of European Society of Hyperthermic Oncology, (ESHO) Munich, 04-07. June

[387] Fiorentini G, deGiorgi U, Turrisi G et al (2006) Deep electro-hyperthermia with radiofrequencies combined with thermoactive drugs in patients with liver metastases from colorectal cancer (CRC): a Phase II clinical study. ICACT 17th, Paris, France, Jan 30–Feb 2 2006

[388] Douwes F (2004) Thermo-Chemotherapie des fortgeschrittenen Pankreaskarzinoms. Ergebnisse einer klinischen Anwendungsstudie. http://www.klinik-st-georg.de/publikationen/pdf/thermo-chemotherapie_des_fortgeschrittenen_pankreaskarzinoms.html

[389] Douwes F, Migeod F, Grote C (2006) Behandlung des fortgeschrittenen Pankreaskarzinoms mit regionaler Hyperthermie und einer Zytostase mit Mitomycin- C und 5-Fluorouracil/Folinsäure. http://www.klinik-st-georg.de/pdf/pankreastherapien.pdf

[390] VeraMed Clinic, Meshede, Germany; Dr.M. Kalden, unpublished data, private information

[391] Renner H, Albrecht I (2007) Analyse der Überlebenszeiten von Patienten mit Pankreastumoren mit erfolgter kapazitativer Hyperthermiebehandlung. Internal Report of Praxis in Klinikum Nord, Nurnberg, Germany, (Prepared by: Mr. Mirko F; May 2007)

[392] Szasz A (2010) Oncothermia from laboratory to Clinical practice, 25th Annual Meeting of Korean Gynaecologic Oncology Group, Jeju, Korea, 29-30. April

[393] Szasz A., Sahinbas H., Dani A.: Electro- hyperthermia for anaplastic astrocytoma and gliobastoma multiforme ICACT 2004, Paris, 9-12. February, 2004

[394] Sahinbas H., Grönemeyer D.H.W., Böcher E., Lange S.: Hyperthermia treatment of advanced relapsed gliomas and astrocytoma, The 9th International Congress on hyperthermic oncology, St. Louis, Missuri, ICHO, April 24-27, 2004

[395] Hager E.D.: Response and survival of patients with gliomas grade III/IV treated with RF capacitive-coupled hyperthermia, ICHO Congress, St. Louis USA 2004

[396] Hager E.D.: Clinical Response and Overall Survival of Patients with Recurrent Gliomas Grade III/IV Treated with RF Deep Hyperthermia – An Update, ICHS Conference, Shenzhen, China, 2004

[397] Sahinbas H, Szasz A: Electrohyperthermia in brain tumors, Retrospective clinical study, Annual Meeting of Hungarian Oncology Society, Budapest November 3-5, 2005

[398] Medical Research Council Brain Tumor Working Party: Randomized Trial of Procarbazine, Lomustine, and Vincristine in the Adjuvant treatment of High-grade Astrocytoma: A Medical Research Council Trial, J. Clin. Oncol. 19:509-518, 2001

[399] Stupp R, Dietrich P-Y, Kraljevic SO et al (2002) Promising survival for patients with newly diagnosed clioblastoma multiforme treated with concomitant radiation plus temi=ozolomide followed by adjuvant temozolomide. J Clin Oncol 20:1375-1382

[400] Stupp R, Mason WP, van den Bent MJ et al (2005) Radiotherapy plus concomitant and adjuvant temozolomide for glioblastoma. The New England J. of Med (352)987-996

[401] Scott CB, Scarantino C, Urtasun R, et al: Validation and predictive power of Radiation Therapy Oncology Group (RTOG) recursive partitioning analysis classes for malignant glioma patients: A report using RTOG 90-06. Int J Radiat Oncol Biol Phys 40:51-55, 1998

[402] Sahinbas H.: EHT bei Kindern mit Hirntumoren und nicht-invasive Messverfahren am beispiel von Hirntumoren, Symposium Hyperthermie, Cologne, 15-16 Oktober 2004

[403] Sahinbas H et al (2006) Retrospective clinical study of adjuvant electro-hyperthermia treatment for advanced brain-gliomas. Deutche Zeitschrifts fuer Onkologie 39:154-160

[404] Fisher PG, Buffler PA: Malignant gliomas in 2005. Where to GO from here?, Editorials, JAMA 293:615-617, 2005

[405] Overgaard J, Nielsen OS, Lindegaard JC (1987) Biological basis for rational design of clinical treatment with combined hyperthermia and radiation. In: Physics and Technology of Hyperthermia, Field SB, Franconi C, (Eds.) NATO ASI Series, E: Applied Sciences, No.127. Martinus Nijhoff Publ. Dordrecht/Boston, pp. 54-79

[406] Fatehi D, van der Zee J, van der Wal E et al (2006) Temperature data analysis for 22 patients with advanced cervical carcinoma treated in Rotterdam using radiotherapy, hyperthermia and chemotherapy: a reference point is needed. Int J Hyperthermia 22:353-363

[407] US National Cancer Act of 1971 signed by then U.S. President Richard Nixon.

Chapter 2

High Temperature Hyperthermia in Breast Cancer Treatment

Mario Francisco Jesús Cepeda Rubio,
Arturo Vera Hernández and Lorenzo Leija Salas

Additional information is available at the end of the chapter

http://dx.doi.org/10.5772/53277

1. Introduction

Globally, breast cancer is the most common type of cancer among women, which comprises 23% of all female cancers that are newly diagnosed in more than 1.1 million women each year. Over 411 000 deaths result from breast cancer annually; this accounts for over 1.6% of female deaths from all causes. Hyperthermia also called thermal therapy or thermotherapy is a type of cancer treatment in which body tissue is exposed to high temperatures. Research has shown that high temperatures can damage and kill cancer cells, usually with minimal injury to normal tissues. Otherwise, ablation or high temperature hyperthermia is defined as the direct application of chemical or thermal therapies to a tumor to achieve eradication or substantial tumor destruction. Many ablation modalities have been used, including cryoablation, ethanol ablation, laser ablation, and radiofrequency ablation. The most recent development has been the use of microwave ablation in tumors. Furthermore, The use of breast cancer mammography screening has allowed detecting a greater number of small carcinomas and this has facilitated treatment by minimally invasive techniques. Currently, physicians test minimally invasive ablation techniques to determine if they will be acceptable substitutes for surgical removal of primary breast tumors. Therefore, numerical electromagnetic and thermal simulations are used to optimize the antenna design and predict heating patterns. A review of different hyperthermia ablative therapies, for breast cancer treatment is summarized in this work. Otherwise, advanced computer modeling in high hyperthermia treatment and experimental model validation will be referred to in this chapter.

1.1. Tumor ablation

Tumor ablation is defined as the direct application of chemical or thermal therapies to a tumor to achieve eradication or substantial tumor destruction. The aim of tumor ablation is to destroy an entire tumor by using heat to kill the malignant cells in a minimally invasive fashion together with a sufficient margin of healthy tissue, to prevent local recurrence. Many ablation modalities have been used, including cryoablation, ethanol ablation, laser ablation, and radiofrequency ablation (RFA). The most recent development has been the use of microwave ablation (MWA) in tumors [1].

Nevertheless the local application of heat to treat patients with malignant tumors is not a novel concept. The Edwin Smith papyrus describes the topical application of hot oil or heated metallic implements that were used approximately 5000 years ago to treat patients with tumors [2]. The use of an electrical current to produce thermal tissue necrosis in patients with breast carcinoma also is not new: Metallic or clay-insulated electrodes were inserted into locally advanced breast tumors in the late 19th century to shrink the tumor and reduce pain and bleeding [3].

1.2. Principles of tissue damage

1.2.1. Radiofrequency ablation

This therapy works by converting radiofrequency waves into heat through ionic vibration. Alternating current passing from an electrode into the surrounding tissue causes ions to vibrate in an attempt to follow the change in the direction of the rapidly alternating current. It is the ionic friction that generates the heat within the tissue and not the electrode itself. The higher the current, the more vigorous the motion of the ions and the higher the temperature reached over a certain time, eventually leading to coagulation necrosis and cell death. The ability to efficiently and predictably create an ablation is based on the energy balance between the heat conduction of localized radiofrequency energy and the heat convection from the circulation of blood, lymph, or extra and intracellular fluid [4]. The amount of radiofrequency produced heat is directly related to the current density dropping precipitously away from the electrodes, thus resulting in lower periphery temperatures. It can be approximated that the heat generated in a region at distance d from the electrode drops as 1/d4. The goal of radiofrequency ablation is to achieve local temperatures that are lethal to the targeted tissue. Generally, thermal damage to cells begins at 42°C; and once above 60°C, intracellular proteins are denatured, the lipid bilayer melts, and irreversible cell death occurs [5].

1.2.2. Microwave ablation

Water molecules are polar, that is, the electric charges on the molecules are asymmetric. The alignment and the charges on the atoms are such that the hydrogen side of the molecule has a positive charge, and the oxygen side has a negative charge. When an oscillating electric charge from radiation interacts with a water molecule, it causes the molecule to flip. Microwave radiation is specially tuned to the natural frequency of water molecules to maximize this interaction. Temperature is a measure of how fast molecules move in a substance, and the vigorous movement of water molecules raises the temperature of water.

Therefore, electromagnetic microwaves heat matter by agitating water molecules in the surrounding tissue, producing friction and heat, thus inducing cellular death via coagulation necrosis [6].

1.3. Ablative devices

1.3.1. Radiofrequency ablation

The different manufacturers employed various strategies to obtain larger ablation zones [7]; there are currently three different manufacturers that offer commercial radiofrequency tumor ablation devices in the USA (Boston Scientific, Rita Medical and Valleylab) and an additional one in Europe (Celon). Two manufacturers (Boston Scientific and Rita Medical) employ multitined electrodes, to increase electrode surface area and volume of tissue heating. For multitined electrodes typically an incremental deployment of the tines in stages is used, with ablation at each deployment stage for a certain amount of time or until the target temperature is achieved to ensure complete ablation of the target volume. Two manufacturers use internal electrode cooling via circulation of water or saline to increase ablation zone size (Valleylab and Celon). By cooling the electrode, the tissue surrounding the electrode is also cooled. The location of maximum temperature is 'pushed' further into the tissue, resulting in a larger ablation zone size. A similar effect is obtained by infusing saline into the tissue via ports in the electrode this method is used by the Starburst Xli^{TM} electrode [8].

1.3.2. Microwave ablation

A variety of probes have been proposed for use in MWA, with the majority being based on a coaxial structure due to the deep-seated location of many tumors and the angular symmetry of the tumor. Initial antennas based upon a coaxial waveguide structure include designs, such as the monopole, dipole and slot antennas, often encased in a polytetrafluoroethylene (PTFE) catheter to minimize adhesion of the probe to desiccated ablated tissue. A number of challenges, characteristics and trade-offs have been identified in the design of MWA probes. Challenges include the reduction of backward heating, minimization of probe diameter and impedance matching of the antenna to the surrounding tissue. Trade-offs in design involve probe diameter versus maximum application of power and ablation power versus ablation time. Early coaxial antennas developed for MWA yielded ablation zones resembling a 'tear drop', as opposed to the desired spherical shape [9]. More recent MWA probes were designed to minimize probe size, maximize ablation zone size, minimize detrimental heating of the feedline and yield more spherical lesions, by minimizing impedance mismatch [10-12].

2. Clinical applications

2.1. Radiofrequency ablation

The first RFA clinical report was published in 1999, Jeffrey *et al.* [13] treated with RFA a small series of five women, aged 38 to 66 years, with locally advanced (stage III) breast cancer or tumors larger than 5 cm. While patients were under general anesthesia and just before surgical resection, a 15-gauge insulated multiple-needle electrode (LeVeen needle electrode; RadioTherapeutics Corp, Mountain View, Calif) was inserted into the tumor under sonographic guidance. The multiple-needle electrode was connected to a RF-2000 generator (Radio Therapeutics Corp), and a return electrode pad (Valley Lab, Boulder, Colo). Radiofrequency energy was applied at a low power by a preset protocol for a period of up to 30 minutes. The ablated area measured 0.8–1.8 cm diameter and non-viable tumor was found within this area in four patients.

Izzo *et al.* [14] used the same RFA electrode in patients with much smaller tumours. Twenty-six women with a mean cancer size of 18 mm underwent RFA and immediate surgical excision. RFA was performed following a predetermined two-phase algorithm. Treatment was initiated at 10 watts of power for 2 minutes, after which, power was increased in 5-watt increments every minute until tissue impedance rose rapidly and power dropped below 10 watts, thus indicating complete coagulative necrosis of the target lesion. After a 30-second pause, a second phase of treatment was applied, again beginning at 10 watts for 2 minutes followed by increases in power of 5 watts per minute until tissue impedance again rose and power rolled off. Power (watts) and impedance (ohms) were monitored continuously during treatment. The maximum power at the time of increase in the tissue impedance preceding power roll off and the total time needed to complete two-phase RFA were recorded. NADH diaphorase histochemical analysis showed a residual cancer focus in an area adjacent to the needle shaft site in one case, while the remaining patients were treated successfully with a complication rate of 4%.

Burak *et al.* [15] treated tumours with a mean diameter of 12 mm, creating an ablation zone of 26–45 mm and reported one case with surviving malignancy. Viability was assessed using cytokeratin 8 / 18 stain. Under ultrasound guidance, 1% lidocaine was injected around the breast tumor for a distance of about 3 cm in all directions surrounding the tumor mass. After a 5–10-minute waiting period, a small skin incision was made with a number 11 surgical blade under aseptic conditions. The 2 cm array RFA probe (Radiotherapeutics, Sunnyvale, CA) was inserted under ultrasound guidance and deployed so that the "prongs" encompassed the breast tumor. Radiofrequency energy was applied over 2 time periods, which were not to exceed a total of 30 minutes. In the first time period, power was set to 10 W and increased in 5 W intervals every 2 minutes until a rapid increase in impedance (ohms) occurred, or when 60 W was reached. If 60 W was obtained, the probe was left in place until impedance or a total period of 15 minutes elapsed. In the second time period, the application began at 10W and the same titration was followed.

Hayashi *et al.* [16] ablated small breast primaries measuring 9 mm median in 22 patients. The median ablated diameter was 35 mm, viability was assessed with NADHdiaphorase and showed eight failures. In three, the site was at the periphery but in five was in a missed untargeted area. Under sterile conditions in the ultrasonography suite, a 15-gauge, 7-array StarBurst radioprobe (RITA Medical Systems, Mountain View, California) was placed directly into the tumor using sonographic guidance (HDI 3000; Phillips Medical, Bothell,

Washington). The prongs were deployed after positioning was confirmed in three dimensions using real-time ultrasound. The probe was connected to the RF generator (RITA model 1500) with a grounding pad placed on each thigh to complete the electrical circuit. The generator was set to automatic, power at 20 W, temperature to 95°C, and ablation time set at 15 minutes. The generator was activated and power was delivered incrementally until the target temperature was attained and held for the set time. The ablation process was monitored with ultrasonography and real time temperature feedback. Vital signs were monitored and if the patient reported significant discomfort, the ablation was temporarily halted. On completion of the procedure, the tines were retracted and the needle withdrawn.

Fornage *et al.* [17] treated 21 breast tumours of < 2 cm and in the subsequent excision specimen all targeted cancer foci were ablated with an average diameter of 3.8 cm. One patient who had received neoadjuvant chemotherapy was found to have a further mammographically and ultrasonically occult viable tumour. A 460-kHz monopolar RF electrosurgical generator specifically designed for use with electrosurgical RF probes (RITA Medical Systems, Mountain View, Calif) was used in this study. The needle-electrode consists of a primary electrode— that is, a 15-gauge stainless-steel cannula with a noninsulated distal tip that acts as an electrode—and secondary electrodes, which are curved, flexible stainless-steel prongs that are contained within and can be deployed outside of the primary electrode. A 50-W model 500 electrosurgical RF generator (RITA Medical Systems) with a disposable, seven-array model 70 Starburst needle electrode (RITA Medical Systems) was used in the first nine patients. Subsequently, a 150-W model 1500 generator (RITA Medical Systems) with a nine-array Starburst XL needle-electrode (RITA Medical Systems) was used in 11 patients. Both types of needle-electrodes were 15 cm long. The arrays on the Starburst XL needle-electrode can be deployed to a length of 5 cm. Thermocouples placed at the tips of four prongs of the seven-array needleelectrode and at the tips of five prongs of the nine-array needle-electrode enabled continuous real-time monitoring of the temperatures at the tips. A laptop computer with proprietary software developed by the manufacturer of the RF ablation equipment was used to graphically display, in real time, the curves of the temperatures at the tips, the power of the generator, and the impedance of the tissues over time.

Marcy *et al.* [18] treated five cancers in four not-fit-for-surgery patients with RFA and had one relapse after 4 months. Percutaneous radiofrequency–lumpectomy was performed under local analgesia (lidocaine, subcutaneous injection), using ultrasound guidance under sterile conditions in the interventional radiology suite. RFA was applied between a large neutral electrode, leading to a high electric field line density in the region of the needle tip, and the 1.5 mm x 1.1 mm non-isolated needle tip ablation electrode. Thermal lesions were always produced with RF power 30 W, at a frequency of 500 kHz, during a 12 min application time as recommended by the manufacturer (Elektrotom 104HF; Thermo-Berchtold Medizinelektronik Gmbh, Tuttlingen, Germany). A controlled interstitial needle perfusion of isotonic sterile saline solution (0.9% NaCl) was applied using an infusion pump (Perfusor Secura FT; Braun, France). The current flows from the uninsulated perfused electrode implanted in the tumour to a grounding pad applied externally to the skin. A feedback system controlling RF power application and saline infusion of the needle maintains power delivery. The RFA probe was designed to create a minimum spherical ablation volume of 3 cm diameter. Thermocoagulation included the tumour plus at least a 5 mm margin. The RFA probe was typically positioned parallel to the overlying skin under ultrasound guidance, and the procedure was carried out during real-time ultrasound monitoring. Ablation zones were visualized as cone-shaped hyperechogenic areas around the needle tip, experiencing the temperature increase. Vital signs were monitored and if the patient reported significant discomfort, the ablation was temporarily halted. On completion of the procedure, the lines were retracted and the needle withdrawn. A small ice pack was placed on the wound for up to 24 h after the procedure for comfort. The patient was discharged home once stable and free of sedative effects.

Susini *et al.* [19] treated three patients who had small breast cancers with RFA and followed them with clinical examination, ultrasound, magnetic resonance imaging (MRI) and core biopsy. After 18 months no relapses were reported. The 18-G Cool tip RF Radionics (Valley Lab, USA) was used to perform RFA, by means of one single electrode, 20-cm length. Local anesthesia was performed using a mixture of lidocaine and naropine injected under the overlying skin, and around the tumor. With ultrasound guidance, the electrode was inserted and its progression was monitored in real-time, allowing the exact positioning of the tip in the center of the lesion. Then, the RF generator was switched on and tissue impedance was measured. The generator produced RF energy through high-frequency (480 kHz) alternating current. When the tissue temperature reached 90°C, ultrasound image showed the "fog effect", in relationship with the vaporization of intracellular water. RF energy was applied for a variable time of 8–12 min.

Oura *et al.* [20] in their series of 52 patients with breast cancers of mean size 1.3 cm. Multifocality, multicentricity and tumour size were thoroughly investigated prior to RFA and patients with multiple malignant areas or large tumours were excluded. Patients were submitted to ultrasound guided RFA and were subsequently followed with clinical examination, ultrasound, MRI and cytology. After a mean follow-up of 18 months no relapses were reported. Operation was performed under general anesthesia in all patients. After the removal of sentinel node(s), RFA started using a Cool-tip RF needle with an uninsulated tip 3 cm in diameter (Valleylab, Boulder, CO). The Cool-tip RF needle was inserted into the tumor from the areola under ultrasound guidance. A total of 20-60 mL of 5% glucose was injected subcutaneously just above the tumor after appropriate insertion of the needle was confirmed. The RFA started at 5 watts, raised the output to 10 watts 1 minute later, and thereafter increased output continuously in increments of 10 watts at 1 minute intervals until either the generator stopped delivering radiofrequency energy due to a 20 ohms or more impedance increase of the ablated tissue from the base line, or the scheduled time which was 30 minutes in the first 29 cases and 15 minutes thereafter when'break'did not occur.

Medina *et al.* (2008) [21] treated Twenty-five patients, aged 42 to 89 years with invasive breast cancer <4 cm (range 0.9–3.8 cm). Under ultrasound guidance, a 17-gauge probe

(Elektrotom 106 HiTT, Berchtold, Germany) was inserted in the center of the tumor. The needle electrode was attached to a 500 kHz monopolar RFA generator. RF energy was applied to the tissue with initial power setting of 30 W, for three cycles of 3 minutes each. The energy was increased with increments of 5 W to a maximum power of 50 W. Radiofrequency was delivered until the tumor was completely hyperechoic with the aim of obtaining a safety margin of 1 cm around the tumor. Of the 25 patients treated, NADPH stain showed no evidence of viable malignant cells in 19 patients (76%), with significant difference between tumors <2 cm (complete necrosis in 13 of 14 cases, 92.8%).

Currently Takayuki [22] *et al.* treated 49 patients, aged 36 – 82 years and tumor size ≤3.0 cm in diameter (range 0.5–3.0 cm) on US examination. Under US guidance, the 17-gauge ValleylabTM RF Ablation System with Cool-tip™ Technology (Covidien, Energy-Based Devices, Interventional Oncology, Boulder, CO) was inserted in the center of the tumor. The needle electrode was attached to a 500-kHz monopolar RF generator capable of producing 200-W power. Tissue impedance was monitored continuously using circuitry incorporated into the generator. RF energy was applied to tissue with an initial power setting of 10 W and subsequently increased with increments of 5 W each minute to a maximum power of 55 W. The power setting was left at this point until power 'rolloff' occurred. Power rolloff implies that there is an increase in the tissue impedance. When this occurs, the power generator will shut off, stopping the flow of current and further tissue coagulation. After waiting 30–60 s, the second phase was started at 75% of the last maximum power until a second rolloff occured. Radiofrequency was applied until the tumor was completely hyperechoic. Following RF ablation, standard tumor resection was achieved with either a wide local excision or mastectomy according to the preference of the patient. Of the 49 treated patients, complete ablation was recognized in 30 patients (61%) by H&E staining and/or NADH diaphorase staining. A summary is presented in tables 1-4.

Authors	Patients	Age range	Tumor Size (cm)
Jeffrey	5	38-66	4-7
Izzo	26	37-78	0.7-3.0
Burak	10	37-67	0.5-2.0
Hayashi	22	60-80	0.5–2.2
Fornage	20	38-80	≤2.0
Marcy	4	79-82	1.8-2.3
Susini	3	76-86	<2.0
Oura	52	37-83	0.5-2.0
Medina	25	42-89	0.9 - 3.8
Takayuki	49	20-90	≤3.0

Table 1. Patient and tumor characteristics in ten studies on radiofrequency ablation for breast cancer

Authors	Electrode Probe	Generator
Jeffrey	15-g multineedle LeVeen	RF-2000 Radio Therapeutics
Izzo	15-g multineedle LeVeen	RF-2000 Radio Therapeutics
Burak	2 cm array probe Radio therapeutics	Not mentioned
Hayashi	15-g, 7 cm array Starburst RITA	RITA-1500 RITA
Fornage	7-array / 15-g, 9 cm array Starburst RITA	RITA-500 / RITA-1500
Marcy	1.5 mm · 1.1 mm non-isolated tip Elektrotom	Elektrotom 104HF
Susini	18-G Cool tip RF Radionics	Not mentioned
Oura	3 cm Cool-tip uninsulated Valleylab	Not mentioned
Medina	17-g Elektrotom 106, Germany	Monopolar 200 W
Takayuki	17-g Valleylab RF Ablation System with Cool-tip	Monopolar 200 W

Table 2. Devices in ten studies on radiofrequency ablation for breast cancer

Authors	Frequency	Feedback control	Temperature (ºC)	Image guided
Jeffrey	480-kHz	Impedance	46.8 - 70.0	Ultrasound
Izzo	480-kHz	Impedance	Not mentioned	Ultrasound
Burak	460 kHz	Impedance	Not mentioned	Ultrasound
Hayashi	460 KHz	NO	95	
Fornage	461 KHz	NO	90 and 95	Ultrasound & Doppler
Marcy	500 kHz	NO	Not mentioned	Ultrasound
Susini	480 kHz	NO	90	Ultrasound
Oura	Not mentioned	Impedance	> 60	Ultrasound
Medina	500 KHz	NO	70 - 80	Ultrasound
Takayuki	500 KHz	Impedance	Not mentioned	Ultrasound

Table 3. Technical settings in ten studies on radiofrequency ablation for breast cancer

Authors	Anesthesia	Fail	Complications
Jeffrey	General	1	0
Izzo	General	1	1
Burak	Local	1	1
Hayashi	Local	3	1
Fornage	General	1	0
Marcy	Local	1	0
Susini	Local	0	0
Oura	General	0	1
Medina	General	6	1
Takayuki	General	18	5

Table 4. Results in ten studies on radiofrequency ablation for breast cancer

2.2. Microwave ablation

Three studies on microwave ablation have been published [23-25]. A pilot safety (phase I) study included ten patients with core needle biopsy-proven invasive breast carcinoma (T1–T3 tumors) [23]. Of the eight patients who responded, 82–97% tumor cell kill was found, confirmed by M30 immunohistochemistry. Image guidance was performed using US. Five to 27 days after treatment patients underwent mastectomy. The same group also published another article in which 21 patients with T1–T2 invasive breast carcinoma underwent microwave ablation [24]. In 68% of the patients, histologic evidence of tumor necrosis was present. Finally, this group published a dose-escalation study [25].

Twenty-five patients with core needle biopsy-proven invasive breast carcinoma (T1–T2 tumors) were included. US provided image guidance; there was no correlation between clinical/ultrasonographic size changes and pathologic tumor response. In 68% of the cases there was evidence of pathologic response using H&E staining. In two cases complete ablation was reached; these patients received the highest temperature dose. Complications mentioned were mild pain during treatment, skin burn, and short-lived erythema of the skin.

2.3. Summary

In RFA several different devices from different manufacturers were used in different ways for varying periods of time and varied protocols, so not surprisingly, they reported quite heterogeneous results. Nevertheless successful cases for different protocols were obtained for smaller tumors with a low failures and complication rate. In addition the clinical MWA is limited to external techniques and currently the greatest amount of interstitial research was conducted in the liver tissue. The generation of an appropriately sized ablation zone, long treatment times, insufficient interoperative imaging modalities and performance in the vicinity of vascular structures are limitations of current devices. An ideal ablative technology would ensure complete destruction of all malignant cells with no significant side effects or complications.

3. Advanced computer modeling in breast cancer hyperthermia treatment

In this section, we present a computer modeling for microwave high hyperthermia in breast cancer treatment. Computational electromagnetic (CEM) or electromagnetic modeling employs numerical methods to describe propagation of electromagnetic waves. It typically involves the formulation of discrete solutions using computationally efficient approximations to Maxwell's equations. There are three techniques of CEM: the finite-difference time-domain (FDTD), the method of moments (MOM), and the finite element method (FEM), which has been extensively used in simulations of cardiac and hepatic radiofrequency (RF) ablation [26]. A FEM model was used in this work because it can provide users with quick, accurate solutions to multiple systems of differential equations and therefore, they are well suited to solve heat transfer problems like ablation [27]. Numerous MWA antenna designs specifically targeted for MWA cardiac and hepatic applications have been reported [20-24], but they have not been used to treat breast cancer. These designs have been focused largely on thin, coaxial-based interstitial antennas [28], which are minimally invasive and capable of delivering a large amount of electromagnetic power. These antennas can usually be classified as one of three types (dipole, slot, or monopole) based on their physical features and radiation properties [29]. On the other hand, several researchers are investigating non-invasive microwave hyperthermia for treatment of breast cancer [30].

3.1. Equations

The frequency-dependent reflection coefficient can be expressed logarithmically as:

$$\Gamma(f) = 10 \cdot \log_{10}\left(\frac{P_r(f)}{P_{in}}\right)[dB] \tag{1}$$

where, Pin is the input power and Pr indicates the reflected power (W). SAR represents the amount of time average power deposited per unit mass of tissue (W/kg) at any position. It can be expressed mathematically as:

$$SAR = \frac{\sigma}{\rho}|E|^2 = [W/Kg] \tag{2}$$

where, σ is tissue conductivity (S/m), ϱ is tissue density (kg/m^3) and E is the electric field [56]. The SAR takes a value proportional to the square of the electric field generated around the antenna and is equivalent to the heating source created by the electric field in the tissue. The SAR pattern of an antenna causes the tissue temperature to rise, but does not determine the final tissue temperature distribution directly. The tissue temperature increment results from both power and time. MW heating thermal effects can be roughly described by Pennes' Bioheat equation [31]:

$$\nabla \cdot (-k\nabla T) = \rho_b C_b \omega_b (T_b - T) + Q_{met} + Q_{ext} \quad (3)$$

where k is the tissue thermal conductivity (W/m°K), ρ_b is the blood density (Kg/m^3), C_b is the blood specific heat (J/Kg°K), ω_b is the blood perfusion rate (1/s). Tb is the temperature of the blood and T is the final temperature. Q_{met} is the heat source from metabolism and Q_{ext} an external heat source. The major physical phenomena considered in the equation are microwave heating and tissue heat conduction. The temperature of the blood is approximated as the core temperature of the body. Moreover, in ex vivo samples, ω_b and Q_{met} can be neglected since no perfusion or metabolism exists. The external heat source is equal to the resistive heat generated by the electromagnetic field.

3.2. Material properties

The computer antenna model used in this work is based on a 50Ω UT-085 semirigid coaxial cable. The entire outer conductor is copper, in which a small ring slot of width is cut close to the short-circuited distal tip of the antenna to allow electromagnetic wave propagation into the tissue. The inner conductor is made from silver-plated copper wire (SPCW) and the coaxial dielectric is a low-loss polytetrafluoroethylene (PTFE). The length of the antenna also affects the power reflection and shape of the SAR pattern. Furthermore, the antenna is encased in a PTFE catheter to prevent adhesion of the antenna to desiccated ablated tissue. Dimensions and thermal properties of the materials and breast tissue, which were taken from the literature [32], are listed in Table 5 and 6.

Parameter	Value
Center conductor diameter	0.51 mm
Dielectric diameter	1.68 mm
Outer conductor diameter	2.20 mm
Diameter of catheter	2.58 mm
Power	10 W
Frequency	2.45 GHz
Electrical Conductivity of breast	0.137 S/m
Thermal conductivity of breast	0.42 W/m K
Specific heat of blood	3639 J/Kg/k
Blood perfusion rate	0.0036 s-1
Electrical conductivity of tumor	3 S/m
Thermal conductivity of tumor	0.5 W/m K

Table 5. Dimensions and properties for the materials and tissue.

Material	Relative permittivity
Inner dielectric oft he coaxial cable	2.03
Catheter	2.60
Breast tissue	5.14
Tumor	57

Table 6. Relative permittivity for the materials and tissue.

Figure 1 shows the axial schematics of each section of the antenna and the interior diameters.

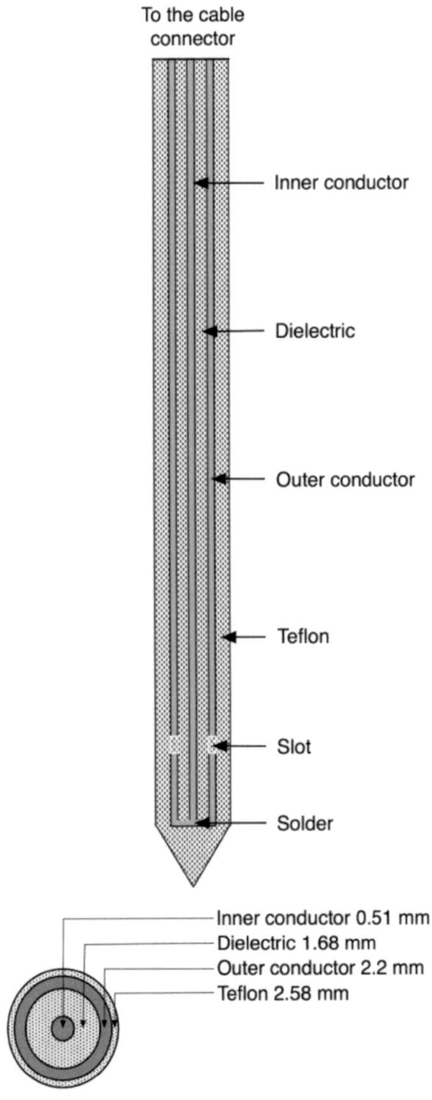

Figure 1. Cross section and axial schematic of the coaxial slot antenna.

A finite element method computer models were developed using COMSOL Multiphysics 4.0 commercial software. One of the models assumed that the coaxial slot antenna was immersed only in homogeneous breast tissue; the other model assumed that the antenna was immersed only in breast cancer. The coaxial slot antenna exhibits rotational symmetry around the longitudinal axis; therefore axisymmetric models, which minimized the computation time, were used. The inner and outer conductors of the antenna were modeled using perfect electric conductor boundary conditions and boundaries along the z axis were set with axial symmetry.

All boundaries of conductors were set to perfect electric conductor (PEC). Boundaries along the *z* axis were set with axial symmetry and all other boundaries were set to low reflection boundaries. Figure 2 shows the geometry of the antenna model with details near its slot; since the model is axisymmetric, only a half of the antenna geometry structure is shown [33].

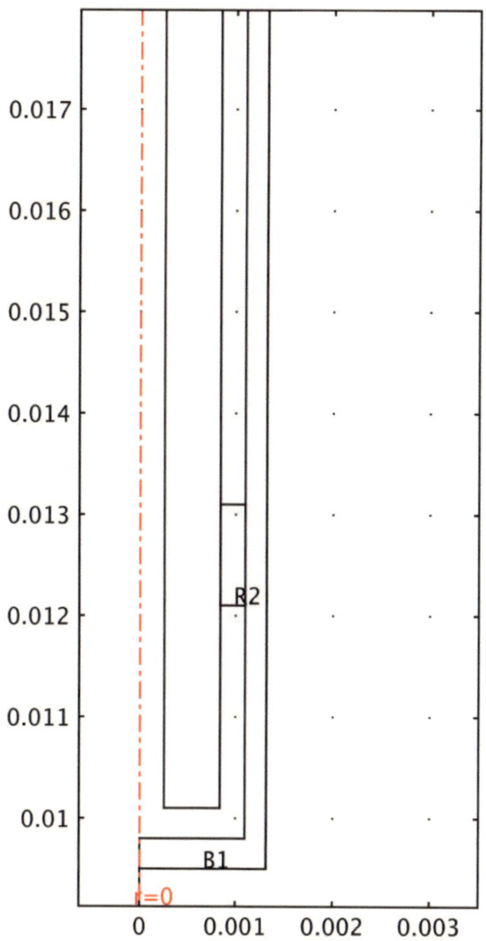

Figure 2. Axisymmetric model in the vicinity of the tip of the coaxial slot antenna. The vertical axis (z) corresponds to the longitudinal axis of the antenna; while the horizontal axis (r) corresponds to radial direction. All units are in meters.

3.3. Results

Figure 3 shows the temperature distribution in normal adipose-dominated tissue [34]. The reflection coefficient calculated for the frequency at 2.45 GHz was -2.82 dB, the maximum temperature was 116.03 ºC, and the ablation zone radius was 53 mm. The isotherm was considered at 60 ºC because ablation is produced above this temperature [35]. Figure 4 shows the temperature distribution in breast cancer tissue. The reflection coefficient calculated for the frequency at 2.45 GHz was -6.38 dB, the maximum temperature was 125.96 ºC, and the ablation zone radius was 92 mm.

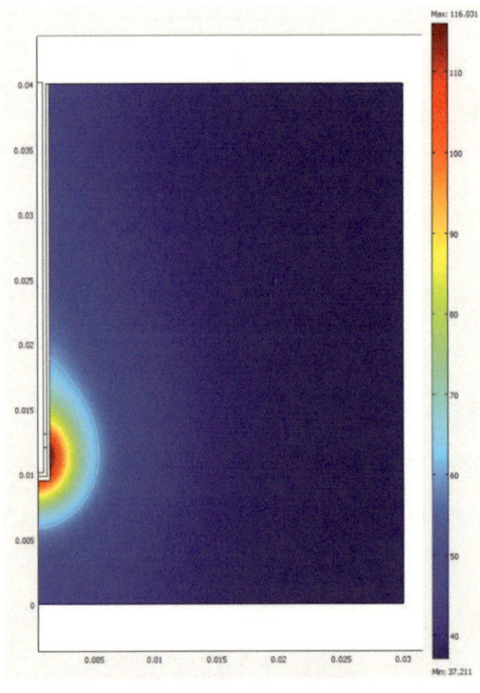

Figure 3. Temperature distribution of normal adipose-dominated breast tissue at a microwave power output of 10 W. The isotherm at 60 ºC is highlighted. The illustration shows half the plane through the symmetry axis. Vertical axis (z) corresponds to the longitudinal axis of the antenna; horizontal axis (r) corresponds to radial direction.

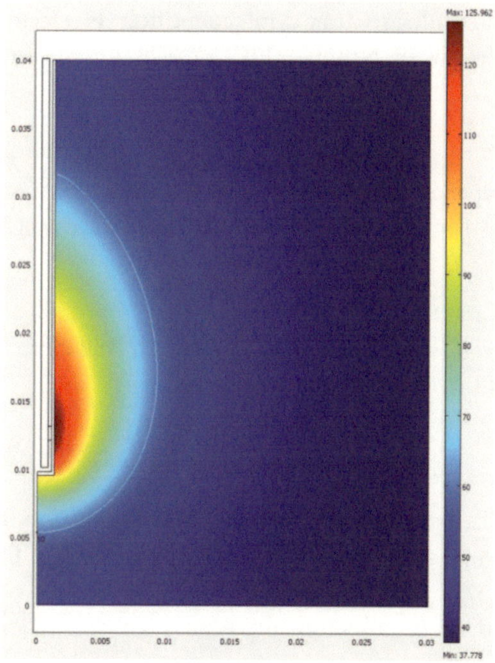

Figure 4. Temperature distribution of breast cancer tissue at a microwave power output of 10 W. The isotherm at 60 ºC is highlighted. The illustration shows half the plane through the symmetry axis. Vertical axis (z) corresponds to the longitudinal axis of the antenna; horizontal axis (r) corresponds to radial direction.

4. Conclusion

In RFA for high temperature hyperthermia therapy in breast cancer several devices from different manufacturers were used in diverse ways for varying periods of time and assorted protocols, therefore exist heterogeneous results. Nevertheless successful cases for were obtained for smaller tumors with a low failures and complication rate. On the other hand the effect of MWA on malignant and normal adipose-dominated tissues of the breast was simulated using an axisymmetric electromagnetic model. This model can analyze the heating patterns using the bioheat equation. The results from computer modeling demonstrated that, effectively, the difference in dielectrical properties and thermal parameters between the malign and normal adipose-dominated tissue could cause the preferential heating on tumor during MWA. Even though electromagnetic high temperature hyperthermia requires further research, it is a promising minimally invasive modality for the local treatment of breast cancer.

Acknowledgement

The project described was supported by Instituto de Ciencia y Tecnología del Distrito Federal. Project Name: "Desarrollo de un sistema automatizado de determinación volumétrica por imágenes ultrasónicas para cuantificar el efecto de la energía térmica aplicada en la ablación del cáncer. Number: PICCO10-78. Agreement: ICYTDF; 340/2010.

Author details

Mario Francisco Jesús Cepeda Rubio,
California State University, Long Beach & Instituto de Ciencia y Tecnología del Distrito Federal (ICyTDF)

Arturo Vera Hernández and Lorenzo Leija Salas
Centro de Investigación y de Estudios Avanzados del Instituto Politécnico Nacional, Department of Electrical Engineering/Bioelectronics, Mexico

5. References

[1] Berber E, Flesher NL, Siperstein AE. Initial clinical evaluation of the RITA 5-centimeter radiofrequency thermal ablation catheter in the treatment of liver tumors. The Cancer Journal 2000; 6:319–329.
[2] Breasted JH. The Edwin Smith surgical papyrus, vol. 54. Chicago: Chicago University Press; 1930.
[3] Rockwell AD. Electro-surgery: benign and malignant tumors. In: Rockwell AD, editor. The medical and surgical uses of electricity. New York: EB Treat & Company 1903; 565–6.
[4] Scudamore C. Volumetric radiofrequency ablation: technical consideration. The Cancer Journal 2000; 6:316–318.
[5] C. J. Simon, D. E. Dupuy, and W. W. Mayo-Smith. Microwave Ablation: Principles and Applications. RadioGraphics 2005; 25(suppl_1): S69 - S83.
[6] Goldberg SN, Gazelle GS. Radiofrequency tissue ablation: physical principles and techniques for increasing coagulation necrosis. Hepatogastroenterology 2001; 48(38), 359–367.
[7] Lobik L, Leveillee RJ, Hoey MF. Geometry and temperature distribution during radiofrequency tissue ablation: an experimental ex vivo model. J. Endourol. 2005; 19(2), 242–247.
[8] O'Rourke, Ann P; Haemmerich, Dieter; Prakash, Punit; Converse, Mark C; Mahvi, David M; Webster, John G. Current status of liver tumor ablation devices. Expert Review of Medical Devices 2007; Volume 4, Number 4, pp. 523-537(15)
[9] Yang D, Bertram JM, Converse MC et al. A floating sleeve antenna yields localized hepatic microwave ablation. IEEE Trans. Biomed. Eng. 2006; 53(3), 533–537.
[10] Brace CL, Laeseke PF, van der Weide DW, Lee FT Jr. Microwave ablation with a triaxial antenna: results in ex vivo bovine liver. IEEE Trans. Microw. Theory 2005; 53(1), 215–220.
[11] Longo I, Gentili GB, Cerretelli M, Tosoratti N. A coaxial antenna with miniaturized choke for minimally invasive interstitial heating. IEEE Trans. Biomed. Eng. 50(1), 82–88.

[12] Stefanie S. Jeffrey, MD; Robyn L. Birdwell, MD; Debra M. Ikeda, MD; Bruce L. Daniel, MD; Kent W. Nowels, MD; Frederick M. Dirbas, MD; Stephen M. Griffey, DVM, PhD. 1999. Radiofrequency Ablation of Breast Cancer First Report of an Emerging Technology. Arch Surg. 2003; 134:1064-1068.

[13] Jeffrey SS, Birdwell RL, Ikeda DM. Radiofrequency ablation of breast cancer: first report of an emerging technology. Arch Surg 1999; 134: 1064–8.

[14] Izzo F, Thomas R, Delrio P. Radiofrequency ablation in patients with primary breast carcinoma: a pilot study in 26 patients. Cancer 2001; 92: 2036–44.

[15] Burak WE, Agnese DM, Povoski SP. Radiofrequency ablation of invasive breast carcinoma followed by delayed surgical excision. Cancer 2003; 98: 1369–76.

[16] Hayashi AH, Silver SF, van der Westhuizen NG. Treatment of invasive breast carcinoma with ultrasound-guided radiofrequency ablation. Am J Surg 2003; 185: 429–35.

[17] Fornage BD, Sneige N, Ross MI et al. 2004. Small (≤2 cm) breast cancer treated with US-guided radiofrequency ablation: feasibility study. Radiology 2004; 231: 215–24.

[18] Marcy PY, Magne N, Castadot P, Bailet C, Namer M. Ultrasoundguided percutaneous radiofrequency ablation in elderly breast cancer patients: preliminary institutional experience. Br J Radiol 2007; 80: 267–73.

[19] Susini T, Nori J, Olivieri S et al. Radiofrequency ablation for minimally invasive treatment of breast carcinoma. A pilot study in elderly inoperable patients. Gynecol Oncol 2007; 104: 304–10.

[20] Oura S, Tamaki T, Hirai I et al. Radiofrequency ablation therapy in patients with breast cancers two centimeters or less in size. Breast Cancer 2007; 14: 48–54.

[21] Medina-Franco H, Soto-Germes S, Ulloa-Gómez JL, Romero-Trejo C, Uribe N, Ramirez-Alvarado CA, Robles-Vidal C. Radiofrequency ablation of invasive breast carcinomas: a phase II trial. Ann Surg Oncol. 2008; 15(6):1689-95.

[22] Kinoshita, T., Iwamoto, E., Tsuda, H. and Seki, K., "Radiofrequency ablation as local therapy for early breast carcinomas," 2010; Breast Cancer.

[23] Gardner RA, Vargas HI, Block JB, et al. Focused microwave phased array thermotherapy for primary breast cancer. Ann Surg Oncol 2002; 9(4):326–332.

[24] Vargas HI, Dooley WC, Gardner RA, et al. Success of sentinel lymph node mapping after breast cancer ablation with focused microwave phased array thermotherapy. Am J Surg 2003; 186(4):330–332.

[25] Vargas HI, Dooley WC, Gardner RA, et al. Focused microwave phased array thermotherapy for ablation of earlystage breast cancer: results of thermal dose escalation. Ann Surg Oncol 2004; 11(2):139–146.

[26] D. Haemmerich, L. Chachati, A.S. Wright, D.M. Mahvi, F.T. Lee Jr and J.G. Webster IEEE Trans Biomed Eng. 2003; 50 493.

[27] J. M. Bertram, D. Yang, M. C. Converse, J. G. Webster and D. M. Mahvi Biomed. Eng. Online. 2006; 5 15.

[28] S. A. Shock, K. Meredith, T. F. Warner, L. A. Sampson, A. S. Wright, T. C. Winter, III, D. M. Mahvi, J. P. Fine, and F. R. Lee, Jr Radiology 2004; 231 143.

[29] J. M. Bertram, D. Yang, M. C. Converse, J. G. Webster and D. M. Mahvi Crit. Rev. Biomed. Eng. 2006; 34 187 (2006)

[30] W.C. Dooley, H.I. Vargas, A. J. Fenn, M. B. Tomaselli and J. K. Harness Ann. Surg. Oncol. 2010; 17 1076.

[31] E. H. Wissler J. Appl. Physiol. 1998; 85 35.

[32] M. Gautherie Ann. N. Y. Acad. Sci. 1980; 335 383.

[33] Cepeda MFJ., Vera A., Leija L., Avila-Navarro, E. & Navarro, E. Coaxial Slot Antenna Design for Microwave Hyperthermia using Finite-Difference Time-Domain and Finite Element Method. The Open Nanomedicine Journal, 2011; Vol. 3, No. 1, pp. (2- 9).

[34] Cepeda MFJ. Estudio y Desarrollo de Aplicadores Coaxiales Tipo Slot de Ablación por Microondas para el Tratamiento Mínimamente Invasivo del Cáncer de Mama. PhD thesis. Centro de Investigación y de Estudios Avanzados del Instituto Politécnico Nacional; 2011.

[35] V. Ekstrand, H. Wiksell, I. Schultz, B. Sandstedt, S. Rotstein and A. Eriksson Biomed. Eng. Online. 2005; 4 41.

Chapter 3

Laser and Radiofrequency Induced Hyperthermia Treatment via Gold-Coated Magnetic Nanocomposites

El-Sayed El-Sherbini and Ahmed El-Shahawy

Additional information is available at the end of the chapter

http://dx.doi.org/10.5772/52375

1. Introduction

Cancer is a disease characterized by unregulated growth of cells. This is caused by damage of deoxyribonucleic acid (DNA) results in mutations to vital genes that control cells divisions *(Albert et al., 2004)*. The most common non-invasive approaches used for cancer treatment represent in chemotherapy, as well as radiotherapy. Chemotherapy uses cytotoxic drugs, which are also known as "anti-cancer" drugs or "anti-neoplastic." On other hand, radiotherapy uses high energy of X-rays which were directed to cancerous tissues to cure or shrink the tumor, as well as to protect the tissue against tumor recurrence. Although chemotherapy and radiotherapy are capable of killing cancerous cell, nevertheless they cause some serious secondary effects including nausea, diarrhea, tiredness and fertility loss *(Johannes et al., 2005)*.The conventional surgery of solid tumors is also an effective therapy for removing of well defined and accessible primary tumors located within nonvital tissue regions. However, this therapy is unsuitable for treatment of ill defined tumors and metastases, as well as tumors that embedded within vital regions *(Hirsch et al., 2003)*.

The current methods for cancer treatment have moderate to severe secondary effects. For this reason, the investigations of new alternatives are essentially. Thermo-therapy is considered one of the most important methods for cancer treatment. In general, the term thermo-therapy refers to both hyperthermia and thermal ablation therapy (*Mriza et al., 2001)*. Hyperthermia therapy is based on the fact that tumor cells are more sensitive to temperature increase than normal tissue cells. It involves tumor heating to temperatures between 41- 42°C inducing almost reversible damage to cells and tissues. For thermal ablation therapy higher temperatures are applied ranging from 50°C to 70°C, leading to destruction of pathologically degenerated cells and irreversible damage resulting in diminishing, disappearing of the tumors or at least growing stop. Thermal methods include radiofrequency ablation (RFA), focused ultrasound thermo-therapy, laser-induced thermal therapy and magnetic thermal ablation *(Hilger et al., 2002)*.

The thermal therapy can provide a minimal invasive alternative to conventional surgical treatment of solid tumors. In addition, the thermal therapeutic procedures are relatively simple to perform and therefore have the potential to improve recovery times and reduce the complication rates and hospital stays *(Hirsch et al., 2003)*. Although, the thermal methods offer several advantages, nevertheless have some of limitations. For example, the tumor volume and speed of ultra-sound thermo therapy is limited by the potential destruction of normal tissue in the near field between the target and the ultrasound probe. Radiofrequency ablation and microwaves approaches suffer from common limitations that are intervening tissue problems. On other wards, the heating effects from these sources are non-specific. In addition, the energy deposition is often much slower with these moieties serving to increase the treatment time and generate less sharp lesion boundaries *(Ko¨hrmann et al., 2002)*.

To overcome these problems, new techniques in the field of nanoscience, nanotechnology and nanomedicine are now developing into treatment approach based on internal heating of tissue such as magnetic fluid hyperthermia (MFH), which in turn based on internal heating sources. In order to achieve the optimal effectiveness, this approach requires photo-thermal convectors to allow heat production within a localized region at lower incident energies. This requires development of particular particles that have highly magnetic properties such as Super-paramagnetic Iron Oxide Nanoparticles Fe_3O_4 (SPIO NPs). During this approach surrounding healthy cells are capable of surviving exposure to temperatures up to around 46.5°C and more readily able to dissipate heat and maintain a normal temperature while the targeted tumor tissues have a higher thermal sensitivity than normal tissue because of experience difficulty in dissipating heat due to the disorganized and compact vascular structure (reduced blood flow), anaerobic metabolism (acidosis), and nutrient depletion. So an irreversible damage to diseased cells occurs at temperatures in a range from approximately 40°C to about 46°C (Yu-Fen *et al., 2008*).

2. Nanomedicine and magnetic nanomaterials

Nanomedicine stands at the boundaries between the physical, the chemical, biological and medical sciences. It originated from the imaginative idea that robots and other related machines at the nanometer scale could be designed, fabricated and introduced into the human body for repairing malignant cells at the molecular level. According to its original vision, nanomedicine is a process including the diagnosis, treatment and prevention of diseases and traumatic injuries, and the preservation and improvement of human health, using molecular tools and molecular knowledge of the human body (*Freitas 2005*). The progress in both nanoscience and nanotechnology makes nanomedicine practical. From a technical viewpoint, nanomedicine consists of the applications of particles and systems at the nanometer scale for the detection and treatment of diseases at the molecular level, and it plays an essential role in eliminating suffering and death from many fatal diseases, such as cancer (*Yih and Wei 2005*). Based on nanofabrication and molecular self-assembly, various biologically functional materials and devices, such as tissue and cellular engineering scaffolds, molecular motors and biomolecules, can be fabricated for sensor, drug delivery and mechanical applications (Royal Society and Royal Academy of Engineering 2004). Nanomedicine has obvious advantages. First, nanoparticles are potentially invaluable tools for investigating cells because of their small size. Second, as their size can be controlled, from that of large molecules to that of small cells, the ability of nanoparticles to escape the vasculature *in vivo* can also be controlled. Third, because of their small size, nanoparticles can circulate systemically in the bloodstream and thus serve in roles such as magnetic resonance enhancement, iron delivery for the production of red blood cells and drug delivery to improve the availability of serum-insoluble drugs (*Whitesides 2005*).

2.1. Status of nanomedicine

Nanomedicine has developed in numerous directions, and it has been fully acknowledged that the capability of structuring materials at the molecular scale greatly benefits the research and practice of medicine. However, nanomedicine is a long-term expectation. Before nanomedicine can be used in clinics, fundamental mechanisms of nanomedicine should be fully investigated, and clinical trials and validation procedures should be strictly conducted. Though, it is possible that some biological entities, such as proteins, DNA and other bio-polymers, could be directly used for biosensor applications, nevertheless some serious issues, such as biocompatibility and robustness, may hinder the progress of these efforts. Though in many areas, such as disease diagnosis, targeted drug delivery and molecular imaging, clinical trials of some nanomedicine products are being made, the clinical applications of these techniques, which require rigorous testing and validation procedures, may not be realized in the near future (Royal Society and Royal Academy of Engineering 2004). At all events, it should be noted that although the applications of nanomaterials in biology and medicine are in an embryo stage, it is the great promise of nanomedicine that has inspired researchers to extensively investigate the interfaces between nanotechnology, biology and medicine (*Satyanarayana, 2005*).

2.2. Magnetic nanomaterials

The magnetic nanomaterials used in biology and medicine generally fall into three categories: zero dimensional nanomaterials such as nanospheres; one-dimensional nanomaterials such as nanowires and nanotubes; and two-dimensional nanomaterials such as thin films. Usually, all the nanospheres, nanorods, nanowires and nanotubes are called nanoparticles, among which, nanorods, nanowires and nanotubes are high aspect-ratio nanoparticles. In most of the biomedical applications, magnetic nanoparticles are suspended in appropriate carrier liquids, forming magnetic fluids, also called ferrofluids. Among the three types of magnetic nanoparticles, magnetic nanospheres are most widely used in biomedicine. To realize their biomedical applications, the magnetic nanospheres should be stably suspended in the carrier liquid, and they should also carry out certain biomedical functions. The magnetic material most often used is iron oxides, and the carrier liquids are usually water, kerosene or various oils. Due to their small size, the magnetic nanoparticles in carrier liquids neither form sediment in the gravitational field or in moderate magnetic field gradients, nor do they agglomerate due to magnetic dipole interaction. However, a stable suspension can only be achieved if the particles are protected against agglomeration due to the van der Waals interaction. Usually this protection can be achieved by one approach is the electric charge stabilization. In this approach, a thin layer of gold is coated on the surface of the nanospheres. Meanwhile, the thin gold layer can also serve as an ideal base on which chemical or biological agents can be functionalized. These molecules generate a repulsive force, preventing the particles from coming into contact and thus suppressing the destabilizing effect of the van der Waals interaction. In practical applications, this approach is often used in combination for the majority of ferrofluids, since this allows the synthesis of suspensions which are stable over years (*Could 2004*).

2.2.1. Magnetic (iron oxide nanoparticles)

Magnetic iron oxide nanoparticles are the most investigated material in biomedical techniques, due to its superior biocompatibility with respect to other magnetic materials, either in form of oxides or pure metals. Several types of iron oxides exist in nature and can be prepared in the laboratory. Nowadays, only maghemite (γ-Fe_2O_3) and magnetite (Fe_3O_4) are able to fulfill the necessary requirements for biomedical applications. These requirements include sufficiently high magnetic moments, chemical stability in physiological conditions and low toxicity, not to mention the easy and economical synthetic procedures available for the preparation of these materials *(Neuberger et al., 2005)*.

The degree of atomic order in the iron oxide lattice, or in other words its degree of crystallinity, as well as the dispersity of the nanoparticles in terms of size and shape are critical parameters that affect their performance in diagnostic and therapeutic techniques as a contrast agent in magnetic resonance imaging (MRI) and hyperthermia, respectively. These parameters are strongly correlated to the approach for their synthesis *(Maenosono et al., 2008)*.

2.2.2. Synthesis of iron oxide nanoparticles

The common existing methods to synthesize the iron oxide nanoparticles are physical, chemical and biological methods. Comparatively, chemical methods, especially wet chemical ones are much simpler and more efficient *(Gupta et al., 2004)*. Several synthetic procedures have been developed to synthesize iron oxide nanoparticles. The simplest, cheapest and most environmentally-friendly procedure is based on the co-precipitation wet chemical method, which involves the simultaneous precipitation of ferrous (Fe^{2+}) and ferric (Fe^{3+}) salts in an alkaline medium *(Kang, 1996)*. So the synthesis of iron oxide nanoparticles with an expected size distribution and stability of suspension is no longer the biggest challenge for researchers. The key issue now is how to achieve the aim of stealth of these nanoparticles in blood circulation and to attach them on desired sites for *in vivo* or *in vitro* applications *(Sun, 2006)*.

Hydrothermal synthesis techniques are an alternative method for the preparation of highly crystalline iron oxide nanoparticles *(Wang et al, 2005)*. In this case a mixture of iron salts dissolved in aqueous media is introduced in a sealed Teflon container and heated above the boiling temperature of water, and consequently the reaction pressure is increased much above atmospheric pressure. The synergistic effect of high temperatures and pressures strongly improves the quality of the nanocrystals and hence their magnetic features. However, and in contrast to the biological technique, there is no straightforward way to control the size and the shape of the final particles and usually polydisperse samples are obtained.

Biological methods, since nanomaterials have comparable dimensions to biological aggregates, bio-related synthesis methods have been explored for novel nanoparticle synthesis. In biological methods, synthesis and assembly of crystalline inorganic materials can be regulated by biological organisms under environmentally benign conditions and desired chemical compositions and phases can be achieved. For example, the nucleation of semiconducting nanoparticles can be initiated in the presence of viruses expressing material-specific peptides. Other examples are the use of porous protein crystals, manipulation of bacteria to produce oxide nanoparticles and selection of metal-specific polypeptides from combinatorial libraries *(Reiss et al. 2004)*. In biological methods, biological entities usually serve as templates for nanoparticles formation. In all cases, the biological entities were used not only to encapsulate the nanoparticles, but to strictly regulate the dimension of the crystals. To prepare magnetic nanoparticles, ferritin can be used which consists of 24 nearly identical subunits. Self-assembly of ferritin will form a spherical cage with a 7.5–8.0 nm-diameter cavity, which can be used for the biological storage of iron in the form of ferrihydrite, an iron (III) oxy-hydroxide? The protein cage is able to withstand relatively high temperatures for biological systems (up to 65 ◦C) and various pH values (~ 4.0–9.0) for certain periods of time. Therefore this protein template is quite strong and will not cause any significant disruption of the quaternary structure.

2.2.3. Classification of iron oxide nanoparticles

There are many categories of iron oxide nanoparticles based on their overall diameter (including iron oxide core and hydrated coating). Iron oxide nanoparticles can be distinctly classified into super-paramagnetic iron oxide nanoparticles (SPIO NPs) between 300 nm and 3.5 μm; standard SPIO (SSPIO) of approximately 60–150 nm; ultra small SPIO (USPIO) of approximately 10–40 nm (*Weissleder et al., 1990)*; monocrystalline iron oxide nanoparticles (MION—a subset of USPIO) of approximately 10–30 nm and cross-linked iron oxides (CLIO) which is a form of MION with cross-linked dextran coating (*Shen et al., 1993)*.

On the other hand, the magnetic materials are characterized by the presence of magnetic dipoles generated by the spinning of some of their electrons. Each of these polarized electrons can be aligned in a parallel or antiparallel fashion with respect to the neighboring ones in the crystal lattice, and this type of interaction is what gives rise to the macroscopic magnetic effect that we can measure. Based on the magnetic response, the magnetic materials can be classified into; diamagnetic, paramagnetic, ferromagnetic, ferrimagnetic, anti-ferromagnetic and super-paramagnetic *(Cozzoli et al., 2006)* as shown in Fig (1).

Diamagnetic materials are characterized by coupled or paired magnetic dipoles, so there is no permanent net magnetic moment per atom. That is to say that these materials have not any interactions or slightly repelled with the magnetic field. The magnetic susceptibility of these materials is negative and independent on temperature.

Paramagnetic materials characterized by randomly oriented (or uncoupled) magnetic dipoles, this can be aligned only in the presence of an external magnetic field along its direction. This type of material has neither coercivity nor remanence, which means that when the external magnetic field is switched off the internal magnetic dipoles randomize again. No extra energy is required to demagnetize the material and hence the initial zero net magnetic moment is spontaneously recovered.

Ferromagnetic materials characterized by individual magnetic dipoles in a crystal, those can align parallel one to the other, hence exhibiting an enhanced collective response even in the absence of an external magnetic field. This is what is known as *ferromagnetism*. Beside strong intensity of magnetization, the fundamental property of ferromagnetic solids is their ability to record the direction of an applied magnetic field. When the magnetic field is removed, the magnetization does not return to zero but retains a record of the applied field.

Ferrimagnetic and anti-ferromagnetic materials, in contrast to the ferromagnetic situation, neighboring magnetic dipoles can align antiparallel in the lattice, which means that they will cancel each other i.e. repulsion of magnetic dipoles . This type of magnetic exchange can lead to two different situations. The first is *ferrimagnetism;* when the two coupled spins show different values, and in that case a net magnetic dipole different than zero will still magnetize the material even in the absence of an external magnetic field. While the second is *anti-ferromagnetism;* when the magnetic dipoles or interacting spins have the same value and hence the material shows a net zero magnetization. The latter case lacks of interest for biomedical applications due to zero net magnetic moment arising in such materials.

Super-paramagnetic materials, bulky sized particles of magnetic materials such as (Fe), (Co) or (Ni), as well as some of their alloys (FePt & FeCo) have ferromagnetic properties due to their multi-domain structures of the particles. In contrast, at the nanometer scale of approximately 14 nm, the multi-domain combined together forming a single domain crystal, which is classified as super -paramagnetic *(Schmidt, 2001)*. Super-paramagnetic iron oxide nanoparticles are special class of paramagnetic materials which combine ferromagnetic and paramagnetic properties due to high magnetic moments which are observed under the effect of a magnetic field, but no remanent magnetic moment will be present when the external magnetic field is removed. This property translates into a significant advantage especially *in vivo* experiments, where the absence of coercivity or in other words the zero net magnetic moment of the nanoparticles after concluding the diagnostic measurement or the therapy will prevent the potential aggregation of the particles that could easily cause the formation of embolisms in the blood vessels (*Thorek et al., 2006)*.The path of magnetization

M as a function of applied field H is called a hysteresis loop or M-H curve as shown in figure (2).

2.2.4. *Characteristics of magnetic nanomaterials for in vivo bio-applications*

When nanoparticles are used for *in vivo* applications, the nanoparticles have to stay with nil or minimal side effects. Therefore, complete characterizations of the particulate system are essentially to make a decision whether the use of nanocarriers systems are appropriate for specific *in vivo* applications or not. The nanoparticles can be described by the following physicochemical properties according to their distribution within the body system: size distribution, surface charge modification ,targeting, cellular uptake, bio-stability, metabolism, toxicity, capacity for protein adsorption, surface hydrophobicity, rate of loading , release kinetics, surface characteristics, density, porosity, degeneration of carrier system, cristallinity, density, mobility and the molecular weight *(Neubergera et al., 2005).*

2.2.4.1. *Size distribution*

Most intravenous administrated nanoparticles are recognized as "foreign" from the body system and are eliminated immediately through macrophages of the mononuclear phagocytosis system (MPS) depending on the size. The size of particles usually refers to the total diameter of the particles including the core and the coating layer. It is well known that, the smallest diameter of capillaries in the body is 4 μm. So, NPs smaller than 4μm are taken up through cells of the reticuloendothelial system (RES) mainly in the liver (60–90%) and spleen (3–10%). While small particles up to 150 nm will be phagocytosed through liver cells. There is a tendency for particles larger than 200 nm to be filtered by the venous sinuses of the spleen, as well as will be captured and withheld in the lungs. In general, the large particles are eliminated faster from the blood, and have short plasma half-life-period compared to the small particles (*Muller et al., 1997).*

2.2.4.2. *Surface charge and protein adsorption*

Particles with large sizes and/or aggregations of small particles such as magnetic nanoparticles (MNPs) may be trapped causing emboli within the capillary bed of the lungs. Therefore, it is important to know the surface charge and aggregation behavior of the particles in the blood circulation system *(Neuberger et al., 2005).*

All bare nanoparticles are unsuitable for *in vivo* applications, where the particle surface would be exposed to a biological environment and oxidized during application. Using bare nanoparticles directly, this could damage its structures and its properties. On the other hand, nanoparticles in solid phase cannot be injected into human body. So, before injection NPs have to be dispersed to hydrophilic solvent via specific interaction between the nanoparticles surface and surfactants *(Harisinghani et al., 2003).*

The surface charge also plays an important role during endocytosis process. There should be a slower uptake for negatively charged particles due to the negative "rejection" effect of the negatively charged cell membrane. However, the endocytosis index *in vitro* is minimal with a zeta potential close to zero. In contrast, Phagocytosis process is increased with a higher surface charge independent of whether the charge is negative or positive. The higher the surface charge the shorter is the residence time of nanoparticles in the circulatory system *(Neuberger et al., 2005)*.

The adsorption of proteins at the particle surface is called *"opsonization"*. This phenomenon results from immediate interaction between nanoparticles with plasma proteins after intravenous injection .The amount of adsorbed proteins is based on the size of the molecules, as well as the surface charge of the particle, where the capacity of protein adsorption increases by increasing size and charge of the particles. The adsorbed protein components play an important role in the biodistribution, degradation and elimination of the nanoparticles. Therefore, the treatment method of the nanoparticles surface must be addressed *(Muller et al., 1997)*.

The surface charge and protein adsorption capability are more related to the surfactants bond to the nanoparticles surface. There is another important role of surfactants on nanoparticles, when the NPs are injected into human body as contrast agents, these nanoparticles must locate the targeting area accurately and rapidly. Appropriate surfactant could achieve such objective. Some experiments *in vitro* already proved folate-mediated nanoparticles composed of ploy ethylene glycol (PEG) / poly ε-caprolactone have potential of tumor cell-selective targeting *(Gee et al., 2003)*.

2.2.4.3. Targeting

All *in vivo* applications require that the NPs should accurately localize to therapeutic sites. All targeting methods could be classified to passive, active and physical targeting. The physical targeting is the localization of the nanoparticles with external assistance, typically by applied magnetic field from outside of the body; the physical targeting has less capability to recognize specific cells or tissues. The passive targeting based only on the disrupted endothelial lining of tumor tissues; enhanced penetration and retention (EPR) allows nanoparticles of smaller size to pass, and accumulate in the tumor. In active targeting, specific targeting functional groups, such as monoclonal antibodies, are immobilized on the particle surface to efficiently increase the chance of uptake by specific cells *(Kelly et al., 2005)*.

2.2.4.4. Cellular uptake

Cellular uptake of nanoparticles is another issue that should be taken into account, when considering their use in diagnostic and therapeutic applications. The cellular uptake of nanoparticles is strongly dependent on particle size as it was proven *in vitro* and *in vivo*. In general, small nanoparticles can go deeper into tissue than larger particles and often penetrate the cell itself *(Leslie-Pelecky, 2007)*. Lewinski et al summarized the situation for many types of nanoparticles *(Lewinski et al., 2008)*.

The cellular uptake of nanoparticles occurs through a process known as endocytosis, which can be generally classified into three processes depending on nanoparticles size. Phagocytosis process which is the predominant mechanism for uptake of large particles, phagocytotic activity increases with size of particles, whereas smaller particles<150 nm can be up-taken by all types of cells through pinocytosis process (cell drinking).The third is non-specific endocytosis or receptor-mediated endocytosis process *(Neuberger et al., 2005)*.Super-paramagnetic iron oxide nanoparticles have been shown to be uptake by a receptor mediated endocytosis process (*Raynal et al., 2004*).

2.2.4.5. Bio-stability

When nanoparticles are introduced into the body, several aspects can compromise its stability. First of all, the physiological media have different ionic strength as compared with the ultrapure water mainly used in laboratories: increasing the ionic strength of aqueous solution will suppress the electric double layer around the charged particles, resulting in a partial or total aggregation of the system. A similar behavior could be observed by the particles once they enter specific body compartments, due to a variation in pH with respect to the media in which the nanoparticles are initially dispersed. In addition, when nanoparticles are injected in the blood circulation system, a nonspecific adsorption of plasma proteins onto nanoparticles surface *"opsonization"* will occur, this phenomenon is more pronounced for nanometer size particles due to two main effects: the high surface to volume ratio, as well as the attractive forces between the nanoparticles such as magnetic nanoparticles. When this phenomenon occurs, a fast clearance of the nanoparticles is observed. To prevent such effects, several synthetic and natural polymers have been introduced to the nanoparticles surface including PEG and dextrin (*Kohler et al., 2004*).

2.2.4.6. Metabolism

The metabolism process of the nanoparticles is another issue that should be taken into account. For example, iron oxide nanoparticles can be present in two different oxidation states: the ferrous Fe (II) form which will be oxidized by endogenous molecular oxygen, resulting in the conversion of ferrous iron to ferric Fe (III). Ferric iron is the preferred physiological oxidation state of iron; Fe (III) is highly reactive and can induce catalytic activity that may result in severe oxidative cell damage. As a result, iron carrier proteins and chelates are used to allow for safe transfer of iron from cell to cell within the body, and for safe intra-cellular storage of excess iron. The natural eventual fate of Fe_3O_4 nanoparticles above approximately 200 nm in diameter is to reside in macrophage-rich tissue, such as the liver and spleen (peak concentration at 2 hours after contrast intake).While particles below 10 nm are removed rapidly through extravasations and renal clearance *(Gupta et al.,* 2004).

2.2.4.7. Biocompatibility

Biocompatibility is one of the most important considerations in the development of biomedical applications of nanomaterials. Most of the magnetic nanowires are compatible with living cells. They can be functionalized with biologically active molecules, and they do not disrupt normal cell functions, such as cell proliferation and adhesion, and gene expression (*Hultgren et al. 2005*).

2.2.4.8. *Toxicity*

The non-cytotoxic, non-immunogenic and biocompatible properties of nanoparticles are important issues for the potential application in nanoimmunology, nanomedicines and nanobiotechnology. When discussing the toxicity of nanoparticles, generalization becomes difficult because their toxicity depends on numerous factors including the dose, chemical composition, method of administration, size, biodegradability, solubility, pharmacokinetics, biodistribution, surface chemistry, design, shape and structure. In general, size, surface area, shape, composition and coating of nanoparticles are the most important characteristics regarding cytotoxicity *(Neuberger et al., 2005).*

Several *in vivo* studies on animals had shown that, with a large dosage of 3,000 μmol Fe based nanoparticles per kg body weight, the histology and serologic blood tests indicated that no side effects occurred after 7 days of treatment *(Lacava et al., 1999).*

To minimize the risks posed by nanoparticles, there are two basic avenues. One is to develop new highly biocompatible nonmaterials with low toxicity such as silica nanoparticles. Another one is the surface modification of nanoparticles with biocompatible chemicals such as PEG, dextrin and chitosan. Thus many great efforts are being made to develop nanoparticles satisfactory for biomedical applications *(Cho, 2009).*

2.2.4.9. *Easy detection*

As almost all biological entities are non-magnetic, magnetic nanoparticles in biological systems can be easily detected and traced. One typical example is the enhancement of the signal from magnetic resonance imaging (MRI) using magnetic nanoparticles. In this technique, a subject is placed in a large, external magnetic field and then exposed to a pulse of radio waves. Changes to the spin of the protons in water molecules are measured after the pulse is turned off. Tiny differences in the way that protons in different tissues behave can then be used to build up a 3D image of the subject (*Koltsov 2004*).

2.2.4.10. *Magnetic manipulation*

Magnetic nanoparticles will rotate under an external uniform magnetic field, and will make translational movements under an external magnetic field gradient. Therefore, magnetic nanoparticles, or magnetically tagged molecules, can be manipulated by applying an external magnetic field. This is important for transporting magnetically tagged drug molecules to diseased sites. The magnetic manipulation of magnetic nanowires and nanotubes is important for applying forces to biological entities, and for nanowires or nanotubes to get into biological entities.

2.2.4.11. *Energy transfer*

Magnetic nanoparticles can resonantly respond to a time-varying magnetic field, transferring energy from the exciting magnetic field to the nanoparticles and the tagged biological entities. This property has been used in hyperthermia treatment of cancer tumors (*Pankhurst et al. 2003*).

2.2.5. *Biomedical applications of iron oxide NPs*

Nanotechnology, dealing with nanoscale objects, has been developed at three major levels: nanomaterials, nanodevices and nanosystems. At present, the nanomaterials level is the most advanced of the three. Nanomaterials are of great importance both in scientific investigations and commercial applications due to their size-dependent physical and chemical properties. Nanomaterials with various shapes have been developed successfully. Common morphologies are quantum dots, nanoparticles/nanocrystals, nanowires, nanorods, nanotubes, etc. It is desirable to have a full range within the nanomaterial family because many applications demand particular nanomaterials with special structures.

Magnetic nanoparticles, being a sub-family of nanomaterials, exhibit unique magnetic properties in addition to other specific characteristics. Their remarkable new phenomena include super-paramagnetism, high saturation field, high field irreversibility, extra anisotropy, and temperature-depended hysteresis, etc. Research investigation has revealed that the finite size and surface effects of magnetic nanoparticles determine their magnetic behavior. For instance, a single magnetic domain forms when the size of a ferromagnetic nanoparticle is less than 15 nm. In other words, an ultrafine ferromagnetic nanoparticle displays a state of uniform magnetization under any field. Thus, at temperatures above the blocking temperature, these nanoparticles show identical magnetization behavior to atomic paramagnets (super-paramagnetism) with an extremely large magnetic moment and large susceptibilities.

Magnetic nanoparticles have found many successful industrial applications. Recently, tremendous research efforts have been stimulated on the usage of magnetic nanoparticles in the field of biomedical and biological applications.

Understanding of biological processes and hence developing biomedical means have been continuously pursued. These aims are one of strong driving forces behind the development of nanotechnology. The interests on magnetic nanoparticles for bio-applications come from their comparable dimensions to biological entities coupled with their unique magnetic behaviors. Though common living organisms are composed of cells of about 10 μm size, the cell components are much smaller and generally in the nanosize dimension. Examples are viruses (20–450 nm), proteins (5–50 nm) and genes (2 nm wide and 10–100 nm long). Synthetic magnetic nanoparticles have controllable dimensions and just a few nanometer-diameter nanoparticles can be synthesized by carefully designing experimental procedures and controlling experimental conditions. With such a nanoscale dimension, it would be possible for magnetic nanoparticles to get close to a biological entity of interest. Moreover, the interaction between magnetic nanoparticles and biological entities can be adjusted by coating nanoparticles with biological molecules, called bio-functionalization. This offers a controllable means of 'tagging' or addressing the binding at nanoscale. The comparable dimensions and magnetic properties of magnetic nanoparticles have prompted the idea of using them as very small probes to spy on the biological processes at the cellular scale without introducing too much interference. Actually, optical and magnetic effects have been treated as the most suitable approaches for biological applications owing to their non-invasive behavior.

In view of the magnetic properties of magnetic nanoparticles, they can be manipulated by an external magnetic field gradient, which is described by Coulomb's law. Magnetic nanoparticles are able to transport into human tissues due to the intrinsic penetrability of magnetic fields into human bodies. This 'action at a distance' opens up many potential bio-applications including transportation of magnetically tagged biological entities, targeted drug delivery, etc. Another important property of magnetic nanoparticles is their resonant response related to a time-varying magnetic field *(Pankhurst et al. 2003)*. Hence energy transfer from the exciting field to the magnetic nanoparticles can be realized. In this way, toxic amounts of thermal energy are able to be delivered via magnetic nanoparticles to the targeted tumors resulting in malignant cell destruction. This process is named hyperthermia, which will be addressed in detail in this chapter. In addition to the site-specific drug delivery and hyperthermic treatment, magnetic nanoparticles have found other versatile bio-applications such as magnetic bio-separation, contrast enhancement of magnetic resonance imaging, gene therapy, enzyme immobilization, magnetic manipulation of cell membranes, immunoassays, magnetic bio-sensing, etc. *(Sun et al. 2005)*. Each application depends upon the relationship between the external magnetic field and the biological system. Magnetic fields with proper field strength are not deleterious to either biological tissues or biotic environments. In a given bio-application, magnetic nanoparticles are usually injected intravenously into the human body and are transported to the targeted region via blood circulation for biomedical diagnostic or treatment. An alternative means is using magnetic nanoparticle suspension for injection *(Berry 2003)*. It has been well accepted that a desirable magnetic medium should not contain nanoparticle aggregation, which will block its own spread. For this reason, stable, uniform magnetic nanoparticle dispersion in either an aqueous or organic solvent at neutral pH and physiological salinity is required. The stability of this magnetic colloidal suspension depends on two parameters: an ultra small dimension and surface chemistry. The particle size should be sufficiently small to avoid precipitation due to gravitation forces while the charge and surface groups should create both steric and coulombic repulsions which stabilize the colloidal suspensions.

The magnetic properties of magnetic nanoparticles are determined by their elemental compositions, crystallinity, shapes and dimensions. Various magnetic nanoparticles have been developed. Therefore, the selection of proper magnetic nanoparticles with the desired properties is the first but crucial step for certain bio-applications. For example, ferromagnetic nanoparticles (e.g. Fe nanoparticles) have a large magnetic moment and they can be the best material candidate in magnetic biosensors because they not only produce a better signal but respond to an applied magnetic field readily. On the other hand, iron oxide nanoparticles with super-paramagnetic behavior do an excellent job when used to enhance the signals in magnetic resonance imaging examinations. With the help of iron oxide nanoparticles a sharpened image with detailed information can be achieved because of the change of behavior of nearby bio-molecules by introduced nanoparticles *(Bystrzejewski et al. 2005)*. For many biomedical applications, magnetic nanoparticles presenting super-paramagnetic behavior (no remanence along with a rapidly changing magnetic state) at room temperature are desirable. Biomedical applications are commonly divided into two major categories: *in vivo* and *in vitro* applications. Consequently, additional restrictions apply on various magnetic nanoparticles for *in vivo* or *in vitro* biomedical applications. It is rather simple for *in vitro* applications of magnetic nanoparticles. The size restriction as well as biocompatibility/toxicity is not so critical for *in vitro* applications, when compared with *in vivo* ones. Therefore, super-paramagnetic composites containing submicron diamagnetic matrixes and super-paramagnetic nanocrystals can be used. Composites with long sedimentation times in the absence of a magnetic field are also acceptable. It was noticed that functionalities may be provided readily for the super-paramagnetic composites because of the diamagnetic matrixes *(Tartaj et al. 2003)*. On the other hand, severe restrictions must be applied for magnetic nanoparticles for *in vivo* biomedical applications. First of all, it is a requisite that the magnetic components should be biocompatible without any toxicity for the bio-systems of interest. This is predominantly determined by the nature of the material (e.g. iron, nickel, cobalt, metal alloy, etc). For instance, cobalt and nickel are highly magnetic materials. However, both of them are rarely used due to their toxic properties and susceptibility to oxidation. Currently, the most commonly employed magnetic nanoparticles in biomedical applications are iron oxides including magnetite (Fe_3O_4), maghemite (γ - Fe_2O_3) and hematite (α-Fe_2O_3). The second requirement for magnetic nanoparticles is their particle sizes. Ultrafine nanoparticles (usually smaller than 100 nm in diameter) have high effective surface area, thus they can be attached to ligand easily. Also the lower sedimentation rate leads to a high stability for colloidal suspensions, and the tissue diffusion can be improved by using nanoparticles in nanometer dimensions. After injection, nanoparticles would be able to remain in the circulation and pass through the capillary systems to reach the targeted organs and tissues without any vessel embolism. Further, the magnetic dipole–dipole interaction among magnetic nanoparticles can be substantially reduced. The third requisite for magnetic nanoparticles is their biocompatible polymer coating which may be done during or after the nanoparticle synthesis. There are several functions of the coating layers: 1) they will prohibit agglomeration of nanoparticles; 2) they prevent structural or elemental changes; 3) unnecessary biodegradation can be stopped; 4) the polymer layer offers a covalent binding or adsorption attachment of drugs to the nanoparticle surface. In summary, for *in vivo* biomedical applications, magnetic nanoparticles must be made of a non-toxic and non-immunogenic material with ultra small particle sizes and high magnetization.

It is no doubt that interdisciplinary research collaboration is badly needed for clinical and biological applications of magnetic nanoparticles *(Berry 2003)*. Research fields involved include chemistry, materials science, cell engineering, clinical tests and other related scientific efforts. In this chapter, an overview of cancer treatment approach as one of biomedical applications of magnetic nanoparticles will be presented

3. Hyperthermia treatment

Another major use of magnetic nanoparticles in therapeutic treatment is hyperthermia treatment for cancers. Gilchrist *et al.* did the experimental investigations for the first time when they heated various tissue samples with γ - Fe_2O_3 of 20–100 nm in diameter by a

1.2MHz magnetic field *(Gilchrist et al. 1957)*. Since then, studies have shown the feasibility of using the hyperthermic effect generated from magnetic nanoparticles by applying a high-frequency AC magnetic field as an alternate therapeutic approach for cancer treatment. Briefly speaking, the hyperthermic effect is generated from the relaxation of magnetic energy of the magnetic nanoparticles which is able to destroy tumor cells effectively *(Levy et al. 2002)*. Hyperthermia is a common cancer therapy in which certain organs or tissues are heated preferentially to temperatures between 41 ◦C and 46 ◦C, artificially induced hyperthermia has been designed to heat malignant cells without destroying the surrounding healthy tissue. When heated to a higher temperature (~56 ◦C), coagulation or carbonization may occur. This 'thermo-ablation' induces a completely different biological response and hence is not considered as hyperthermia. A classical hyperthermia not only causes almost reversible damage to cells and tissues, but also enhances radiation injury of tumor cells *(Jordan et al. 1999)*. For modern clinical hyperthermia trials, moderate temperatures (42–43 ◦C) are normally selected to optimize the thermal homogeneity in the target area. It is true that the heating effect will change the dose-dependent behavior of treated cells. However, the exact mechanism of thermal dose-response in hyperthermia is still unknown. There are great difficulties in identifying the individual cell as the target for hyperthermia. Instead, hyperthermia affects most bio-molecules including proteins and receptor molecules. On the other hand, DNA damage by irradiation has been well understood due to the highly specific interaction. As far as the underlying physics of the heating effect in hyperthermia is concerned, magnetic heating via magnetic nanoparticles essentially is determined by their sizes and magnetic properties *(Mornet et al. 2004)*.

Magnetic nanoparticles can be divided into two major categories: multi-domain and single-domain nanoparticles, which possess different heating effects. Multi-domain nanoparticles usually have larger dimensions and contain several sub-domains with definite magnetization direction for each. When they are exposed to a magnetic field, a phenomenon called 'domain wall displacements' occurs. This is featured by growth of the domain with magnetization direction along the magnetic field axis and shrinkage of the other. Figure 2 above, depicts this irreversible phenomenon. It can be seen that the magnetization curves for increasing and decreasing magnetic field do not coincide, and the area within the hysteresis loop represents the heating energy, named 'hysteresis loss', due to the AC magnetic field. For single-domain nanoparticles, since there is no domain wall, no hysteresis loss occurs leading to no heating. When exposed to an external AC magnetic field, rotation of magnetic moments from super-paramagnetic nanoparticles is assisted by the supplied energy which overcomes the energy barrier. Then these nanoparticles undergo N´eel relaxation in which their moments relax to their equilibrium orientation. Simultaneously, heat is generated during this relaxation by thermal dissipation. The N´eel relaxation time tN is related to the temperature, and can be described as:

$$t_N = t_0 e\ KV/kT \qquad (1)$$

Where $t_0 \approx 10^{-9}$ s, T is the temperature and k is the Boltzmann constant. For both multi- and single-domain nanoparticles, rotational Brownian motion in a carrier also generates heat.

This rotation is caused by the torque exerted on the magnetic moment by the AC magnetic field. The Brown relaxation time t_B is described as:

$$t_B = 3\eta v_B/kT \tag{2}$$

Where η is the viscosity of the carrier, and v_B is the frequency for maximal heating via Brown rotation, corresponding to the hydrodynamic volume of the particle, and it is given by the equation $2\pi v_B t_B = 1$.

The heating capacity of magnetic nanoparticles is expressed by specific absorption rate SAR, also called specific power loss (SPL), both of them have the same physical meaning, which determines the heating ability of magnetic nanoparticles in the presence of magnetic field, and can be defined as the amount of heat generated per unit gram per unit time. SAR values are usually expressed in watts per gram of magnetic material (W/g), also can be expressed in volumetric units (W/m^3).The heat generated per unit volume can be obtained by multiplying the SAR value by the density of the nanoparticles. It has been well documented that the orientation and magnetized domains of magnetic nanoparticles are dependent on their intrinsic features (elemental composition, crystallinity, magneto anisotropy, shape, dimension, etc.) and micro-structural features (impurities, grain boundaries, vacancies, etc). In magnetic hyperthermia treatment, after heat conducts into the area with diseased tissues, the surrounding temperature can be maintained above the therapeutic threshold of 42 °C for about half an hour to destroy the cancer. It is of great importance for hyperthermia to minimize the heat effect on healthy cells. Assisted by magnetic nanoparticles, it is possible to heat the specific area while unacceptable coincidental heating of healthy tissue is avoided. Although the hyperthermia treatment for cancer has been demonstrated with therapeutic efficacy in animal models, however, there have been no reports of successful hyperthermia treatment for human patients. The major reasons are the necessities of an adequate amount of magnetic nanoparticles and sufficiently high magnetic field which are not safe for human treatments. To date, laboratory research efforts on hyperthermia treatment for animals have all used magnetic field conditions which are not clinically acceptable. In most instances, hyperthermia treatments with a reduced amount of magnetic nanoparticles and reduced field strength or frequency cannot be effective due to the reduction of heat generated. Simulations suggest a sufficient level with heat deposition rate of $100mWcm^{-3}$ to destroy cancer cells effectively in most circumstances. The practical frequency and strength of the external AC magnetic field are 0.05–1.2MHz and 0–15 kAm^{-1}, respectively. On the other hand, sufficient magnetic materials are needed to enrich around the cancer tissues to generate enough heat for hyperthermia treatment. Direct injection of ferrofluid into the tumor tissues is able to introduce a large amount of magnetic materials for heat generation. Antibody targeting and intravascular administration offer better preference heating, but the problem here is the small quantity. It is estimated that about 5–10 mg of magnetic material concentrated in each cm^3 of tumor tissues is able to generate enough heat for tumor cell destruction in human bodies. Magnetite (Fe_3O_4) and maghemite (γ -Fe_2O_3) nanoparticles are two common types used in hyperthermia treatments owing to their appropriate magnetic properties and their excellent biocompatibilities. Several examples will be given here.

The history of using magnetic particles for selective heating of the tumors started in 1957 when Gilchrist et al used particles of a few mm in size for inductive heating of lymph nodes in dogs *(Gilchrist et al., 1957)*. More than 20 years later, Gordon et al used a magnetic fluid ('dextran-magnetites' with a core size of up to ~ 6 nm) for inducing hyperthermia *(Jordon et al., 1979)*. Injection of micro-scaled ferromagnetic particles into renal carcinomas of rabbits and subsequent heating was reported by Rand and co-workers *(Rand et al., 1981)*. Magnetic nanoparticles used in a different approach termed as ferromagnetic embolization. In this technique, the MNPs were injected into the main feeding artery of the tumor; this injection resulted in aggregates of MNPs which in turn embolized the feeding artery and hence necrosis of the tumor cells. This technique seems to be especially well suited for the treatment of hepatic malignancies due to the differences in blood supply between hepatic tumor cells and normal liver parenchyma *(Archer et al., 1990)*. Direct injection of dextran-coated magnetite NPs with a core size of ~ 3 nm into tumors was first reported in 1997 *(Jordan et al., 1997)*. Other groups in Japan developed "magnetic cationic liposomes" (MCLs) with improved adsorption and accumulation properties within tumors and demonstrated the efficacy of their technique in several animal tumor models: rat glioma *(Le et al., 2001)*. Hilger et al injected colloidal suspensions of coated MNPs (particle sizes of ~10 nm and 200 nm) into human carcinomas implanted into mice *(Hilger et al., 2002)*. Ohno et al inserted stick-type carboxymethyl cellulose magnetite containing NPs into gliomas and described as a three-fold prolongation of survival time *(Ohno et al., 2002)*. Moroz and co-workers concluded from their data that for a given tumor iron concentration, larger tumors heat at a greater rate than small tumors due to the poorer tissue cooling and better heat conduction in the necrotic regions of large tumors *(Moroz et al., 2002)*. Tanaka et al used MCLs in melanoma in combination with immunotherapy *(Tanaka et al., 2005)* and used for prostate cancer treatment *(Kawai et al., 2005)*. Yan *et al.* demonstrated the use of Fe_2O_3 nanoparticles combined with magnetic fluid for hyperthermia treatment on human hepatocarcinoma SMMC-7721 cells *in vitro* and xenograft liver cancer in nude mice (2005). Their experiments verified the significantly inhibitory effect of magnetic ferrofluid in weight and volume on xenograft liver cancer. After infiltrating magnetic ferrofluid into the target tissues, a time-varied magnetic field was applied and its energy was transformed to heat energy by the magnetic nanoparticles resulting in a temperature rise to 42–45 °C. This generated heat is able to kill malignant tumor cells without injuring the normal cells nearby. The growth and apoptosis of SMMC-7721 cells treated with the ferrofluids containing Fe_2O_3 nanoparticles at various concentrations (2, 4, 6 and 8 mg/ml) were examined by MTT, flow cytometry (FCM) and transmission electron microscopy (TEM) after 30–60 minute treatments. It was observed that Fe_2O_3 nanoparticles-based ferrofluid could significantly inhibit the proliferation and increase the ratio of apoptosis of SMMC-7721 cells. These dose-dependent inhibitions were 26.5 %, 33.53 %, 54.4 %, 81.2 %, and 30.26 %, 38.65 %, 50.28 %, 69.33 %, for inhibitory rate and apoptosis rate, respectively. It was also observed from animal experiments that the tumors became smaller and smaller as the dosage of magnetic ferrofluid increased. The weight and volume inhibitory ratios were 42.10 %, 66.34 %, 78.5 %, 91.46 %, and 58.77 %, 80.44 %, 93.40 %, 98.30 %, respectively. In a comparison of the control and experimental groups, each group exhibited significant difference. According to histological examination, many brown uniform spots are located at the stroma in the margin of the tumors, which are identified as iron oxide nanoparticles. Although interstitial hyperthermia following direct injection of nanoparticles has been proven successful in many animal models, nevertheless only one of these approaches has been successfully translated from research to clinical stage for prostate cancer treatment either by iron oxide against RF ,this clinical studies were performed by Johannsen 2005.

Fumiko et al 2004 developed magnetite cationic liposomes (MCLs) and applied them to local hyperthermia as a mediator. MCLs have a positive charge and generate heat under an alternating magnetic field (AMF) by hysteresis loss. In this study, the effect of hyperthermia using MCLs was examined in an in vivo study of hamster osteosarcoma. In this study, three-week-old Syrian female hamsters were purchased from Japan SLC, Inc., Shizuoka, Japan, and used for the animal study. After that MCLs were injected into the osteosarcoma and then subjected to an AMF. The results revealed that, the tumor was heated at over 42°C, but other normal tissues were not heated as much. Complete regression was observed in 100% of the treated group hamsters, whereas no regression was observed in the control group hamsters. At day 12, the average tumor volume of the treated hamsters was about 1/1000 of that of the control hamsters. In the treated hamsters, no regrowth of osteosarcomas was observed over a period of 3 months after the complete regression. These results suggest that this treatment is effective for osteosarcoma.

One of recent and novel study was applied by El Sherbini et al (2011). The aim of this experimental study is to evaluate the effect of magnetic resonance on magnetic nanoparticles, this *in -vivo* experiments in which hyperthermia is induced in female Swiss albino mice weighing 20.0 to 29.2g median, 26.3g implanted with subcutaneous *Ehrlich* carcinoma cells under magnetic resonance imaging. The strategy of this study was based on preparation, characterization of super-paramagnetic magnetic iron oxides nanoparticles and evaluation of magnetic resonance hyperthermia (MRH) technique in presence of super-paramagnetic nanoparticles and an alternating magnetic field (AMF).

Preparation of tumors bearing mice and iron oxide magnetic nanoparticles followed the method described by Elsherbini et al (2011). The prepared SPIO nanoparticles were suspended in glycerin medium to increase the stability especially *in vivo* conditions. The prepared suspension was stable for several months due to the high viscosity of glycerin. The influence of the SPIO nanoparticles concentration on the total amount of specific heat energy dose (SED) was studied in a preliminary study. The mean values of the total cumulative specific energy dose were monitored for different concentrations of SPIO nanoparticles in the tumors. The mean values reported of SED Jgm^{-1} were [282.1±13.8 for (200μg), 462.7±10.0 for (400μg), 663.7±13.0 for (600μg), 864.1±16.6 for (800μg) and 1087 ±18 for (10^3μg)] as shown in figure (3). The quantitative analysis revealed that, the SED values were directly proportional to the concentrations of the injected nanoparticles inside the tumors.

The results of heat deposition rate HDR inside the tumor revealed that, the mean values of HDR were [0.157 for (200μg), 0.259 for (400μg), and 0.367 for (600μg), 0.478 for (800μg) and 0.604 for (10^3μg)] as shown in figure (4). These values varied considerably between the different concentrations of SPIO nanoparticles with highly significant *p* value $p < .007$. The temperature changes were recorded in the intra-tumoural SPIO nanoparticles accumulation. The results revealed that the maximum temperatures achieved were [40.11±1.52°C for (200µg), 42.36±1.54°C for (400µg), 44.43±2.0°C for (600µg), 46.8±1.5°C for (800µg) and 48.6±1.0 °C for (10^3µg)] as shown in figure (5).The time taken to maximum temperature TMT was recorded as [40±2.5 min for 200&400µg, 30±2.0 min for 600µg, 25±5.0 min for 800µg and 20± 5.0 min for 10^3µg] as shown in figure (6). The statistical analysis revealed that the TMT values were inversely proportional to the concentrations of the injected nanoparticles inside the tumors. *In vivo* experiments for magnetic resonance hyperthermia demonstrated that the use of SPIO nanoparticles combined with magnetic resonance for hyperthermia treatment on Ehrlich carcinoma. The experiments revealed that after treatment sessions, magnetic resonance images verified degree of apoptotic cells presented by dark signal intensity in the center of the tumor in all mice on T1 weighted images; the centers of the lesions were asymmetrical and non-homogenous when compared to magnetic resonance images before treatment, as well as the images showed variations in signal intensity in the abdominal regions attributed to the distribution of the SPIO nanoparticles over the treatment sessions as shown in figure (7). As well as the experiments verified the significantly inhibitory effect of SPIO nanoparticles in volume on Ehrlich tumor. Significant volume differences between mice in all groups under experiments are shown in figure (8). It worth mentioning that, histopathology examination was further used to confirm MR results.

Plasmonic photo-thermal therapy (PPTT).Gold nanoshells belong to a prospective class of optical adjustable nanoparticles with a dielectric silica core encased in a thin metallic gold shell (Hirsch, et al 2006). The absorption cross-section of a solid nanoshell is high enough to provide a competitive nanoparticle technology with application of indocyanine green dye, a typical photothermal sensitizer used in laser cancer therapy (Gupta, et al 2007).

On the other hand, there are several *in vitro* experiments concerning application of gold nanoparticles and core shell NPs to PPTT of cancer cells, while number of *in vivo* studies is quite limited (Loo, et al, 2005). The first account of the use of gold nanoparticles in hyper-thermal therapy was published in 2003. Halas et al used gold -on-silica nanoshells to treat breast carcinoma cells using the HER2 antibody *(Hirsch et al., 2003)*. Another study using pulsed laser and gold nanospheres was performed in 2003 by Lin and co-workers for selective and highly localized photothermolysis of targeted lymphocytes cells. Lymphocytes incubated with gold nanospheres conjugated to anti-bodies were exposed to nanosecond laser pulses (Q-switched Nd: YAG laser, 565 nm wavelength, 20 ns duration) .The results showed that 100 laser pulses at an energy of 0.5 J/cm^2 were sufficient to induce cell death. While adjacent cells just a few micrometers away without nanoparticles remained viable *(Pitsillides et al., 2003)*. In the same year, Zharov et al performed similar studies on the photo-thermal destruction of K562 cancer cells. They further detected the laser induced- bubbles and studied their dynamics during the treatment using a pump–probe photo thermal imaging technique *(Zharov et al., 2003)*. O'Neal et al 2004 reported *in vivo* impressive results by showing selective photo-thermal ablation in mice using near infrared-absorbing NPs *(O' Neal et al., 2004)*. Another *in vivo study was applied on* a murine model using NIR light against gold nanoshells (*Loo et al., 2004*).

In a study by El- Sayed and co-workers conjugated gold nanoparticles of approximately 40 nm to anti-epithelial growth factors receptors (EGFR) antibodies and targeted to types of human head and neck cancer cells, the nanoparticles induce cancer cell damage at 19 W/cm^2 after the irradiation with argon Ar^+ laser at 514 nm for 4 min, while healthy cells do not show the loss of cell viability under the same treatment *(El Sayed et al., 2005).*

Huang et al also described the photo-thermal destruction of cancer cells using bio-functionalized gold nanorods. The nanorods were conjugated to anti- EGFR (specific antibody to the malignant cell types used), and then incubated with a non-malignant epithelial cell line (HaCat), as well as two malignant oral epithelial cell lines (HOC313 clone8 and HSC3). Following laser irradiation, the results revealed that the malignant cells were destroyed at about half the laser fluence needed to kill the nonmalignant cells. The efficient destruction of the malignant cells was evidently due to the preferential attachment of the anti-EGFR-gold nanorod conjugates to the over-expressed EGFR on the surface of the malignant cell *(Huang et al., 2006).*

In 2006, El-Sayed and co-workers conjugated gold nanorods to anti-EGFR antibodies specifically bind to the head and neck cancer cells, these labeled cells subjected to laser irradiation (Ti: Sapphire laser, CW at 800 nm) which was maximally overlapped with the surface plasmonic resonance absorption band of the nanorods. Under laser exposure for 4 min, it was found that the cancer cells required half the laser energy (10 W/cm^2) to be photo-thermally damaged as compared to the normal cells (20 W/cm^2) *(El Sayed et al., 2006).*

In 2007, Huff and co-workers conjugated folate ligands with oligo-ethylene-glycol onto gold nanorods by *in situ* dithio-carbamate formation; the folate conjugated gold nanorods were selectively bound to KB cancer cells (a tumor cell line derived from oral epithelium) which led to photo-thermal damage on cell membranes following laser irradiation *(Huff et al., 2007).* Another study from the same group showed that under laser irradiation membrane blebbing occurred due to the influx of calcium ion Ca^{2+} into the cells *(Tong et al., 2007).*

Attempts using gold nanocages for PPPT have also been made recently. In the *in vitro* studies by Li and co-workers conjugated gold nanocages of approximately 30 nm to anti-EGFR to target A431 cells. At laser energy density of 40 W/cm^2, almost all immunonanocage treated cells were damaged *(Li et al., 2008).* Other *in vitro* studies by Xiaohug and co-workers using gold nanocages of approximately 45 nm conjugated to HER-2 and near infrared femtosecond Ti: Sapphire pulsed laser to treat Sk-BR-3 breast cancer cells *(Xiaohua et al., 2010).*

Paul and Tuan reported the application of liposome-encapsulated gold nanoshells for in vitro photo-induced hyperthermia in human mammary carcinoma cells. In addition to evaluating their effects in vitro, the authors compared the application liposome-encapsulated gold nanoshells and free-standing gold nanoshells for NanoPhotoTherapy (NPT). NPT-induced hyperthermia was performed using a 785-nm near-infrared light from a diode laser and the in vitro effects were evaluated using nucleic acid molecular probes by fluorescence microscopy. Additionally, they monitored the effectiveness of NPT by detecting apoptosis via capase-9 activity. The experiments clearly showed that liposomal delivery enhanced the intracellular bioavailability of gold nanoshells and thus is able to induce a higher degree of cell death more effectively than free-standing gold nanoshells.

Single-walled carbon nanotubes (SWNTs) have a high optical absorbance in the near-infrared (NIR) region. In this special optical window, biological systems are known to be highly transparent. The optical properties of SWNTs provide an opportunity for selective photo thermal therapy for cancer treatment. Specifically, SWNTs with a uniform size about (0.81 nm) and a narrow absorption peak at 980 nm are ideal candidates for such a novel approach. In a study by Feifan et al, SWNTs are conjugated to folate, which can bind specifically to the surface of the folate receptor tumor markers. Folate- SWNT (FA-SWNT) targeted tumor cells were irradiated by a 980 nm laser. Results in *vitro* and *in vivo* experiments revealed that FA-SWNT effectively enhanced the photo thermal destruction on tumor cells and noticeably spared the photo thermal destruction for non targeted normal cells. Thus, SWNTs, combined with suitable tumor markers, can be used as novel nanomaterials for selective photo thermal therapy for cancer treatment. The authors used the mammary tumor model with EMT6 cells in the female Balb/c mice to investigate the *in vivo* effects of FA-SWNT. The mouse tumors with or without FA-SWNT were treated by the 980-nm laser. To determine the effects of NIR optical excitation of SWNTs inside tumors, the authors measured the temperature on the tumor surface during the irradiation by the 980-nm laser with an infrared thermal camera. In one experimental mouse, irradiation of tumors with a power density of 1 W/cm2 with FA-SWNT (1 mg/kg) for 5 min caused a surface temperature elevation of 63 °C. Without FASWNT, the tumor irradiated at the same light dose caused a surface temperature elevation of 54 °C. Experiments with other animals yielded similar results. These findings clearly show that FA-SWNT could effectively enhance the tumor photo thermal therapy.

Kim et al achieved close to 90% cancer cell destruction in vitro using FeNi@Aumagnetic-vortex microdiscs (MDs), on the application of only a few tens of hertz AMF for just 10min. This confirms that operation of MFH at lower frequencies is possible and for effective heat generation can be achieved using core–shell type of structures. Likewise, in yet another demonstration, a gold coating of approximately 0.4 to 0.5 nm thickness around SPIONs resulted in a four- to five-fold increase in the amount of heat released (the highest value of 976W/g in ethanol at 430 Hz frequency) in comparison with SPIONs on application of low frequency oscillating magnetic fields (44–430 Hz). This study was done by Mohamed et al 2010. In addition, the SPIONs@Au were found to be not particularly cytotoxic to mammalian cells. (MCF-7 breast carcinoma cells and H9c2 cardiomyoblasts) in *in vitro* studies were done by Pollert et al 2010. When similar heating experiments were carried out using stable water suspensions of La0.75Sr0.25MnO3 cores covered by silica (conc. of Mn=3.39 mg/ml), highest SAR of 130 W/g Mn at 37 °C was reached for the applied amplitude and frequency of 8.7 kAm−1, 480 kHz respectively.

In this context, a study was done by Elsherbini and co-workers, 2011. The group evaluated two different approaches in the nanotechnology era for inducing hyperthermia in subcutaneous Ehrlich carcinoma cells. The first called Optical Resonance Hyperthermia (ORH) technique in presence of gold nanospheres and green diode laser, as shown in fig (9). While the second technique called Magneto-Optical Resonance Hyperthermia (MORH), in presence of gold-iron oxide core shell nanoparticles with green, near infra-red diode laser, and magnetic field, as shown in fig (10). This approach was performed under magnetic resonance imaging guidance. The results revealed that, all mice treated by the first technique, the tumors were still as the same as before the treatments, as well as the rate of tumors growth were very slow if compared with the control mice. In contrast more than 50% of the mice treated with the second technique revealed a complete disappearance of the tumor, as shown in figure (11). So the study have demonstrated that a pair of synthetic nanospheres can work together more effectively for inducing hyperthermia than individual nanospheres, whereby more than .So, this simple, non-invasive method shows great promise as a treatment technique for clinical setting.

There are two main advantages of the plasmonic photothermal therapy technique. Firstly, there is the benefit of photostability compared with the photosensitizer dyes used in photodynamic therapy, which suffer from photobleaching as well as diffusion under laser irradiation. Secondly, there is the advantage of absorption and scattering cross-sections of gold nanoparticles, which are significantly superior to the absorbing dyes conventionally used in biological systems. Mie theory estimates that the optical cross-sections of gold nanospheres are typically four to five orders of magnitude higher than those of conventional dyes.

In spite of much progress having been made using the plasmonic photothermal therapy technique for cancer treatment in a laboratory setting, there are still many factors which must be taken into account before this method may be taken to a clinical setting, and they need to be studied further. First of all, the distribution of the elevated temperature under plasmonic photothermal therapy treatment is related to absorption of light by nanospheres acting as point wise local heat sources and by thermal diffusion over surrounding tissues. At the practical level, plasmonic photothermal therapy needs to provide an appropriate temperature increment, ΔT, gold nanosphere concentration, laser power density, duration of laser exposure, optimization of absorption and scattering cross-sections of nanospheres, as well as penetration of the laser light into the area of interest. It should be noted that the biological effects have a nonlinear dependence on changes in particle concentration and laser power density, which is defined by the type of tissue and thermoregulation ability of the living organism.

Although interstitial hyperthermia following direct injection of nanoparticles has been proven successful in many animal models, nevertheless only one of these approaches has been successfully translated from research to clinical stage for prostate cancer treatment either by iron oxide against RF ,this clinical studies were performed by Johannsen 2005. The aim of this pilot study was to evaluate whether the technique of magnetic fluid hyperthermia can be used for minimally invasive treatment of prostate cancer. This paper presents the first clinical application of interstitial hyperthermia using magnetic nanoparticles in locally recurrent prostate cancer. Treatment planning was carried out using computerized tomography (CT) of the prostate. Based on the individual anatomy of the prostate and the estimated specific absorption rate (SAR) of magnetic fluids in prostatic tissue, the number and position of magnetic fluid depots required for sufficient heat deposition was calculated while rectum and urethra were spared. Nanoparticle suspensions were injected transperineally into the prostate under transrectal ultrasound and flouroscopy guidance. Treatments were delivered in the first magnetic field applicator for use in humans, using an alternating current magnetic field with a frequency of 100 kHz and variable field strength (0–18 kAm^{-1}). Invasive thermometry of the prostate was carried out in the first and last of six weekly hyperthermia sessions of 60 min duration. CT-scans of the prostate were repeated following the first and last hyperthermia treatment to document magnetic nanoparticle distribution and the position of the thermometry probes in the prostate. Nanoparticles were retained in the prostate during the treatment interval of 6 weeks. Using appropriate software (AMIRA), a non-invasive estimation of temperature values in the prostate, based on intra-tumoural distribution of magnetic nanoparticles, can be performed and correlated with invasively measured intra-prostatic temperatures. Using a specially designed cooling device, treatment was well tolerated without anesthesia. In the first patient treated, maximum and minimum intraprostatic temperatures measured at field strength of 4.0–5.0 kAm^{-1} were 48.5^{0}C and 40.0^{0}C during the 1st treatment and 42.5^{0}C and 39.4^{0}C during the 6th treatment, respectively. These first clinical experiences prompted us to initiate a phase I study to evaluate feasibility, toxicity and quality of life during hyperthermia using magnetic nanoparticles in patients with biopsy-proven local recurrence of prostate cancer following radiotherapy with curative intent. To the authors' knowledge, this is the first report on clinical application of interstitial hyperthermia using magnetic nanoparticles in the treatment of human cancer.

Akihiko et al have developed a novel hyperthermic treatment modality using magnetic materials for metastatic bone tumors. The purpose of this study is to show the results of novel hyperthermia for metastatic bone tumors. This novel hyperthermic treatment modality was used for 15 patients with 16 metastatic bone lesions. In seven lesions, after curettage of the metastatic lesion followed by reinforcement with a metal intra-medullary nail or plate, calcium phosphate cement (CPC) containing powdery Fe_3O_4 was implanted into the cavity. In one lesion, prosthetic reconstruction was then performed after an intralesional tumor excision. For the remaining eight lesions, metal intra-medullary nails were inserted into the affected bone. Hyperthermic therapy was started at 1 week postoperatively. To comparatively evaluate the radiographic results of patients who underwent hyperthermia (HT group), the authers also assessed eight patients who received a palliative operation without either radiotherapy or hyperthermia (Op group), and 22 patients who received operation in combination with postoperative radiotherapy (Op + RT group). In HT group, all patients had an acceptable limb function with pain relief without any complications. On radiographs, 87, 38, and 91% were, respectively, considered to demonstrate an effective treatment outcome in HT group, Op group, and Op + RT group. The patients in HT group showed a statistically better radiographic outcome than the patients in Op group (P = 0.0042). But when compared between HT group and Op + RT group, there were no significant difference (P = 0.412). This first series of clinical hyperthermia using magnetic materials achieved good local control of metastatic bone lesion.

Study by Manfred et al 2007, or by using laser against gold nanoparticles, for instance Yusheng et al 2009 used core shells (silica as a core with a diameter 110nm and an outer gold shell with thickness 15 nm) to mediate laser surgery stimulation for prostate cancer treatment. The goal of this paper is to present an integrated computer model using a so-called nested-block optimization algorithm to simulate laser surgery and provides transient temperature field predictions. In particular, this algorithm aims to capture changes in optical and thermal properties due to nanoshell inclusion and tissue property variation during laser surgery. Numerical results show that this model is able to characterize variation of tissue properties for laser surgical procedures and predict transient temperature field comparable to that measured by in vivo magnetic resonance temperature imaging (MRTI) techniques. Note that the computational approach presented in the study is quite general and can be applied to other types of nanoparticle inclusions.

In conclusion, this is a brief review on different approaches for inducing hyperthermia cancer treatment relevant to nanomedicine

Author details

El-Sayed El-Sherbini
National Institute of Laser Enhanced Science (NILES), Cairo University, Egypt

Ahmed El-Shahawy
Children Cancer Hospital, Cairo, Egypt

4. References

Albert B, Bray D, Hopkin K, Johnson A, Lewis J, Raff M, Roberts K and Walter P: *Essential Cell Biology*, Second Ed. New York and London: Garland Science, 2004.

Akihiko M, Katsuyuki K, Takao M, Ken S, Haruhiko S,Toru W, Shinichi M, Katsuya M, Kenji T, Atsumasa U: *Novel hyperthermia for metastatic bone tumors with magnetic materials by generating an alternating electromagnetic field.* Clin Exp Metastasis, 2007, 24:191–200 DOI 10.1007/s10585-007-9068-8.

Archer S and Gray B: *Comparison of portal vein chemotherapy with hepatic artery chemotherapy in the treatment of liver micro- metastases*. J. Am. Surgery, 1990; vol159: pp325–329.

Berry C: *Progress in functionalization of magnetic nanoparticles for applications in biomedicine.* Journal of Physics D: Applied Physics, 2009, 42(22): p. 224003.

Bystrejewski M, Huczko A. and Lange H: Arc plasma route to carbon-encapsulated magnetic nanoparticles for biomedical applications, *Sensors and Actuators B*, 2005, 109, 81–5.

Cho W, Jeong J, Choi M, Han B, Kim S, Kim H, Lim Y and Chung B: *Acute toxicity and pharmacokinetics of 13 nm-sized PEG-coated gold nanoparticles*. J. Appl. Pharmacology, 2009; vol 236: PP16–24.

Could P: *Nanoparticles probe biosystems*, Materials Today, 2004,7 (2), 36–43.

Cozzoli P, Pellegrino D, Manna L: *Synthesis, properties and perspectives of hybrid nanocrystal structures*. Chemical Society Reviews, 2006; vol 35 (11): pp1195-1208.

El-Sayed M and Huang X: *Surface Plasmon Resonance Scattering and Absorption of anti-EGFR Antibody Conjugated Gold Nanoparticles in Cancer Diagnostics: Applications in Oral Cancer*. Nano Letters. April, 2005.

EI-Sayed M, Huang X and Qian W: *Cancer cell imaging and photo thermal therapy in the near-infrared region by using gold nanorods*. J. Am. Chem. Soc, 2006; vol128: pp2115–2120.

El-Sherbini A, Mahmoud S, Mohamed A, Ahmed A and Hesham S: *Magnetic nanoparticles-induced hyperthermia treatment under magnetic resonance imaging*. J. Magnetic Resonance Imaging, 2011; vol 29:pp272-280.

El-Sherbini A, Mahmoud S, Mohamed A, Ahmed A and Hesham S: *Laser and Radiofrequency Induced Hyperthermia Treatment via Gold-Coated Magnetic Nanocomposites*. J. international Nanomedicine, 2011; volume 6 (September): pp1-10.Indexed on pubMed .Link (http//www.ncbi.nlm.nih.gov/pubMed/2211449).

Feifan Z, Da Xing ,Zhongmin Ou , Baoyan W Daniel E, Resasco and Wei R: *Cancer photo thermal therapy in the near-infrared region by using single-walled carbon nanotubes, 2009*.Journal of Biomedical Optics 14(2), 021009.

Freitas R: *What is nanomedicine*? Nanomedicine: Nanotechnology, Biology, and Medicine, 2005, 1, 2–9.

Fumiko M, Masashige S, Hiroyuki H, Tadahiko K, Takashi S and Takeshi K: *Hyperthermia using magnetite cationic liposome for hamster osteosarcoma*. J. BioMagnetic Research and Technology, 2004; vol 2: p3.

Gee S, Hong Y: *Synthesis and aging effect of spherical magnetite (Fe_3O_4) nanoparticles for biosensor application*. Journal of applied physics, 2003; vol 93(102):pp7560-7562.

Gilchrist R, Shorey W, Hanselman R, Parrott J, Taylor C and Medal R: *Selective Inductive Heating of Lymph Nodes*. J. Annals of Surgery, 1957; vol 146:pp596–606.

Gupta A: *Synthesis and surface engineering of iron oxide nanoparticles for biomedical application*. J. Biomaterials, 2004; vol 26:pp3995-4021.

Harisinghani M and Barentsz J: *Noninvasive Detection of Clinically Occult Lymph-Node Metastases in Prostate Cancer*. The New England journal of Medicine, 2003; vol 348(25): pp 2491-2499.

Hilger I, Hiergeist R, Hergt R, Winnefeld K, Schubert H and Kaiser A: *Thermal ablation of tumors using magnetic nanoparticles: An in vivo feasibility study*. J. Invest Radiology, 2002; vol 37: pp 580–586.

Hirsch L, Stafford J, Bankson A, Sershen S, Rivera B and Halas N: *Nanoshells-mediated near-infrared thermal therapy of tumors under magnetic resonance guidance*. PNAS, November11, 2003; vol 100(23):pp13549-13554.

Hirsch L, Gobin A, Lowery A, et al. *Metal nanoshells*. Ann Biomed

Eng. 2006; 34:15–22.

Huang X, El-Sayed I, QianW and El-Sayed M: *Cancer cell imaging and photo-thermal therapy in the near-infrared region by using gold nanorods*. Journal of the American Chemical Society, 2006; vol 128: pp 2115-20.

Huff T, Tong Y, Zhao M, Hansen J, Cheng X and Wei A: *Hyperthermic effects of gold nanorods on tumor cells*. J .Nanomedicine, 2007: vol 2: pp 125–132.

Hultgren A, Tanase M, Felton E, Bhadriraju K, Salem A, Chen Cand Reich D: *Optimization of yield in magnetic cell separations using nickel nanowires of different lengths*, Biotechnology Progress, 2005 21, 509–15.

Johannsen M, Gneveckow U, Eckelt L, Feussner A, Waldo Fner N, Scholz R, Deger S, Wust P and Jordan A: *Clinical hyperthermia of prostate cancer using magnetic nanoparticles: Presentation of a new interstitial technique*. Int. J. Hyperthermia, April 2005:pp1-11.

Jordan A, Scholz R, Wust P, Fahling H, Krause J, Wlodarczyk W, Sander B, Vogl T and Felix R: *Effects of magnetic fluid hyperthermia (MFH) on C3H mammary carcinoma in vivo*. Int .J .Hyperthermia, 1997; vol 13:pp587–605.

Jordan A, Scholz R, Wust P, Fahling H and Felix R: *Magnetic fluid hyperthermia: cancer treatment with AC magnetic field induced excitation of biocompatible super paramagnetic nanoparticles*. J. Mag Mat, 1999; vol 201: pp 413 – 419.

Kang, Y: *Synthesis and characterization of nanometer-size Fe_3O_4 and gamma-Fe_2O_3 particles* .J. Chemistry of Materials, 1996; vol 8(9): pp 2209-2215.

Kawai N, Ito A, Nakahara Y, Futakuchi M, Shirai T, Honda H, Kobayashi T and Kohri K: *Anticancer effect of hyperthermia on prostate cancer mediated by magnetite cationic induction in transplanted syngenic rats*. Prostate, 2005; vol 64: pp 373-381.

Kelly K, Allport J, Tsourkas A, Shinde-Patil V, Josephson L and Weissleder R: *Detection of vascular adhesion molecule-1 expression using a novel multimodal nanoparticles*. Circ. Res, 2005; vol 96:pp327–336.

Kim D, Rozhkova E, Ulasov I, Bader S, Rajh T, Lesniak M and Novosad V: *Biofunctionalized magnetic-vortex microdiscs for targeted cancer-cell destruction*, Nat. Mater,2009, 9,165–171.

Kohler N, Fryxell G and Zhang M: *Bi-functional poly (ethylene glycol) silane immobilized on metallic oxide-based nanoparticles for conjugation with cell targeting agents*. Journal of the American Chemical Society, 2004; vol 126 (23): PP7206-7211.

Ko¨hrmann K, Michel M, Gaa J, Marlinghaus E and Alken P: *Urology*, 2002; vol 167: pp 2397–2403.

Koltsov D and Perry M. Magnets and nanometres: mutual attraction, *Physics World*, (2004), 17(7), 31–5.

Lacava Z and Azevedo R: *Toxic effects of ionic magnetic fluids in mice*. J. Magnetism and Magnetic Materiala, 1999: vol 194 (1-3):pp90-95.

Le B, Shinkai M, Kitade T, Honda H, Yoshida J, Wakabayashi T and Kobayashi T:*Preparation of tumor-specific magnetoliposomes and their application for hyperthermia*. J. Chem Eng Japan, 2001; vol 34:pp66–72.

Leslie-Pelecky D: *Nano-toxicology: In Biomedical Applications of Nanotechnology*. New Jersey: Wiley- Interscience, 2007:pp227-234.

Levy L, Sahoo Y, Kim K, Bergey E and Prasad P: Nan chemistry: synthesis and characterization of multifunctional monoclinic for biological applications, *Chemistry of Materials*, 2002, 14, 3715–21.

Lewinski N, Colvin V, Drezek R: *Cytotoxicity of nanoparticles.* J .Small, 2008; vol 4:pp26–49.

Li X, Au L, Zheng D, Zhou F, Li ZY and Xia Y: *A quantitative study on the photo thermal effect of immuno gold nanocages targeted to breast cancer cells.* J.ACS Nano, 2008; vol 2 (8):pp1645–52.

Loo C, Lin A, Hirsch L, Lee M, Barton J, Halas N, West J and Drezek R: *Nanoshells-enabled photonics-based imaging and therapy of cancer.* J. Technology Cancer Res. Treat, 2004; vol 3:pp33-40.

Loo C, Lowery A, Halas N, West J and Drezek R: *Immunotargeted nanoshells for integrated cancer imaging and therapy.* Nano Lett.2005; 5:709–711.

Maenosono S, Suzuki T and Saita S: *Super paramagnetic FePt nanoparticles as excellent MRI contrast agents.* J. Magnetism and Magnetic Materials, 2008; vole 320(9): pp L79-L83.

Manfred J, Burghard T, Kasra T, Chie H, Norbert W, Regina S, Andreas J, Stefan A and Peter W: *Thermotherapy of prostate cancer using magnetic nanoparticles: Feasibility, Imaging ,Three-dimensional Temperature distribution.* J. European Urology, 2007; vol 52:pp653- 662.

Mirza A, Fornage B, Sneige N, Kuerer M, Newman L, Ames F and Singletary S: *Radiofrequency ablation of solid tumors.* J. Cancer, 2001 vol 7: pp 95–102.

Mohammad F, Balaji G, Weber A , Uppu R and Kumar C: *Influence of gold nanoshell on hyperthermia of superparamagnetic iron oxide nanoparticles.* Phys. Chem. C, 2010, 114, 19194–19201.

Moroz P, Jones SK and Gray B: *The effect of tumor size on ferromagnetic embolization hyperthermia in a rabbit liver tumor model.* Int. J. Hyperthermia, 2002; vol18:pp129–140.

Mornet S, Vasseur S, Grasset F and Duguet E: Magnetic nanoparticle design for medical diagnosis and therapy, *Journal of Materials Chemistry*, (2004), 14, 2161–75.

Muller R, Luck M and Harnisch S: *Intravenously injected particles: surface properties and interaction with blood proteins-the key determining the organ distribution.* Journal of scientific and clinical applications of Magnetic Carriers, Plenum Press, 1997: p 135.

Neuberger T and Schopf B: *Super paramagnetic nanoparticles for biomedical applications: possibilities and limitations of a new drug delivery system.* J. Magnetism and Magnetic Materials, 2005; vol 293: pp 483-496.

Ohno T, Wakabayashi T, Takemura A, Yoshida J, Ito A, Shinkai M, Honda H and Kobayashi T: *Effective solitary hyperthermia treatment of malignant glioma using stick type CMC-magnetite. In vivo study.* J. Neuro-Oncol, 2002; vol 56:pp233–239.

O'Neal D, Hirsch L, Halas N, Payne J, and West L: *Photo-thermal tumor ablation in mice using near infrared absorbing nanoparticles.* J.Cancer Lett, 2004; vol 209:pp171–176.

Pankhurst Q, Connolly J, Jones Sand Dobson J. Applications of magnetic nanoparticles in biomedicine, Journal of Physics D: Applied Physics, (2003), 36, R167–R181.

Paul M. and Tuan Vo-Dinh: *Photothermal Treatment of Human Carcinoma Cells Using Liposome-Encapsulated Gold Nanoshells.* Nanobiotechnology, 2005. DOI: 10.1385/Nano: 1:3:245

Pitsillides C, Joe E, Wei X, Anderson R and Lin C: *Selective cell targeting with light absorbing micro-particles and nanoparticles*. J. Biophysics, 2003; vol 84(6):pp4023–4032.

Pollert E, Kaman O, Veverka P, Veverka M , Marysko M, Záveta K, Kacenka M, Lukes I, Jendelová P, Kaspar P, Burian M and Herynek V: *Core–shell La1−xSrxMnO3 nanoparticles as colloidal mediators for magnetic fluid hyperthermia*. Philos. Trans. R. Soc. A, 2010, 368, 4389–4405.

Rynal I, Prigent P, Peyramaure S and Corot C: *Macrophage endocytosis of super paramagnetic iron oxide nanoparticles*. J. Investigative radiology, 2004; vol 39(1): pp 56-63.

Rand R, Snow H and Brown W: *Thermo magnetic Surgery for Cancer*. J. Surgical Research, 1981; vol 33:pp177–183.

Reiss B, Mao C, Solis J, Ryan K, Thomson T and Belcher A: Biological routes to metal alloy ferromagnetic nanostructures, *Nano Letters*, (2004), 4, 1127–32.

Schmidt H: *Nanoparticles by chemical Synthsis, processing to materials and innovative Applications*, Appl, organometal. J. Chem, 2001; vol 15: pp 331-343.

Satyanarayana M: the flow of innovation continues, *Monthly Feather*, NCI Alliance for Nanotechnology in Cancer, August 2005.

Shen T, Weissleder R, Papisov M, Bogdanov A and Brady T: *Monocrystalline iron oxide nanocompounds (MION): Physicochemical properties*. J.Magn. Reson. Med, 1993; vol 29:pp599–604.

Sun L, Hao Y, Chien C and Searson P: *Tuning the properties of magnetic nanowires*, Journal of Research and Development, 2005, 49(1) , 79–102.

Sun S: *Recent Advances in Chemical Synthesis, self-Assemply, and Applications of FePt Nanoparticles*. Journal of Advanced Materials, 2006; vol 18:pp393-403.

Tanaka K, Ito A, Kobayashi T, Kawamura T, Shimada S, Matsumoto K, Saida T and Honda H:*Intratumoral injection of immature dendritic cells enhances antitumor effect of hyperthermia using magnetic nanoparticles*. Int. J Cancer, 2005; vol 116: pp 624–633.

Tartaj P, Morales M, Veintemillas S, Gonz′alez-Carre˜no T. and Serna C: The preparation of magnetic nanoparticles for applications in biomedicine, *Journal of Physics D: Applied Physics*, (2003), 36, R182–R197.

Thorek D, Chen A, Czupryna J and Tsourkas: *Super paramagnetic Iron Oxide Nanoparticles Probes for Molecular Imaging, Annals of Biomedical Engineering,* January 2006; vol 34, No1:pp. 23–38.

Tong L, Zhao Y, Huff T, Hansen M, Wei A and Cheng J: *Gold nanorods mediate tumor cell death by compromising membrane integrity*.J.Adv. Mater, 2007; vol 19: pp 3136–3141.

Wang X: *A general strategy for nanocrystal synthesis*.J. Nature, 2005, vol 437(7055): pp 121-124.

Weissleder R and Stark D: *Super-paramagnetic iron oxide: Pharmacokinetics and toxicity.* American Journal of roentgen-logy, 1989; vol 152(1):pp167-173.

Whitesides G: *Nanoscience, nanotechnology, and chemistry*, Small, (2005), 1(2), 172–9.

Xiaohua H: *Gold nanoparticles: Optical properties and implementations in cancer diagnosis and photo thermal therapy*. Journal of Advanced Research, 2010; vol 1: pp 13–2.

Yu-Fen H, Kwame S, Suwussa B, Huan-Tsung C and Weihong T: *selective photo thermal therapy for mixed cancer cells using Aptamer-conjugated nanorods*. Langmuir J, 2008; vol 24: pp 11860-11865.

Yih T and Wei C. *Nanomedicine in cancer treatment*, Nanomedicine: Nanotechnology, Biology, and Medicine, (2005), 1, 191–2.

Yusheng F, David F, Andrea H, Jon B, Marissa N and Anil Shetty R: *Nanoshells-mediated laser surgery simulation for prostate cancer treatments*. J. Engineering with Computers, 2009; vol 25:pp3–13.

Zharov V, Galitovsky V and Viegas M: *Photo thermal detection of local Thermal effects during selective nano photothermolysis*. J. Appl Phys Lett, 2003; vol 83:pp4897- 9.

Chapter 4

Diffusion of Magnetic Nanoparticles Within a Biological Tissue During Magnetic Fluid Hyperthermia

Mansour Lahonian

Additional information is available at the end of the chapter

http://dx.doi.org/10.5772/52305

1. Introduction

Hyperthermia is one of many techniques used in oncology. It uses the physical methods to heat certain organ or tissue delivering an adequate temperature in an appropriate period of time (thermal dose), to the entire tumor volume for achieving optimal therapeutic results. Thermal dose has been identified as one of the most important factors which, influences the efficacy of hyperthermia [Perez and Sapareto (1984)]. Although there are definite prescriptions for temperature (generally 43 °C) and time (usually 60 *min*), variations in the temperature and time of delivery are frequent throughout the treatment sessions [Perez and Sapareto (1984), Jordan *et al.* (1999), Jordan *et al.* (2001), Overgaard *et al.* (2009)].

The effectiveness of hyperthermia treatment is related to the temperature achieved during the treatment. An ideal hyperthermia treatment should selectively destroy the tumor cells without damaging the surrounding healthy tissue. [Andrä *et al.* (1999), Lagendijk (2000), Moroz *et al.* (2002), Maenosono and Saita (2006), Lin and Liu (2009)]. Therefore, the ability to predict the temperature distribution inside as well as outside the target region as a function of the exposure time, possesses a high degree of importance.

In the past fifteen years, MFH has drawn greater attention due to the potential advantages for cancer hyperthermia therapy. In MFH, a nanofluid containing the MNPs is injected directly into the tumor. An alternating magnetic field is then applied to the target region, and then MNPs generate heat according to Néel relaxation and Brownian rotation losses as localized heat sources [Jordan *et al.* (1999), Jordan *et al.* (2001), Thiesen and Jordan (2008)]. The heat generated increases the temperature of the tumor. In general, the cancerous cells possess a higher chance to die when the temperature is above 43 °C whereas healthy cells will be safe at this temperature [Andrä *et al.* (1999), Moroz *et al.* (2002)].

Two techniques are currently used to deliver the MNPs to the tumor. The first is to deliver particles to the tumor vasculature [Matsuki and Yanada (1994)] through its supplying artery; however, this method is not effective for poorly perfused tumors. Furthermore, for a tumor with an irregular shape, inadequate MNPs distribution may cause under-dosage of heating in the tumor or overheating of the normal tissue. The second approach, is to directly inject MNPs into the extracellular space in the tumors. The MNPs diffuse inside the tissue after injection of nanofluid. If the tumor has an irregular shape, multi-site injection can be exploited to cover the entire target region [Salloum *et al.* (2008a)].

The nanofluid injection volume as well as infusion flow rate of nanofluid are important factors in dispersion and concentration of the MNPs, within the tissue. A successful MFH treatment is substantially dependent on the MNPs distribution in the tissue [Bagaria and Johnson (2005), Salloum *et al.* (2008a), Salloum *et al.* (2008b), Lin and Liu (2009), Bellizzi and Bucci (2010), Golneshan and Lahonian (2011a)].

2. Heat dissipation of MNPs

In MFH, after introducing the MNPs into the tumor (Figure 1), an alternating magnetic field is applied. This causes an increase in the tumor temperature and subsequent tumor regression. The temperature that can be achieved in the tissue strongly depends on the properties of the magnetic material used, the frequency and the strength of the applied magnetic field, duration of application of the magnetic field, and dispersion of the MNPs within the tissue.

2.1. Mechanisms of heat dissipation of MNPs

To turn MNPs into heaters, they are subjected to an oscillating electromagnetic field, where the field's direction changes cyclically. There are various theories which explain the reasons for the heating of the MNPs when subjected to an oscillating electromagnetic field [Brusentsova *et al.* (2005), Jo´zefczak and Skumiel (2007), Kim *et al.* (2008), Golneshan and Lahonian (2010), Golneshan and Lahonian (2011c)].

There exist at least four different mechanisms by which magnetic materials can generate heat in an alternating field [Nedelcu (2008)]:

1. Generation of eddy currents in magnetic particles with size >1μ,
2. Hysteresis losses in magnetic particles >1μ and multidomain MNPs,
3. Relaxation losses in 'superparamagnetic' single-domain MNPs,
4. Frictional losses in viscous suspensions.

Relaxation losses in single-domain MNPs fall into two modes: rotational (Brownian) mode and Néel mode. The principle of heat generation due to each individual mode is shown in Figure 2.

In the Néel mode, the magnetic moment originally locked along the crystal easy axis rotates away from that axis towards the external field. The Néel mechanism is analogous to the hysteresis loss in multi-domain MNPs whereby there is an 'internal friction' due to the

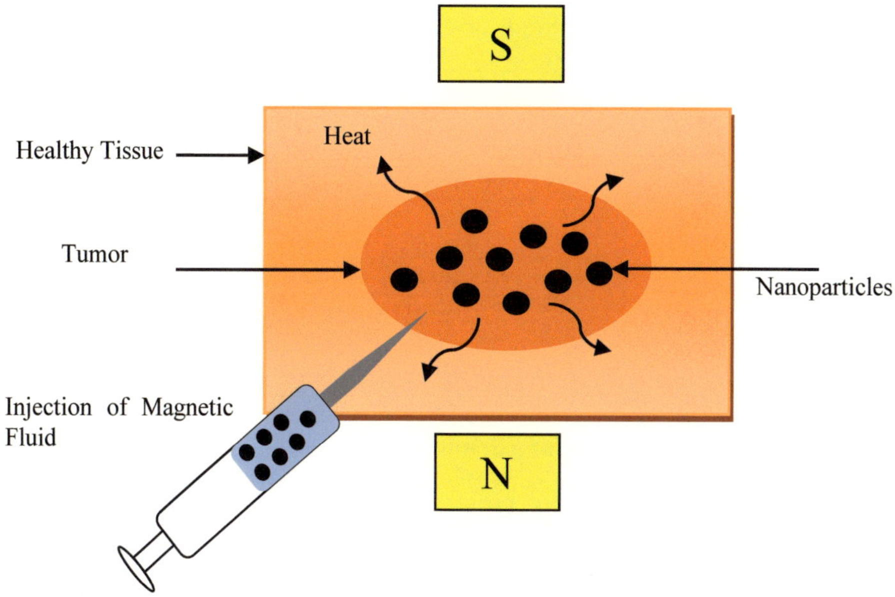

Figure 1. Schematic of magnetic fluid hyperthermia process.

movement of the magnetic moment in an external field that results in heat generation. In the Brownian mode, the whole particle oscillates towards the field with the moment locked along the crystal axis under the effect of a thermal force against a viscous drag in a suspending medium. This mechanism essentially represents the mechanical friction component in a given suspending medium [Nedelcu (2008)].

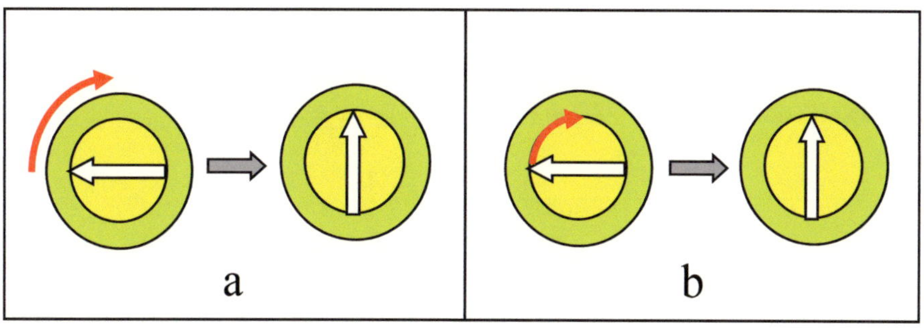

Figure 2. Relaxation mechanisms of MNPs in Magnetic Fluid. a) Brownian relaxation, entire particle rotates in fluid; b) Néel relaxation, direction of magnetization rotates in core. The structure of MNP: core (inner), shell (outer). The arrow inside the core represents the direction of magnetization.

Power dissipation of MNPs in an alternating magnetic field is expressed as [Rosensweig (2002), Nedelcu (2008)]:

$$P = \pi\mu_0 x_0 H_0^2 f \frac{2\pi f\tau}{1 + (2\pi f\tau)^2} \tag{1}$$

where μ_0 ($4\pi.10^{-7}\,T.m/A$) is the permeability of free space, x_0 is the equilibrium susceptibility, H_0 and f are the amplitude and frequency of the alternating magnetic field and τ is the effective relaxation time, given by:

$$\tau^{-1} = \tau_N^{-1} + \tau_B^{-1} \tag{2}$$

where τ_N and τ_B are the Néel relaxation and the Brownian relaxation time, respectively. τ_N and τ_B are written as:

$$\tau_N = \frac{\sqrt{\pi}}{2}\tau_0\frac{exp(\Gamma)}{\sqrt{\Gamma}} \tag{3}$$

$$\tau_B = \frac{3\eta V_H}{kT} \tag{4}$$

where the shorter time constant tends to dominate in determining the effective relaxation time for any given size of particle. τ_0 is the average relaxation time in response to a thermal fluctuation, η is the viscosity of medium, V_H is the hydrodynamic volume of MNPs, k is the Boltzmann constant, 1.38×10^{-23} J/K, and T is the temperature. Here, $\Gamma = KV_M/\,kT$ where K is the magnetocrystalline anisotropy constant and V_M is the volume of MNPs. The MNPs volume V_M and the hydrodynamic volume including the ligand layer V_H are written as:

$$V_M = \frac{\pi D^3}{6} \tag{5}$$

$$V_H = \frac{\pi(D+2\delta)^3}{6} \tag{6}$$

where D is the diameter of MNP and δ is the ligand layer thickness.

The equilibrium susceptibility x_0 is assumed to be the chord susceptibility corresponding to the Langevin equation ($L(\xi) = M/M_s = \coth\xi - 1/\xi$), and expressed as:

$$x_0 = x_i\frac{3}{\xi}\left(\coth\xi - \frac{1}{\xi}\right) \tag{7}$$

where $\xi = \mu_0 M_d H V_M/kT$, $H = H_0 cos(\omega t)$, $M_s = \phi M_d$, and ϕ is the volume fraction of MNPs. Here, M_d and M_s are the domain and saturation magnetization, respectively. The initial susceptibility is given by:

$$x_i = \frac{\mu_0 \phi M_d^2 V_M}{3kT} \tag{8}$$

Generally, the practical range of frequency and amplitudes are often described as $50 - 1200\ kHz$ and $0\text{–}15\ kA/m$ and the typical magnetite dosage is $\sim 10\ mg$ magnetite MNPs per gram of tumor as reported in clinical studies [Jordan *et al.* (1997), Jordan *et al.* (2001), Pankhurst *et al.* (2003), Lahonian and Golneshan (2011)].

2.2. Heating rate of aqueous dispersions of MNPs

Based on the theory mentioned in previous section, Lahonian and Golneshan (2011) calculated the power dissipations for aqueous dispersion of mono-dispersed equiatomic face centred cubic iron-platinum (FCC FePt) MNPs varying the diameter of MNP in adiabatic condition. For comparison, also the power dissipations for magnetite (Fe_3O_4), and maghemite (γ-Fe_2O_3) have been estimated. In Table 1, physical properties of each magnetic material are shown [Maenosono and Saita (2006)].

In practice, the magnetic anisotropy may considerably vary due to the shape contributions of MNPs. For simplicity, however, the shape effect is not taken into account in the above mentioned model.

It has been pointed out that hysteresis losses are important especially for magnetic single domain particles with high magneto-crystalline anisotropy [Hergt *et al.* (1998)]. However, the hysteresis losses are not considered, because MNPs are assumed as super-paramagnetic in their study.

Figure 3 shows comparative power dissipation for aqueous mono-dispersions of the various MNPs listed in Table 1, assuming $\tau_0 = 10^{-9}\,s$ and $\phi = 2 \times 10^{-5}$. Induction and frequency of applied magnetic field were fixed at $B_0 = \mu_0 H_0 = 50\,mT$ and $300\,kHz$. The carrier liquid is pure water in all cases. Surface ligand layer thickness is assumed to be $\delta = 1\,nm$. On these conditions, FCC FePt MNPs yield the largest power dissipation. Most operative sizes of each MNPs, D_{max}, which give a maximum heating rate, are $10.5\,nm$ for FCC FePt MNPs, $19\,nm$ for magnetite and $23\,nm$ for maghemite. The maghemite MNPs also have large power dissipation as well as magnetite MNPs. The typical size ranges of standard magnetic nanofluid are $D = 8 - 10\,nm$, and generally the stability of magnetic colloid becomes impaired when $D > 20\,nm$ due to the spontaneous magnetization [Golneshan and Lahonian (2010), Lahonian and Golneshan (2011), Golneshan and Lahonian (2011b).

Figure 4 shows the dependence of power dissipation on induction of applied magnetic field, for fixed $f = 300\,kHz$. Note that B_0 is varied as 30, 50, and $80\,mT$. Increasing B_0 earns a raise for power dissipation [Lahonian and Golneshan (2011)].

Figures 5, 6 and 7 show the dependence of power dissipation on the frequency (f), the surface ligand layer thickness (δ), and the volume fraction (ϕ) respectively. Increasing f earns a raise and a gradual decrease, respectively, in the power dissipation and D_{max}. The power dissipation decreases and increases with increasing δ and ϕ, respectivly. Also, the gradual decrease in D_{max} with decreasing δ is observed [Lahonian and Golneshan (2011)].

Material	M_d kA/m	K kJ/m^3	c_p $J/(kg.K)$	ρ kg/m^3
FCC FePt	1140	206	327	15200
Magnetite	446	9	670	5180
Maghemite	414	4.7	746	4600

Table 1. Physical properties of various MNPs [Maenosono and Saita (2006)]

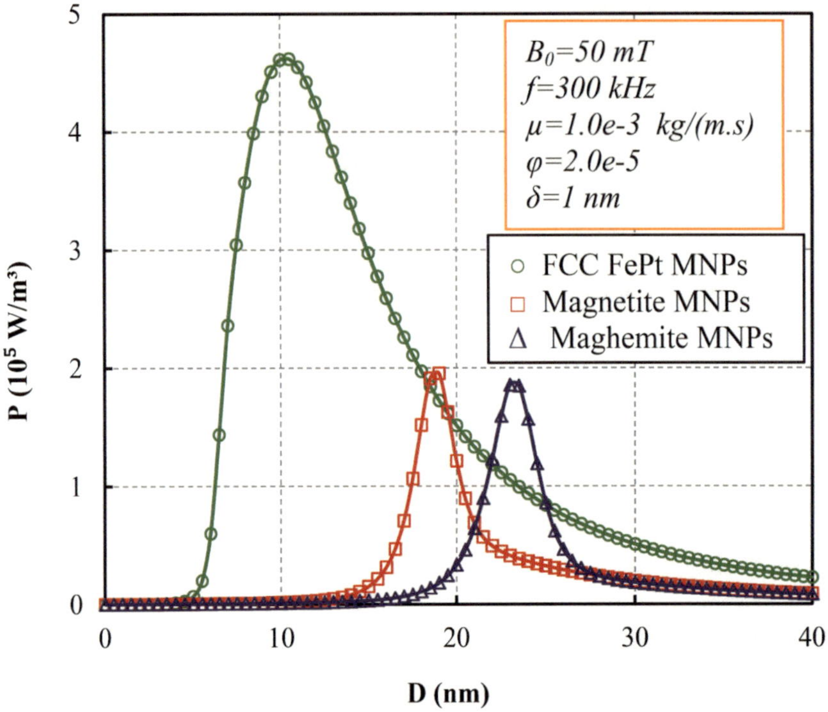

Figure 3. Power dissipations as a function of particle diameter for various MNPs [Lahonian and Golneshan (2011)].

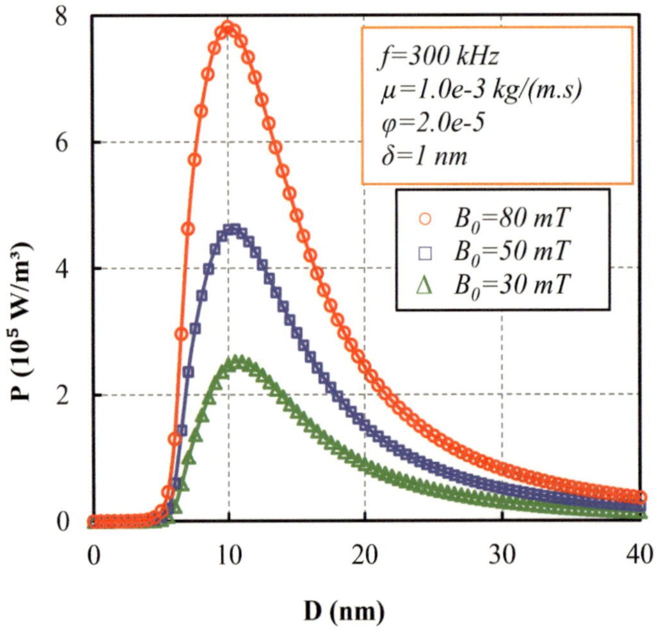

Figure 4. Dependence of power dissipation on B_0 [Lahonian and Golneshan (2011)].

Figures 4 to 7 show that dispersion and concentration of MNPs inside the tissue are important factors in heat dissipation of MNPs and temperature distribution inside the tumor and its surrounding healthy tissue. Also, the effect of concentration of MNPs is comparable with the effects of induction and frequency of the magnetic field on the maximum power dissipation. Therefore, study of the MNPs diffusion and concentration, possesses a high degree of importance.

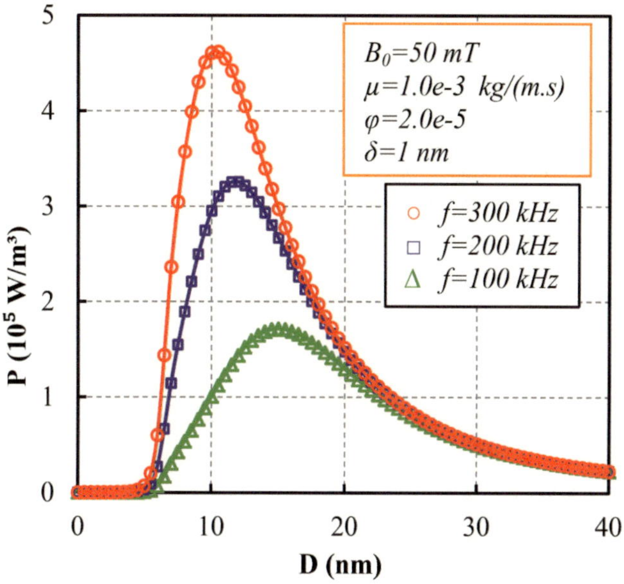

Figure 5. Dependence of power dissipation on f [Lahonian and Golneshan (2011)].

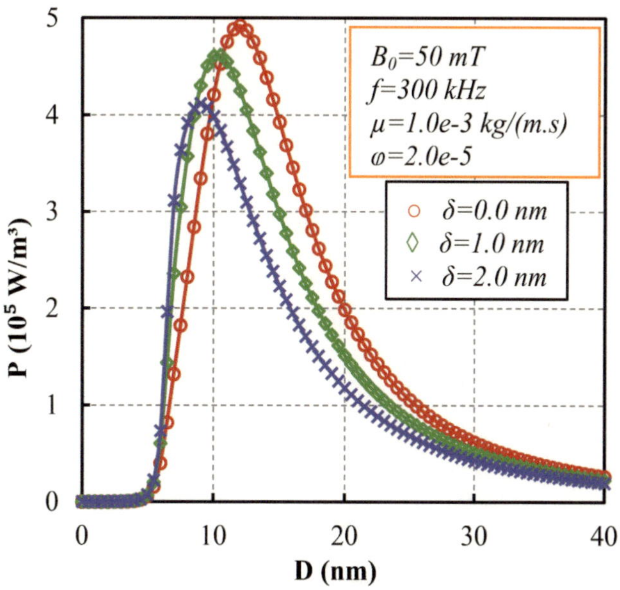

Figure 6. Dependence of power dissipation on δ [Lahonian and Golneshan (2011)].

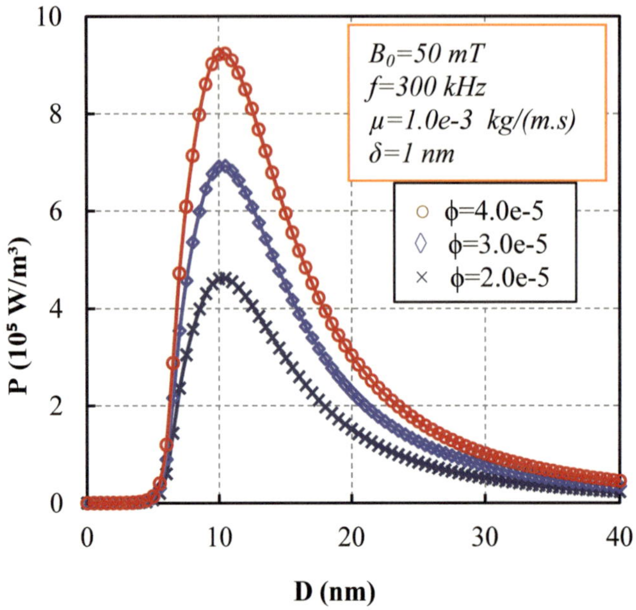

Figure 7. Dependence of power dissipation on ϕ [Lahonian and Golneshan (2011)].

3. Diffusion of MNPs within the biological tissue

The relationship among the MNPs distribution, the blood perfusion, the infusion flow rate, the injection volume of nanofluid, and the tissue structure are not well understood. It is difficult to devise a treatment protocol that enables the optimum distribution of temperature elevation in the tumor. Hence, it is important to quantify the MNPs distribution and heating pattern following the injection regarding the above mentioned factors [Salloum *et al.* (2008b)].

Diffusion in isotropic tissues, can be modeled as [Nicholson (2001)]:

$$\frac{\partial C}{\partial t} = \mathrm{D}^{*}\nabla^{2}C + S/\varepsilon \tag{9}$$

where C, D^{*}, S, ε and t are the volume average concentration of the species, effective diffusivity, mass source density, porosity of the tissue and time, respectively. The effective diffusivity, however, is related to the tortuosity of the tissue, λ, and the diffusivity in the absence of the porous medium, D through the following relation:

$$D^{*} = D/\lambda^{2} \tag{10}$$

Therefore an increase in the tortuosity and a decrease in the porosity have significant effects on reducing the effective mass diffusivity.

Experimental study of Salloum *et al.* (2008a) in a tissue-equivalent agarose gel, showed that the particle concentration was not uniform after the injection and were confined in the vicinity of the injection site. Also the particle deposition was greatly affected by the injection rate and amount. Furthermore, the shape of the distribution tended to be more irregular with higher infusion flow rate.

Due to difficulties in experimental studies, to understand the actual spatial distribution of the MNPs after being injected into the tumor, some numerical simulations have been down.

Diffusion of MNPs inside the tissue was simulated by Golneshan and Lahonian (2011a). A square region with side of 2 cm was chosen as the domain of the analysis (Figure 8). Water-based ferrofluid with a concentration of 3.3% by volume and a particle size of 10 nm magnetite MNPs was used in their work. Based on the density of magnetite (5240 kg/m^3) and the given ferrofluid concentration, each 0.1 cc of ferrofluid contains 17.3mg of solid iron oxide [Golneshan and Lahonian (2010)]. The ferrofluid infusion flow rates were chosen equal to $\dot{V} = 10, 20$ and 30 $\mu l/min$ and ferrofluid injection volumes were chosen equal to $V = 0.1, 0.2$ and 0.3 cc. Porosity and effective diffusivity were chosen to be equal to $\varepsilon = 0.1$ and $D^* = 2.5 \times 10^{-10}\ m^2/s$ respectively [Nicholson (2001), Golneshan and Lahonian (2010)].

Figure 9 shows the concentration of ferrofluid in the tissue for $V = 0.2\ cc$ and $\dot{V} = 20\ \mu l/min$, for different time intervals after the end of ferrofluid injection. Results show that the concentration of ferrofluid is maximum at the injection site, and decreases rapidly with increasing distance from it. Also, concentration of ferrofluid decreases at the injection area with time and increases in the surrounding of injection site [Golneshan and Lahonian (2011a)].

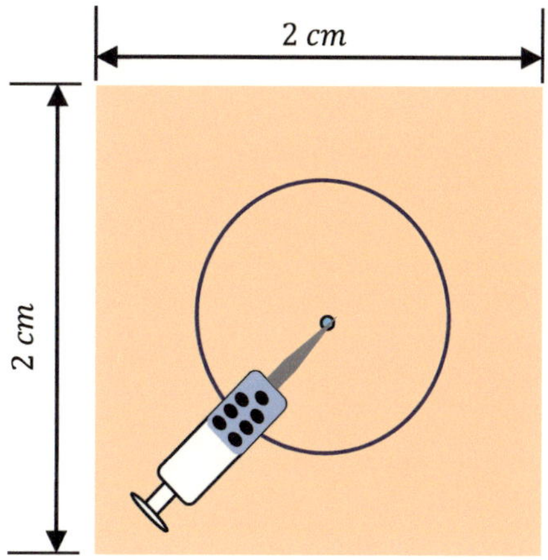

Figure 8. Simulation domain of tissue and injection site.

Figure 10 shows volume fraction of MNPs in the tissue for different ferrofluid injection volumes, $\dot{V} = 20\ \mu l/min$, at 20 minutes after the end of ferrofluid injection [Golneshan and Lahonian (2011a)].

Figure 11 shows the concentration of ferrofluid in the tissue for $V = 0.2\ cc$, and different infusion flow rates, just 20 minutes after the end of ferrofluid injection. Results show that the increasing infusion flow rate, increases concentration of ferrofluid in the vicinity of the injection site while decreasing the concentration in the layers far from the injection site [Golneshan and Lahonian (2011a)].

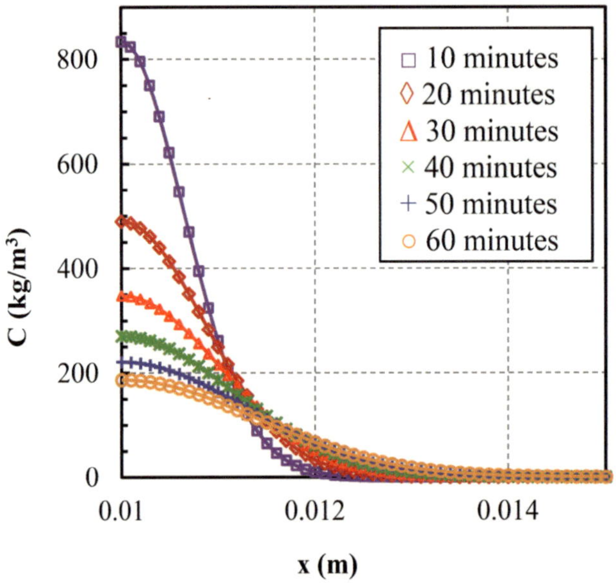

Figure 9. Concentration of ferrofluid in the tissue, for different time intervals after the end of ferrofluid injection ($V = 0.2\ cc$ and $\dot{V} = 20\ \mu l/min$) [Golneshan and Lahonian (2011a)].

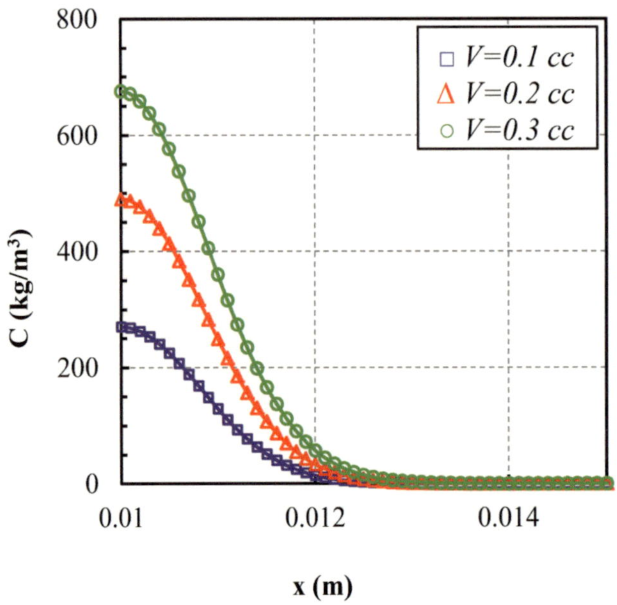

Figure 10. Ferrofluid concentration for $\dot{V} = 20\ \mu l/min$, and different ferrofluid injection volumes, just 20 minutes after the end of ferrofluid injection [Golneshan and Lahonian (2011a)].

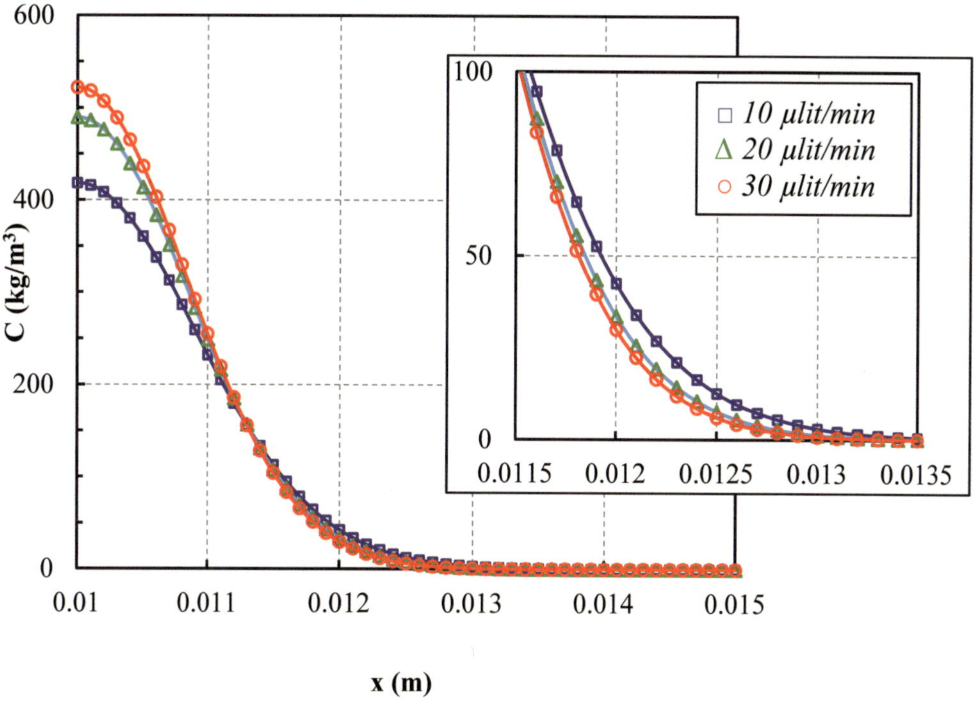

Figure 11. Concentration of ferrofluid in the tissue for $V = 0.2\ cc$, and different infusion flow rates, just 20 minutes after the end of ferrofluid injection [Golneshan and Lahonian (2011a)].

Figure 12 shows the concentration of ferrofluid in the tissue for $V = 0.2\ cc$, and different infusion flow rates, just 20 minutes after the end of ferrofluid injection. Results show that the increasing infusion flow rate, increases concentration of ferrofluid in the vicinity of the injection site but decreases the concentration in the layers far from the injection site [Golneshan and Lahonian (2010), Golneshan and Lahonian (2011a)].

4. Diffusion of MNPs in a biological tissue for mono and multi-site injection for irregular tumors

Golneshan and Lahonian (2011a) studied diffusion of MNPs in a biological tissue for irregular tumors. A $2 \times 2\ cm$ tissue with an irregular tumor inside, was chosen as the domain of the analysis (Figures 13a).

They considered multi-site injection as shown in Figure 13d and divided the irregular tumor almost into four equal sections. In each injection site, one fourth the amount of $0.2\ cc$ ferrofluid was injected. Figure 14 shows the concentration of ferrofluid for infusion flow rate of $\dot{V} = 20\ \mu l/min$, at the end of ferrofluid injection [Golneshan and Lahonian (2011a)].

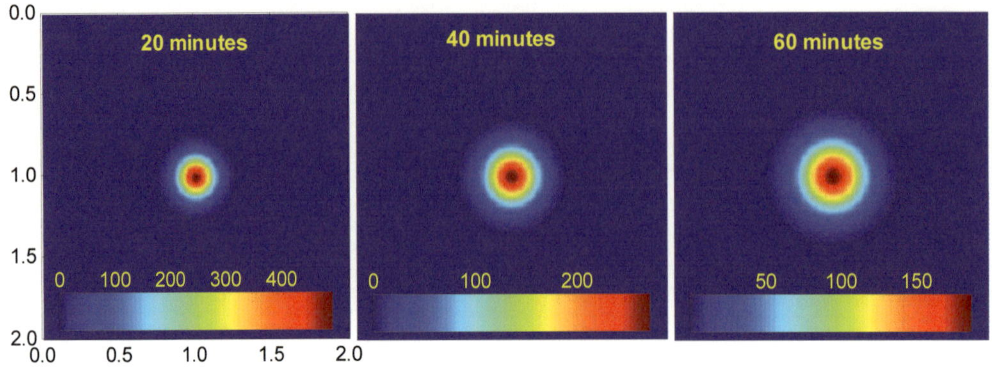

Figure 12. Concentration of ferrofluid in kg/m^3 in the tissue for $V = 0.2\ cc$, $\dot{V} = 20\ \mu l/min$, at 20, 40 and 60 minutes after the end of ferrofluid injection [Golneshan and Lahonian (2011a)].

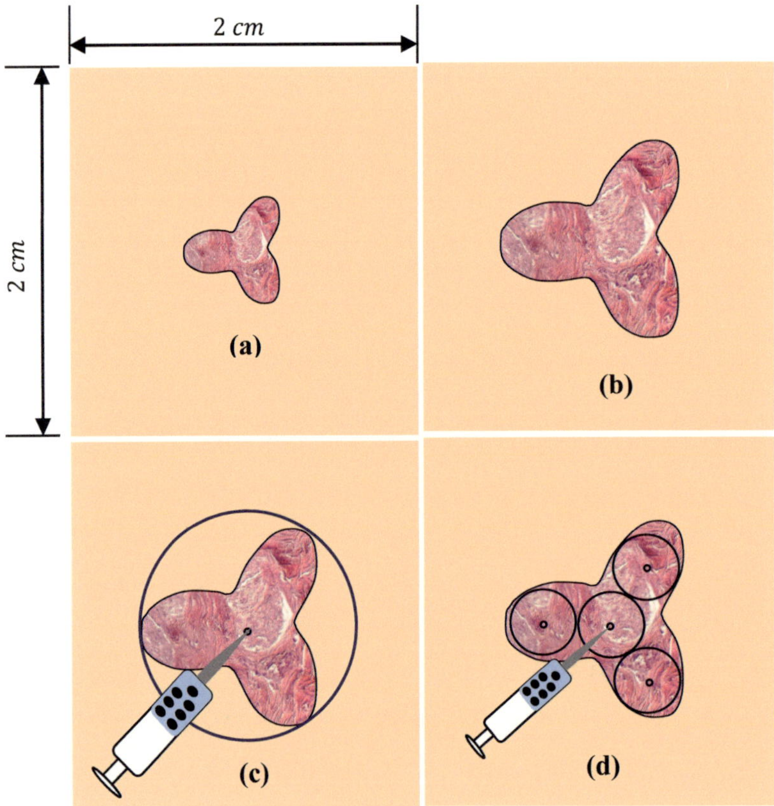

Figure 13. a: The tissue and an irregular tumor, b: Zoomed irregular tumor c: Mono-site injection, d: Multi-site injection [Golneshan and Lahonian (2011a)].

Figure 15 shows the concentration of ferrofluid in kg/m^3 in the tissue for mono and multi-site injection of $V = 0.2\ cc$ ferrofluid injection volume and infusion flow rate of $\dot{V} = 20\ \mu l/min$, at 10, 20, and 30 minutes after the end of ferrofluid injection. Ten minutes after

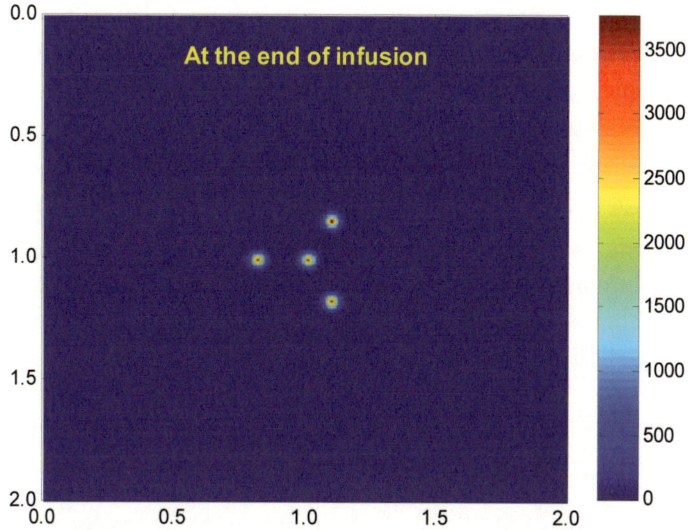

Figure 14. Concentration of ferrofluid in kg/m^3 for multi-site injection, at the end of injection process [Golneshan and Lahonian (2011a)].

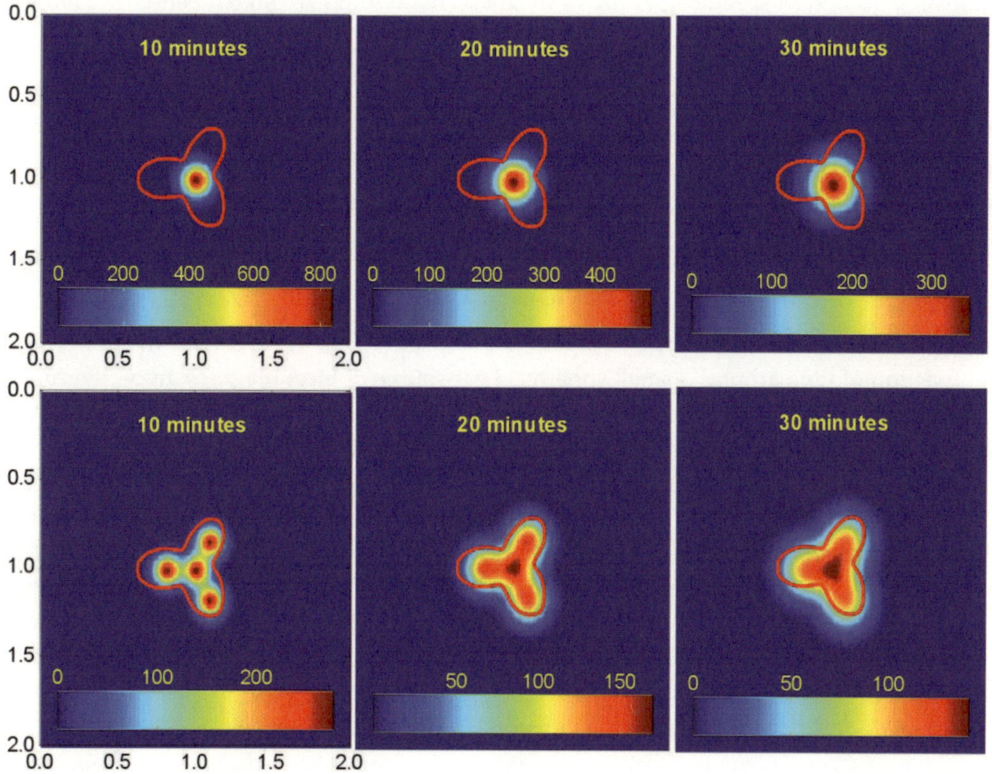

Figure 15. Concentration of ferrofluid in kg/m^3 in the tissue for $V = 0.2\ cc$, $\dot{V} = 20\ \mu l/min$, at 10, 20 and 30 minutes after the end of ferrofluid injection. Up row: Mono-site injection, Down row: Multi-site injection [Golneshan and Lahonian (2011a)].

the injection, the maximum concentration of ferrofluid happens at the injection sites, decreasing rapidly with increasing the distance from the injection sites. At this stage, nearly clear boundaries are seen between diffused ferrofluid for each injection regions. As ferrofluid diffuses more and more, these boundaries are disappeared. Thirty minutes after the injection, the ferrofluid is spread all over the tomour [Golneshan and Lahonian (2011a)].

Comparison between mono-site and multi-site injections in Figures 15 show that diffusion of ferrofluid in the tissue for a multi-site injection is much more uniform and covers all points inside the tumor 30 minutes after the end of injection process. Furthermore, no substantial concentration gradient is seen between the center and the boundary of the tumor at this time for the multi-site injection case [Golneshan and Lahonian (2011a)].

5. Conclusion

Results showed and clarified that increasing the magnetic nanofluid injection volume, increases the concentration of MNPs inside the tissue. Also, increasing magnetic nanofluid infusion flow rate increased the concentration of MNPs in the center of the tumor only. For irregular tumors, the effect of multi-site injection was investigated. Results showed that multi-site injection of specific quantity of magnetic nanofluid provided a better distribution of MNPs inside the tumor, in contrast to mono-site injection.

Author details

Mansour Lahonian
Mechanical Engineering Department, Engineering School, Kurdistan University, Sanandaj, Iran

6. References

Andrä W, C G D'Ambly, R Hergt, I Hilger, W A Kaiser (1999). Temperature distribution as function of time around a small spherical heat source of local magnetic hyperthermia. *J Magn Magn Mater* 194:197–203.

Bagaria H G, and D T Johnson (2005). Transient solution to the BHE and optimization for magnetic fluid hyperthermia treatment *Int J Hyperther* 21(1): 57–75.

Bellizzi G, O M Bucci (2010). On the optimal choice of the exposure conditions and the nanoparticle features in magnetic nanoparticle hyperthermia *Int J Hyperther* 26:389-403.

Brusentsova T N, N A Brusentsov, V D Kuznetsov, V N Nikiforov (2005). Synthesis and investigation of magnetic properties of Gd-substituted Mn–Zn ferrite nanoparticles as a potential low-TC agent for magnetic fluid hyperthermia *J Magn Magn Mater* 293: 298-302.

Golneshan A A, M Lahonian (2010). Diffusion of magnetic nanoparticles within spherical tissue as a porous media during magnetic fluid hyperthermia using lattice Boltzmann method *International Congress on Nanoscience and Nanotechnology* 9-11 November, shiraz iran.

Golneshan A A, M Lahonian (2011a). Diffusion of magnetic nanoparticles in a multi-site injection process within a biological tissue during magnetic fluid hyperthermia using lattice Boltzmann method *Mech Res Commun* 38: 425– 430.

Golneshan A A, M Lahonian (2011b). Effect of heated region on temperature distribution within tissue during magnetic fluid hyperthermia using lattice Boltzmann method *Journal of Mechanics in Medicine and Biology* 11(2):457–469.

Golneshan A A, M Lahonian (2011c). The effect of magnetic nanoparticle dispersion on temperature distribution in a spherical tissue in magnetic fluid hyperthermia using the lattice Boltzmann method *Int J Hypertherm* 27(3):266–274.

Hergt R, W Andrä, C G d'Ambly, I Hilger, W A Kaiser, U Richter, H-G Schmidt (1998). Physical limits of hyperthermia using magnetite fine particles *IEEE T Magn* 5: 3745–3754.

Jo´zefczak A, A Skumiel (2007). Study of heating effect and acoustic properties of dextran stabilized magnetic fluid *J Magn Magn Mater* 311: 193–196.

Jordan A, R Scholz, K Maier-Hauff, M Johannsen, P Wust, J Nadobny, H Schirra, H Schmidt, S Deger, S Loening, W Lanksch, R Felix (2001). Presentation of a new magnetic field therapy system for the treatment of human solid tumors with magnetic fluid hyperthermia *J Mag Mag Mater* 225: 118-126.

Jordan A, R Scholz, P Wust, H Fähling, J Krause, W Wlodarczyk,B Sander, T Vogl, R Felix (1997). Effect of magnetic fluid hyperthermia on C3H mammary carcinoma in vivo *Int J Hypertherm* 13:587–605.

Jordan A, R Scholz, P Wust, H Schirra, T Schiestel, H Schmidt, R Felix (1999). Endocytosis of dextran and silan-coated magnetite nanoparticles and the effect of intracellular hyperthermia on human mammary carcinoma cells in vitro *J Magn Magn Mater* 194: 185–196.

Kim D H, D E Nikles, D T Johnson, C S Brazel (2008). Heat generation of aqueously dispersed CoFe2O4 nanoparticles as heating agents for magnetically activated drug delivery and hyperthermia *J Magn Magn Mater* 320: 2390– 2396.

Lagendijk J J W (2000). Hyperthermia treatment planning *Phys Med Biol* 45:R61–R76.

Lahonian M. A A Golneshan (2011). Numerical study of temperature distribution in a spherical tissue in magnetic fluid hyperthermia using lattice Boltzmann method *IEEE Trans Nanobio* 10(4): 262-268.

Lin Ch T, Liu K Ch (2009). Estimation for the heating effect of magnetic nanoparticles in perfused tissues *Int Commun Heat Mass* 36: 241–244.

Maenosono S, S Saita (2006). Theoretical assessment of FePt nanoparticles as heating elements for magnetic hyperthermia *IEEE T Magn* 42: 1638–1642.

Matsuki H, T Yanada (1994). Temperature sensitive amorphous magnetic flakes for intra-tissue hyperthermia *Mat Sci Eng A-Struct* 181/A182: 1366–1368.

Moroz P, S K Jones, B N Gray (2002). Magnetically mediated hyperthermia: Current status and future directions *Int J Hyperther* 18: 267–284.

Nedelcu G (2008). Magnetic nanoparticles impact on tumoural cells in the treatment by magnetic fluid hyperthermia *Digest J Nanomat Biost* 3(3): 103–107.

Nicholson C (2001). Diffusion and related transport mechanism in brain tissue *Rep Prog Phys* 64: 815–884.

Overgaard J, D Gonzalez, M C C H Hulshof, G Arcangeli, O Dahl, O Mella, S M Bentzen (2009). Hyperthermia as an adjuvant to radiation therapy of recurrent or metastatic malignant melanoma. A multicentre randomized trial by the European Society for Hyperthermic Oncology *Int J Hyperther* 25: 323-334.

Pankhurst QA, J Connolly, S K Jones, J Dobson (2003). Application of magnetic nanoparticles in biomedicine *J Phys D Appl Phys* 36:R167–R187.

Perez C A, S A Sapareto (1984). Thermal dose expression in clinical hyperthermia and correlation with tumor response/controll *Cancer Res* 44: 4818-4825.

Rosensweig R E (2002). Heating magnetic fluid with alternating magnetic field *J Magn Magn Mater* 252: 370-374.

Salloum M, R H Ma, D Weeks, L Zhu (2008a). Controlling nanoparticle delivery in magnetic nanoparticle hyperthermia for cancer treatment: Experimental study in agarose gel *Int J Hyperther* 24: 337–345.

Salloum M, R H Ma, L Zhu (2008b). An in-vivo experimental study of temperature elevations in animal tissue during magnetic nanoparticle hyperthermia *Int J Hyperther* 24: 589-601.

Thiesen B, A Jordan (2008). Clinical applications of magnetic nanoparticles for hyperthermia *Int J Hyperther* 24: 467-474.

Chapter 5

Hyperthermia Tissue Ablation in Radiology

Ragab Hani Donkol and Ahmed Al Nammi

Additional information is available at the end of the chapter

http://dx.doi.org/10.5772/52274

1. Introduction

Hyperthermia is part of thermal medicine, in which increasing body or tissue temperature used for the treatment of diseases. It can be traced back to the earliest practice of medicine. Cultures from around the world can point to ancient uses of hot therapy for specific medical applications. As mentioned in the foregoing books, cauterization is the first application of hyperthermia in medicine. Cauterization can be done by heat, or by chemicals such as caustics. Al-Zahrawi - an ancient Arabic scientist- generally preferred the former for the use of cauterization in treatment of diseases (1). Depending on the nature of the disease, the patient's temperament and the weather condition, different kinds of metals such as bronze, iron and gold could be used. The important considerations in the procedure include the shape of the cautery, the site of cauterization and the number of exposures. Many of the cauteries were taken from the Greeks, but Al-Zahrawi takes an independent line while describing cauterization for hare-lip, entropion, pulmonary disease, pre-anal fistula, dislocation of femur, back pain, headache, ptosis, perianal fistulae, humeral dislocation, sciatica and face swellings (fig 1).

Modern research in thermal medicine aims to understand molecular, cellular and physiological effects of temperature manipulation and the "stress" response, as well as to develop effective and safe equipment for clinical application and temperature monitoring. As a result, today there are a growing number of clinical applications of thermal therapy that benefit patients with a variety of diseases. Remarkable progress in engineering, radiology and physics over the past decades has led to the implementation of clinical trials that are revealing the true potential of hyperthermia for the treatment of different disease. Hyperthermia ablation (e.g. by radiofrequency electric current, microwaves, laser, or ultrasound), whereby localized heating destroys tissue is now used worldwide for tumors treatment and many other important medical applications. In most circumstances thermal ablation is used under guidance of different radiological modalities such as ultrasound (US), computed tomography (CT) or magnetic resonance imaging (MRI). Thermal ablation is a

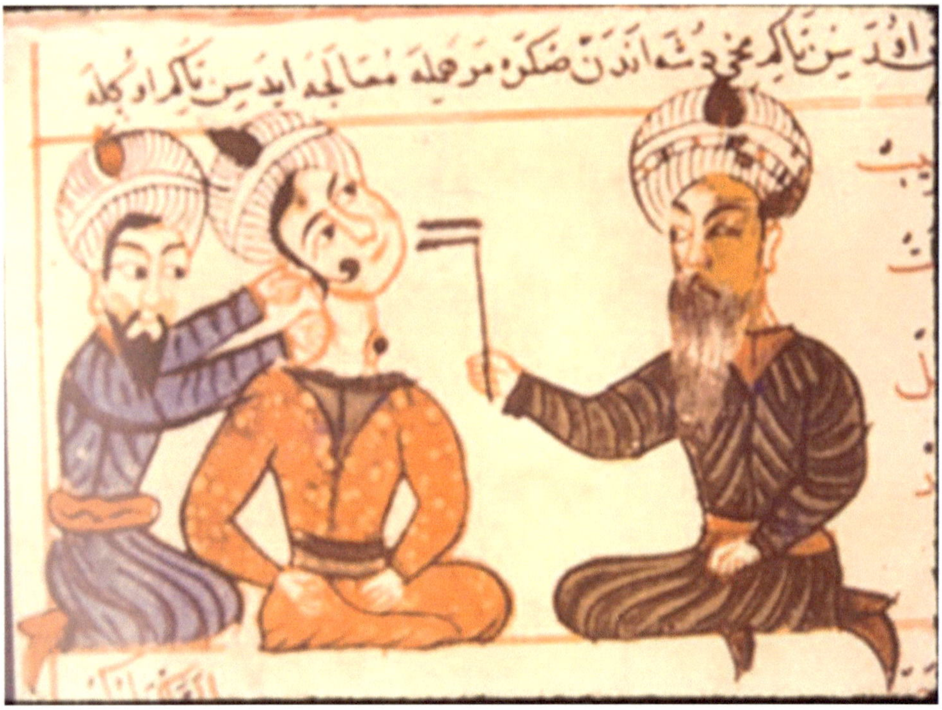

Figure 1. Technique of Cauterization by fire for a patient with neck swelling (1)

minimally invasive procedure that significantly reduces risks and speeds recovery. So, it provides an excellent safe alternative to major surgery. The primary advantage of percutaneous radiofrequency thermal ablation is a reduction in the need for post-operative hospitalization and a reduced duration of convalescence. In this chapter, we will review the recent application of hyperthermia medicine in treatment of different disease under the guidance of different radiological modalities. In this chapter, we will provide a clearer picture of the intimate relation between hyperthermia, radiology and medical imaging. We will discuss the multiple facets of tumor growth and the tumor microenvironment that can be impacted by heat during hyperthermia medicine. We will emphasize the approved clinical application of hyperthermia in management of growing number of patients with a variety of diseases. We also discuss other experimental and investigational trial studies that can be used effectively in the future for management of other clinical conditions. Also we will emphasize the adjuvant role of thermal therapy in combination with radiotherapy and chemotherapy in management of cancer. Finally, we will elaborate the exciting new generation of clinical trials of heat-activated drug delivery.

2. Various energy sources of hyperthermia

Various energy sources including laser, ultrasound, microwaves, and radiofrequency electric current are being investigated as minimally invasive, and potentially non-invasive therapies. There are two types of thermal ablation: radiofrequency (RFA) and microwave.

Both are minimally invasive techniques that treat lesions by applying intense heat through a small probe inserted directly into the tumor. Hyperthermia can be either superficial, produced by a microwave generator, or regional, produced by a radiofrequency applicator with multiple antennas, which emanate a deep focalized heating, saving the skin, or interstitial heating. In all these systems the radiations are non-ionizing, in which the energy presents a heterogeneous distribution inside the tissues, depending on their thermal characteristics and on blood perfusion. Radiofrequency ablation (RFA) involves percutaneous or intra-operative insertion of an electrode into a lesion under ultrasonic or CT guidance. Radiofrequency energy is emitted through the electrode and generates heat, leading to coagulative necrosis of the tissue.

3. Rational of tissue necrosis (ablation) in hyperthermia medicine

Modern research in thermal medicine aims to understand molecular, cellular and physiological effects of temperature manipulation and the "stress" response, as well as to develop effective and safe equipment for clinical application and temperature monitoring. Multiple facets of tumor growth and the tumor microenvironment, including vascular perfusion, heat shock protein expression, endothelial/stromal cells, hypoxia, immune cells, pro-inflammatory cytokines, are impacted by heat and these effects may underlie remarkable successes being obtained in a surge of clinical trials throughout the world. Thermal ablation whereby tissue is destroyed by localized heating or freezing, is now used worldwide for treatment of many benign and malignant tumors and several other important medical applications (2-4).

The main actions of hyperthermia in the neoplastic tissues are the following:

- Greater heat sensitivity of neoplastic tissues to hyperthermia, due to its chronic ischemia, hypoxia and acid pH;
- Lethal effect of temperature of 42-43 °C on tumor cells, depending on the application time;
- Temporary growth stabilization of tumor cells after a moderate hyperthermia (39-41 °C);
- Prolonged action of temperature, due to lower thermal dissipation, caused by a chronic ischemia inside the tumor, as a result of its reduced vessel regulation mechanisms;
- Alterations in the neoplastic cell cycle, which lead to the blocking of mitosis, due to a disruption in the S phase;
- Marked action on the core of the tumor, less sensitive to radiation because of ischemia, hypoxia and low pH;
- action in favor of apoptosis mechanisms.

4. Common clinical application of hyperthermia therapy:

Today there are a growing number of clinical applications of thermal therapy that benefit patients with a variety of diseases. Several studies have been published reporting efficacy of RFA in treatment of many different clinical conditions.

Several studies have been published reporting successful use of radiofrequency ablation in the following conditions: as an alternative to surgical resection for debulking of primary and metastatic malignant neoplasms, removal of primary or metastatic malignant neoplasms, treatment of distant metastases of medullary thyroid carcinoma, treatment of metastatic gastrointestinal stromal tumors (GIST) with limited progression, treatment of osteoid osteoma, as a less invasive alternative to surgical resection of the tumor ,treatment of soft tissue sarcoma of the trunk or extremities in symptomatic persons with disseminated metastases and many other condition.

There is growing research and experimental and investigational studies interest in the use of hyperthermia for treatment of many other clinical conditions. But these studies need to improve its clinical outcomes to be implemented in the practical life. Examples of these studies include; curative treatment of primary or metastatic malignant neoplasms (e.g., breast cancer, kidney cancer including renal angiomyolipoma, lung cancer, and pancreatic cancer) in persons who are able to tolerate surgical resection, treatment of malignant bile duct obstruction due to insufficient evidence in the peer-reviewed literature. Treatment of Barrett's esophagus, treatment of hepatic tumors, treatment of benign prostatic hypertrophy (transurethral needle ablation or TUNA) ,cardiac catheter thermal ablation is now standard of care for a variety of cardiac arrhythmia types (irregular heart beat rhythm) ,endometrial ablation is clinically used to treat endometrial bleeding ,intravascular heating can eliminate varicose veins with laser or radiofrequency current, laser and other thermal methods treat excessive subcutaneous fat, which can contribute to obesity and metabolic disorders including diabetes. Hyperthermia can also be used to activate cytotoxic effects of chemotherapy within tumors, thereby sparing normal tissue, when the drugs are encapsulated in thermally sensitive nanoparticles. As a result of these and other clinical applications, combined with a rapidly expanding research base, interest in thermal medicine is rapidly growing, attracting the attention of laboratory and clinical researchers, physicians, engineers, physicists and biotechnologists

4.1. Radiofrequency ablation of osteoid osteoma

Osteoid osteoma, a benign tumor of the bone. It is the third most common primary benign bone tumor, representing approximately 10–12% of benign bone tumors . It generally affects children and young adults. Approximately 80% of patients are between 5 and 24 years of age, with a male: female ratio of 3:1. Clinically, pain is the most common presenting symptom and is described as severe, sharp, boring, and typically worse at night, and improves with nonsteroidal anti-inflammatory drugs [5]. The growth potential of these benign lesions is limited, with a maximum diameter rarely exceeding 15 mm. However, the inflammatory response leads to the characteristic severe pain. The consequences of these lesions include growth deformities when tumors are located in the long bones and scoliosis when the posterior elements of the spine are involved [6]. Patients who cannot tolerate the symptoms or nonsteroidal anti-inflammatory drugs require intervention for pain relief and/or to prevent growth disturbance. Traditionally, surgical resection was the treatment of choice. During open surgery the nidus of the tumor is often difficult to visualize and to prevent recurrence a wide resection margin may be required. This results in many complications such as hematoma, infection, and fracture. In addition, surgical treatment may require a long period of hospitalization, a period during which the patient cannot bear weight on the affected limb resulting in delayed resumption of physical activity [7]. The optimal method of treatment for osteoid osteoma would involve minimization of bone removal with avoidance of grafting and fixation while ensuring complete destruction of the tumor nidus in a single session. During the past two decades, many attempts have been made to minimize bone removal to decrease the risk of postoperative complications. Percutaneous resection utilizing CT guidance to guide trephines and drills has been described. However, the complication rates are as high as 24% and include fractures, muscular haematomas, paraesthesia, skin burns, transient paresis, and osteomyelitis [8]. Radiofrequency ablation has proved to be an effective method for the treatment of many malignant and benign tumors. RF ablation for the treatment of osteoid osteoma was first described in a four-patient series in 1992 [9]. Since the promising results of Rosenthal et al in the management of osteoid osteoma with RF ablation a large number of studies evaluating RF ablation of osteoid osteoma have been reported in the peer-reviewed medical literature. Most of these studies found very high technical success rates (100%) and good primary success rates with a single session of ablation ranging from 76% to 100% (fig 2 and fig 3). Today, percutaneous CT-guided RF ablation is an effective and safe minimally invasive procedure for the treatment of osteoid osteoma in all ages. It has high technical and clinical success rates (10-12)

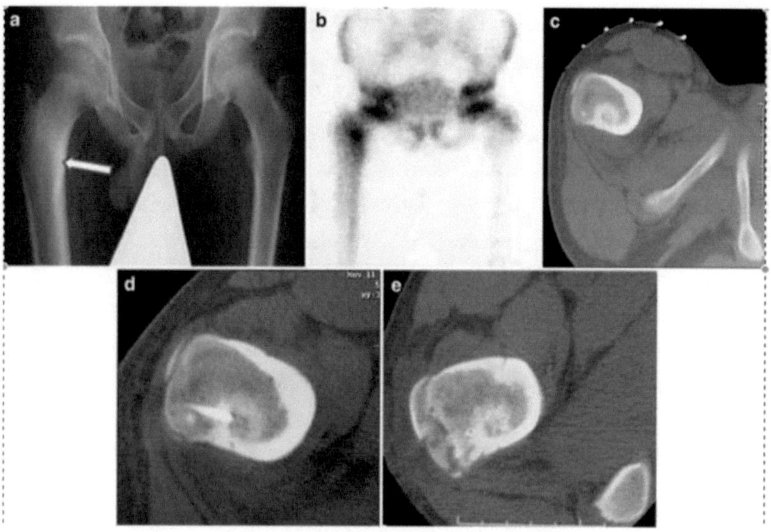

Figure 2. Technique of RFA of osteoid osteoma in a 12-year-boy with chronic right hip pain. a Radiograph of the pelvis shows an ill-defined area of dense sclerosis in the medial aspect of the proximal femoral shaft (arrow). b Bone scan shows active uptake at the site of the dense sclerosis consistent with the diagnosis of osteoid osteoma. c CT scan shows the nidus located deep to the cortex and surrounded by dense new bone. The radiopaque markers on the skin surface are for planning the skin entry point. d Axial 1-mm CT slice shows the correct position of the tip of the RF electrode within the centre of the nidus. e Follow-up CT after 15 months shows sclerosis within the nidus (12)

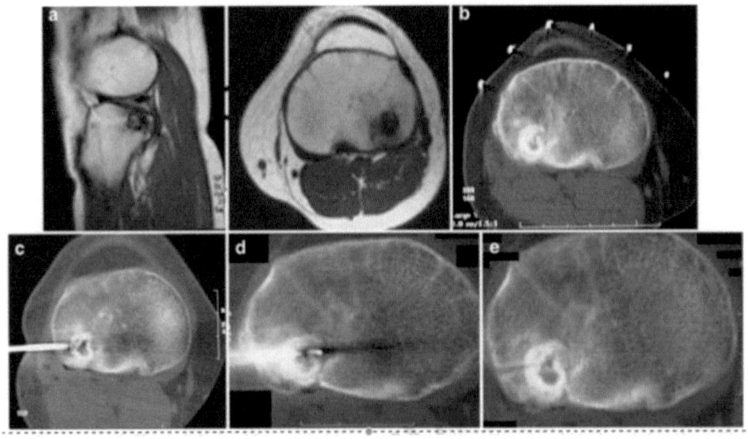

Figure 3. RFA of osteoid osteoma in a 14-year-old girl. a MR images shows a small, well-defined lesion in the proximal tibial epiphysis. b CT during percutaneous RF ablation shows a radiolucent nidus with central calcification surrounded by a dense rim of sclerosis. Note markers for planning the skin entry point. c CT shows the bone biopsy probe tip at the margin of the nidus . d CT shows the tip of the RF electrode within the nidus after slight withdrawal of the penetrating cannula. e Control image obtained immediately after the intervention shows the biopsy tract with no bleeding(12)

4.2. Radiofrequency ablation of pulmonary tumors

Radiofrequency ablation has been advocated as an alternative to resection in persons with lung nodules who cannot be treated surgically because of medical problems, multiple tumors, or poor surgical risk. There are, however, no adequate prospective clinical studies that demonstrate that RFA of lung metastases is as effective as surgical (cold knife) resection in curative resection of malignant neoplasms. An important concern is that RFA does not allow for examination of surgical margins to ensure that cancer is completely resected. Le and Petrik considered RFA as a promising technique for the treatment of early states (state I and stage II) non-small cell lung cancer (13). An assessment by the National Institute for Health and Clinical Excellence (NICE, 2006) concluded: "Current evidence on the safety and efficacy of percutaneous radiofrequency ablation for primary and secondary lung cancers shows that there are no major safety concerns with this procedure. There is evidence that the treatment can reduce tumor bulk; however, this evidence is limited and is based on heterogeneous indications for treatment. The procedure should therefore be used only with special arrangements for consent, audit and clinical governance (14). "The Food and Drug Administration (FDA) has issued a Public Health Notification as clarification for healthcare providers that no RFA devices are specifically approved for use in partial or full ablation of lung tumors (15). Radiofrequency ablation devices are minimally invasive tools used for general removal of soft tissue, such as those that contain cancer cells. It is an image-guided technique that heats and destroys cancer cells. Imaging techniques such as ultrasound and computed tomography (CT) are used to help guide a needle electrode into a cancerous tumor. High-frequency electrical currents are then passed through the electrode, creating heat that destroys the abnormal cells.

4.3. Radiofrequency ablation of pancreatic cancer

Radiofrequency ablation has been used as a treatment of pancreatic cancer for a number of years in Japan. Current evidence of effectiveness of RFA for pancreatic cancer consists of case reports and a phase II (safety) study; the latter concluded that RFA was a relatively safe treatment for pancreatic cancer. However, this evidence is insufficient to draw conclusions about the effectiveness of RFA for this indication. Girelli et al (2010) examined the feasibility and safety of RFA as a treatment option for locally advanced pancreatic cancer. A total of 50 patients with locally advanced pancreatic cancer were studied prospectively. Ultrasound-guided RFA was performed during laparotomy. The main outcome measures were short-term morbidity and mortality. The tumor was located in the pancreatic head or uncinate process in 34 patients and in the body or tail in 16; median diameter was 40 (inter-quartile range [IQR] of 30 to 50) mm. Radiofrequency ablation was the only treatment in 19 patients; it was combined with biliary and gastric bypass in 19 patients, gastric bypass alone in 8, biliary bypass alone in 3 and pancreatico-jejunostomy in 1. The 30-day mortality rate was 2 %. Abdominal complications occurred in 24 % of patients; in half they were directly associated with RFA and treated conservatively. Three patients with surgery-related complications needed re-operation. Reduction of RFA temperature from 105 degrees C to 90 degrees C resulted in a significant reduction in complications (10 versus 2 of 25 patients; $p = 0.028$). Median post-operative hospital stay was 10 (range of 7 to 31) days. The authors concluded that RFA of locally advanced pancreatic cancer is feasible and relatively well tolerated, with a 24 % complication rate. This was a feasibility and safety study; it did not provide any data on the effectiveness of RFA in treating pancreatic cancer (16).

4.4. Radiofrequency ablation of renal tumors

Several authorities have noted that RFA of renal tumors is a promising investigational alternative to partial or total nephrectomy. Studies performed have focused on the technical feasibility of RFA of renal tumors. Prospective clinical studies are needed to determine if RFA of renal cell carcinomas improve survival and are as effective as total or partial nephrectomy (17-18)

An assessment conducted by the National Institute for Clinical Excellence in 2010 reached the following conclusions about RFA of renal tumors: " A meta-analysis of 47 studies (non-randomized comparative studies and case series) including a total of 1375 tumors treated by RFA ($n = 775$) or cryoablation ($n = 600$) reported local tumor progression (defined as radiographic or pathological evidence of residual disease after initial treatment, regardless of time to recurrence) in 13% (100/775) and 5% (31/600) of tumors respectively at a mean 19-month follow-up ($p < 0.001$). The meta-analysis reported progression to metastatic disease in 2% (19/775) of tumors treated by RFA and 1% (6/600) of tumors treated by cryoablation®(p = not significant)" (19). Another assessment of the evidence for RFA of kidney cancer prepared by the Canadian Coordinating Office for Health Technology Assessment (20) reached the following conclusions: "RFA is emerging as a useful alternative to nephrectomy in the management of some types of kidney cancer. It appears to be useful for smaller, non-central tumors, and for cases where surgery is contraindicated. A disadvantage is the possibility of residual cancer that cannot be detected by diagnostic imaging during follow-up. There are no results from randomized trials, and the period of follow-up for patients who have had the procedure is short. Only with longer follow-up evaluations (five years to 10 years) will relevant comparison with radical and partial nephrectomy be possible."

Furthermore, Hinshaw and Lee stated that RFA, cryoablation, microwave ablation, and laser ablation have all shown promise for the treatment of renal cell carcinomas (RCC), with high local control and low complication rates for RFA and cryoablation. However, the clinical trial data remain early, and survival data are not yet available for a definitive comparison with conventional surgical techniques for removal of RCC (21). Mahnken noted that the increasing number of clinical reports on RFA of the kidney show the promising potential of renal RFA for minimally invasive tumor treatment. Due to its technical benefits, RFA seems to be advantageous when compared to cryoablation or laser ablation. However, there are no long-term follow-up or comparative data proving an equal effectiveness to surgery (22) .

In a systematic review on focal therapy for kidney cancer, Kutikov and colleagues stated that most cryoablations are performed using a laparoscopic approach, whereas RFA of the localized small renal masses (SRM) is more commonly administered percutaneously. Pre-treatment biopsy is performed more often for lesions treated by cryoablation than RFA with a significantly higher rate of indeterminate or unknown pathology for SRMs undergoing RFA versus cryoablation ($p < 0.0001$). Currently available data suggest that cryoablation results in lower re-treatments ($p < 0.0001$), less local tumor progressions ($p < 0.0001$) and may be associated with a decreased risk of metastatic progression compared with RFA. It is unclear if these differences are a function of the technologies or their application. The extent to which focal ablation altars the natural history of SRMs has not yet been established. The authors concluded that currently, data on the ability of interventions for SRMs to affect the natural history of these masses are lacking. They stated that prospective randomized evaluations of available clinical approaches to SRMs are needed (23). A Cochrane systematic evidence review (24) of surgical management of localized renal cell carcinoma found that the main source of evidence for the current practice of laparoscopic excision of renal cancer is drawn from case series, small retrospective studies and very few small-randomized controlled trials. "The results and conclusions of these studies must therefore be interpreted with caution." The authors of the systematic evidence review did not identify any randomized trials meeting the inclusion criteria reporting on the comparison between open radical nephrectomy with laparoscopic approach or new modalities of treatment such as RFA or cryoablation. Three randomized controlled trials compared the different laparoscopic approaches to nephrectomy (transperitoneal versus retroperitoneal) and found no statistical difference in operative or peri-operative outcomes between the two treatment groups. There were several non-randomized and retrospective case series reporting various advantages of laparoscopic renal cancer surgery such as less blood loss, early recovery and shorter hospital stay.

Sooriakumaran and co-workers examined the presentation, management and outcomes of patients with renal angiomyolipoma (AML) over a period of 10 years. These investigators evaluated retrospectively 102 patients (median follow-up of 4 years); 70 had tuberous sclerosis complex (TSC; median tumor size of 3.5 cm) and the other 32 were sporadic (median tumor size of 1.2 cm). Data were gathered from several sources, including radiology and clinical genetics databases. The 77 patients with stable disease were followed-up with surveillance imaging, and 25 received interventions, some more than one. Indications for intervention included spontaneous life-threatening hemorrhage, large AML (10 to 20 cm), pain and visceral compressive symptoms. Selective arterial embolization (SAE) was performed in 19 patients; 10 received operative management and 4 had a RFA. Selective arterial embolization was effective in controlling hemorrhage from AMLs in the acute setting (n = 6) but some patients required further intervention (n = 4) and there was a significant complication rate. The reduction in tumor volume was only modest (28 %). No complications occurred after surgery (median follow-up of 5.5 years) or RFA (median follow-up of 9 months). One patient was entered into a trial and treated with sirolimus (rapamycin). The authors concluded that the management of AML is both complex and challenging, especially in those with TSC, where tumors are usually larger and multiple. Although SAE was effective at controlling hemorrhage in the acute setting it was deemed to be of limited value in the longer-term management of these tumors. Thus, novel techniques such as focused ablation and pharmacotherapies including the use of anti-angiogenic molecules and mammalian target of rapamycin inhibitors, which might prove to be safer and equally effective, should be further explored (25).

4.5. Radiofrequency ablation of bone metastases

Radiofrequency ablation has also been used to treat bone metastases. However, there are no adequate clinical studies reported in the literature on the use of RFA of metastatic lesions to bone. In a review of the evidence on RFA of tumors, Wood et al concluded "more rigorous scientific review, long-term follow-up, and randomized prospective trials are needed to help define the role of RFA in oncology" (26). Rhim noted that although RFA represents a paradigm shift in local therapy for many commonly seen tumors, more sophisticated strategies to enhance the therapeutic effectiveness are needed and more randomized, controlled trials to estimate its clinical benefit are warranted (27).

4.6. Radiofrequency ablation of breast cancer

On of the first attempt to use hyperthermia in tratment of breast cancer was in 2001 by Hilger et al (28). They studied the parameters for the minimally invasive elimination of breast tumors by using a selective application of magnetite and exposure of the breast to an alternating magnetic field. Temperature elevations based on magnetite mass (7–112 mg) and magnetic field amplitude (1.2–6.5 kA/m; frequency, 400 kHz) . They observed that a mean temperature of 71°C ± 8 was recorded in the tumor region at the end of magnetic field exposure of the mice. Typical macroscopic findings included tumor shrinkage after heating. Histologically nuclear degenerations were observed in heated malignant cells. They concluded that magnetic heating of breast tumors is a promising technique for future interventional radiologic treatments. Agnese and Burak stated that ablative therapies, including RFA have been shown promise in the treatment of small cancers of the breast. However, more research is needed to ascertain the effectiveness of these techniques when they are used as the sole therapy and to determine the long-term local recurrence rates and survival associated with these treatment strategies (29). van der Ploeg et al in 2007 reviewed the literature on the use of RFA for the treatment of small breast carcinoma. The authors concluded that RFA is a promising new tool for minimally invasive ablation of small carcinomas of the breast. They noted that a large randomized control study is needed to ascertain the long-term advantages of RFA compared to the current breast conserving therapies (30).

4.7. Radiofrequency ablation of a parathyroid adenoma

One of the methods of nonsurgical parathyroid ablation is percutaneous thermal ablation, such as laser or radiofrequency ablation. Percutaneous laser and radiofrequency ablation of parathyroid adenomas has been limited to case reports and small-series cases [31–32]. The ultimate utility of thermal ablation has yet to be determined but because it continues to be refined, it does hold promise as a method for treatment of parathyroid disease when surgery is not indicated. RFA can be a therapeutic alternative for patients with contraindications for surgery. Usually after percutaneous ultrasound guided RFTA of the adenoma of the parathyroid gland, the serum parathormone levels and the serum calcium levels dropped back to normal in most of patients (fig 4). Recurrent hyperparathyroidism is rare following transcatheter ablation of mediastinal parathyroid adenomas. When it occurs it is usually early and resistant to further attempts at ablation (33)

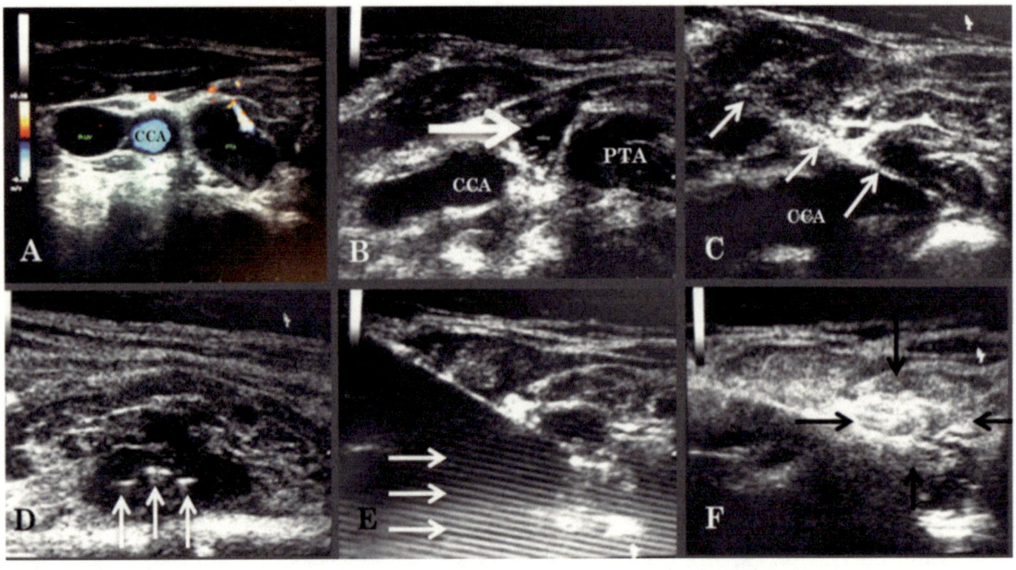

Figure 4. Radiofrequency ablation of parathyroid adenoma .A, Transverse sonogram of neck shows 15x10-mm right inferior parathyroid adenoma (PTA) .B; Sonogram of the neck after inflation of 5 ml saline (white arrow) to separate the PTA from the right common carotid artery (CCA). C ; Sonogram shows 25-gauge needle (arrows) inserted into parathyroid adenoma . D; Sonogram shows fans (arrows) of the radiofrequency probe within the PTA . E ; Sonogram during RFA of PTA shows reverberation artifacts (arrows) posterior to the needle) . F; Sonogram at the total RFA of the PTA, The ablated gland (arrows) appears echogenic.

4.8. RFA in management of Barrett's esophagus

Barrett's esophagus (BE) is defined as the presence of specialized intestinal metaplasia within the esophagus, and it is the pre-malignant precursor of esophageal adenocarcinoma. Esophageal cancer is one of the most deadly gastrointestinal cancers with a mortality rate over 90 %. The principal risk factors for esophageal adenocarcinoma are gastroesophageal reflux disease (GERD) and its sequela, BE. Gastroesophageal reflux disease usually leads to esophagitis. However, in a minority of patients, ongoing GERD leads to replacement of esophageal squamous mucosa with metaplastic, intestinal-type Barrett's mucosa. In the setting of continued peptic injury, Barrett's mucosa can give rise to esophageal adenocarcinoma (34). A new method of endoscopic ablation of BE is balloon-based, bipolar RFA (Stellartech Research Coagulation System; BARRx, Inc, Sunnyvale, Calif), also known as Barrett's endoscopy. This technique requires the use of sizing balloons to determine the inner diameter of the targeted portion of the esophagus. This is followed by placement of a balloon-based electrode with a 3-cm long treatment area that incorporates tightly spaced, bipolar electrodes that alternate in polarity. The electrode is then attached to a radiofrequency generator and a preselected amount of energy is delivered in less than 1 second at 350 W. In a review of evidence on ablative techniques for BE, Johnston stated that it is not clear which of the numerous endoscopic ablative techniques available -- photodynamic therapy, laser therapy, multi-polar electrocoagulation, argon plasma coagulation, endoscopic mucosal resection, RFA or cryotherapy -- will emerge as superior for treatment of BE. In addition, it has yet to be determined whether the risks associated with ablation therapy is less than the risk of BE progressing to cancer. Whether ablation therapy eliminates or significantly reduces the risk of cancer, eliminates the need for surveillance endoscopy, or is cost-effective, also remains to be seen. Comparative trials that are now underway should help to answer these questions (35). Hubbard and Velanovich stated that endoscopic endoluminal RFA using the Barrx device (Barrx Medical, Sunnyvale, CA) is a new technique to treat BE. This procedure has been used in patients who have not had anti-reflux surgery. This report presented an early experience of the effects of endoluminal ablation on the reflux symptoms and completeness of ablation in post-fundoplication patients. A total of 7 patients who have had either a laparoscopic or open Nissen fundoplication and BE underwent endoscopic endoluminal ablation of the Barrett's metaplasia using the Barrx device. Pre-procedure, none of the patients had significant symptoms related to GERD. One to 2 weeks after the ablation, patients were questioned as to the presence of symptoms. Pre-procedure and post-procedure, they completed the GERD-HRQL symptom severity questionnaire (best possible score, 0; worst possible score, 50). Patients had follow-up endoscopy to assess completeness of ablation 3 months after the original treatment. All patients completed the ablation without complications. No patients reported recurrence of their GERD symptoms. The median pre-procedure total GERD-HRQL score was 2, compared to a median post-procedure score of 1. One patient had residual Barrett's metaplasia at 3 months follow-up, requiring re-ablation. The authors concluded that this preliminary report of a small number of patients demonstrated that endoscopic endoluminal ablation of Barrett's metaplasia using the Barrx device is safe and effective in patients who have already undergone anti-reflux surgery. There appears to be no disruption in the fundoplication or recurrence of GERD-related symptoms. Nevertheless, they stated that studies with longer-term follow-up and with more patients are needed (36).

Ganz et al evaluated the safety and effectiveness of endoscopic circumferential balloon-based ablation by using radiofrequency energy for treating BE that contains high-grade dysplasia (HGD). Patients with histologic evidence of intestinal metaplasia (IM) that contained HGD confirmed by at least 2 expert pathologists were included in this study. A prior endoscopic mucosal resection (EMR) was permitted, provided that residual HGD remained in the BE region for ablation. Histologic complete response (CR) end points: (i) all biopsy specimen fragments obtained at the last biopsy session were negative for HGD (CR-HGD), (ii) all biopsy specimens were negative for any dysplasia (CR-D), and (iii) all biopsy specimens were negative for IM (CR-IM). A total of 142 patients (median age of 66 years, IQR 59 to 75 years) who had BE HGD (median length of 6 cm, IQR 3 to 8 cm) underwent circumferential ablation (median of 1 session, IQR 1 to 2 sessions). No serious adverse events were reported. There was 1 asymptomatic stricture and no buried glands. Ninety-two patients had at least 1 follow-up biopsy session (median follow-up of 12 months, IQR 8 to 15 months). A CR-HGD was achieved in 90.2 % of patients, CR-D in 80.4 %, and CR-IM in 54.3 %. The authors concluded that endoscopic circumferential ablation is a promising modality for the treatment of BE that contains HGD. In this multi-center registry, the intervention safely achieved a CR for HGD in 90.2 % of patients at a median of 12 months of follow-up. Major drawbacks of this study were a non-randomized study design, absence of a control arm, a lack of centralized pathology review, ablation and biopsy technique not standardized, and a relatively short-term follow-up (37) .

Shaheen et al examined if endoscopic RFA could eradicate dysplastic BE and decrease the rate of neoplastic progression. In a multi-center, sham-controlled trial, these researchers randomly assigned 127 patients with dysplastic BE in a 2:1 ratio to receive either RFA (ablation group) or a sham procedure (control group). Randomization was stratified according to the grade of dysplasia and the length of BE. Primary outcomes at 12 months included the complete eradication of dysplasia and intestinal metaplasia. In the intention-to-treat analyses, among patients with low-grade dysplasia, complete eradication of dysplasia occurred in 90.5 % of those in the ablation group, as compared with 22.7 % of those in the control group ($p < 0.001$). Among patients with high-grade dysplasia, complete eradication occurred in 81.0 % of those in the ablation group, as compared with 19.0 % of those in the control group ($p < 0.001$). Overall, 77.4 % of patients in the ablation group had complete eradication of intestinal metaplasia, as compared with 2.3 % of those in the control group ($p < 0.001$). Patients in the ablation group had less disease progression (3.6 % versus 16.3 %, $p = 0.03$) and fewer cancers (1.2 % versus 9.3 %, $p = 0.045$). Patients reported having more chest pain after the ablation procedure than after the sham procedure. In the ablation group, 1 patient had upper gastrointestinal hemorrhage, and 5 patients (6.0 %) had esophageal stricture. The authors concluded that in patients with dysplastic BE, RFA was associated with a high rate of complete eradication of both dysplasia and intestinal metaplasia and a reduced risk of disease progression (38). As stated by the authors, this study has several limitations: (i) these investigators used eradication of intestinal metaplasia and dysplasia, along with neoplastic progression, as surrogate markers for death from cancer, even though long-term data demonstrating an association between eradication of intestinal metaplasia and a decreased risk of cancer are sparse, (ii) the study duration was 1 year. Although other data suggest that reversion to neosquamous epithelium after RFA is durable, it is unclear if the results of the study will persist, (iii) because of stratified randomization according to the degree of dysplasia and the 2:1 ratio for assignment of patients to the ablation group and the control group, the number of patients in some groups was small, (iv) since this study did not compare RFA with other interventions, such as photodynamic therapy and esophagectomy, these researchers can not determine which of these interventions is superior, (v) whether these findings can be generalized to community-practice settings is unknown. Furthermore, the risk of subsquamous intestinal metaplasia following ablative therapy is a concern for all ablative techniques. However, the malignant potential of subsquamous intestinal metaplasia is unknown. In this study, subsquamous intestinal metaplasia was quite common in patients (25.2 %) before enrollment and, similar to previous reports, was low after RF ablation (5.1 %). Although the biopsy regimen in this study was aggressive, it is possible that some patients had undetected subsquamous intestinal metaplasia. Finally, because these investigators sought to define the efficacy of RFA for the spectrum of dysplasia, they enrolled patients with both low-grade dysplasia and high-grade dysplasia. However, the implications of these 2 diagnoses are markedly different. Low-grade dysplasia implies a risk of progression to cancer of less than 1 % per patient-year, whereas the risk associated with high-grade dysplasia may be higher by a factor of 10. In making decisions about the management of pre-cancerous conditions, clinicians, patients, and policy-makers consider possible benefits and risks of competing strategies. Because high-grade dysplasia has a more ominous natural history than low-grade dysplasia (or non-dysplastic intestinal metaplasia), greater risks and costs are tolerable. For less severe disease, the safety profile and associated costs become increasingly important. Detailed consideration of these trade-offs is beyond the scope of this study. Regardless, both of the dysplasia subgroups showed high rates of reversion to squamous epithelium after RFA and reduced rates of disease progression with few serious adverse effects, suggesting that the application of ablative therapy in patients with low-grade dysplasia is worth further investigation and consideration (38).

In the accompanying editorial, Bergman stated that it is still too early to promote RFA for patients with non-dysplastic BE. Dr. Bergman also asked the following questions: (i) is complete response after ablation maintained over time, thus reducing the risk of progression to high-grade dysplasia or cancer?, (ii) will ablation improve patients' quality of life and decrease costs, as compared with the surveillance strategy?, and (iii) can we define a stratification index predicting disease progression or response to therapy? The author noted that "[w]e run the risk of losing the momentum to enroll patients in a trial that is required at this stage: a randomized comparison of endoscopic surveillance and radiofrequency ablation for non-dysplastic Barrett's esophagus. Such a study might truly revolutionize the management of this condition and answer the question as to whether radiofrequency ablation is great just for some or justified for many" (39). Furthermore, the American College of Gastroenterology's updated guidelines for the diagnosis, surveillance and therapy of BE , Wang and Sampliner states that "further evaluation of the most recent technology; radiofrequency ablation is awaited. Cryotherapy is beginning clinical trials and older technologies are becoming more refined (e.g., photodynamic therapy with the development of new agents). Documentation of the frequency and duration of the surveillance protocol after endoscopic ablation therapy requires careful study" (40).

4.9. RFA of esophageal neoplasm

Yeh and Triadafilopoulos noted that a wide variety of endoscopic mucosal ablative techniques have been developed for early esophageal neoplasia. However, long-term control of neoplasic risk has not been demonstrated. The authors explained that most studies show that specialized intestinal metaplasia may persist underneath neo-squamous mucosa, posing a risk for subsequent neoplastic progression (41). Shaheen noted that the pathogenesis of BE is poorly understood. Given that some patients will have repeated bouts of severe erosive esophagitis and never develop BE, host factors must play an important role. The author stated that the utility of neoadjuvant radiation and chemotherapy in those with adenocarcinoma, although they are widely practiced, is not of clear benefit, and some authorities recommend against it. Ablative therapies, as well as endoscopic mucosal resection, hold promise for those with superficial cancer or high-grade dysplasia. The author noted that most series using these modalities feature relatively short follow-up; longer-term studies are needed to better ascertain the effectiveness of these treatments (38).

Pedrazzani et al evaluated the effectiveness of 90 W argon plasma coagulation (APC) for the ablation of BE that is considered to be the main risk factor for the development of esophageal adenocarcinoma. They found that high power setting APC showed to be safe. The effects persist at a mean follow-up period of 2 years with a comparable cost in term of complications with respect to standard power settings. The authors stated, however, that further studies with greater number of patients are required to confirm these results and to assess if ablation reduces the incidence of malignant progression (42). Hage et al stated that although endoscopic removal of BE by ablative therapies is possible in the majority of patients, histologically complete elimination can not be achieved in all cases. Persistent BE may still harbor molecular aberrations and must therefore be considered still to be at risk of progression to adenocarcinoma (43).

4.10. RFA of thyroid metastasis

Guidelines on thyroid cancer from the National Comprehensive Cancer Network (NCCN, 2010) state that distant metastases from recurrent or persistent medullary thyroid carcinoma that are causing symptoms (e.g., those in bone) could be considered for palliative resection, RFA, or other regional treatment. The guidelines state that these interventions may also be considered for asymptomatic distant metastases (especially for progressive disease) but observation is acceptable, given the lack of data regarding alteration in outcome (44). Monchik and colleagues evaluated the long-term effectiveness of RFA and percutaneous ethanol (EtOH) injection treatment of patients with local recurrence or focal distant metastases of well-differentiated thyroid cancer (WTC). A total of 20 patients underwent treatment of biopsy-proven recurrent WTC in the neck. Sixteen of these patients had lesions treated by ultrasound-guided RFA (mean size, 17.0 mm; range of 8 to 40 mm), while 6 had ultrasound-guided EtOH injection treatment (mean size, 11.4 mm; range of 6 to 15 mm). Four patients underwent RFA treatment of focal distant metastases from WTC. Three of these patients had CT-guided RFA of bone metastases (mean size, 40.0 mm; range of 30 to 60 mm), and 1 patient underwent RFA for a solitary lung metastasis (size, 27 mm). Patients were then followed with routine ultrasound, whole body scan, and/or serum thyroglobulin levels for recurrence at the treatment site. No recurrent disease was detected at the treatment site in 14 of the 16 patients treated with RFA and in all 6 patients treated with EtOH injection at a mean follow-up of 40.7 and 18.7 months, respectively. Two of the 3 patients treated for bone metastases were disease-free at the treatment site at 44 and 53 months of follow-up, respectively. The patient who underwent RFA for a solitary lung metastasis was disease-free at the treatment site at 10 months of follow-up. No complications were experienced in the group treated by EtOH injection, while 1 minor skin burn and 1 permanent vocal cord paralysis occurred in the RFA treatment group. The authors concluded that RFA and EtOH ablation show promise as alternatives to surgical treatment of recurrent WTC in patients with difficult reoperations. They stated that further long-term follow-up studies are needed to ascertain the precise role these therapies should play in the treatment of recurrent WTC (45).

4.11. RFA of Soft tissue masses

Radiofrequency ablation devices have been cleared by the FDA for the general indication of soft tissue cutting, coagulation, and ablation by thermal coagulation necrosis. This clearance was based only on bench testing or animal testing performance data. Guidelines from the National Comprehensive Cancer Network (NCCN, 2010) include recommendations for RFA of the trunk and extremities in metastatic soft tissue sarcoma. The guidelines include metastasectomy with RFA as an alternative method for control of metastatic lesions in limited metastases. The guidelines also include RFA as options for symptomatic patients with disseminated metastases. "The guidelines are intentionally nonspecific about this group of options, because many different issues are factored into this decision (e.g., patient performance status, patient preferences, specific clinical problems from the metastases, treatment availability.)" (46).

4.12. RFA of gastrointestinal stromal tumors

Pawlik et al at MD Anderson Cancer Center reported a series with 36 non-GIST sarcoma patients and 31 GIST patients who received RFA and/or surgical resection of liver metastases. (47). When surgical resection was possible, that was the first choice (35 patients). RFA was used in combination with surgical resection of the largest lesions in 18 cases. RFA was used alone in 13 cases. Those patients treated with RFA alone, or in combination with surgical resection, had a significantly higher rate of recurrence (90.9%) than did patients who underwent resection alone (57.1%). However, this difference probably reflects a selection bias, since RFA was never used for patients whose tumors were resectable. Patients who were treated with RFA either alone or as a combined modality with resection also had a shorter disease-free interval (7.4 months) than patients who underwent resection alone (18.6 months). Avritscher et al reported three advanced GIST patients whose focal liver progression was successfully treated with RFA. The patients remained progression-free at 8, 15, and 16 months after ablation (48) .

In an ASCO poster presentation, Dileo et al reported treating 9 patients with percutaneous CT-guided RFA for single or limited site(s) of progressing disease (8 liver lesions and 1 soft tissue lesion). Thee were no complications from the RFA procedure. With median follow-up of 4.2 months (range 1-11 months), all patients had their lesions completely ablated. Five patients developed systemic progression, while 4 patients remain stable on continued treatment with imatinib (median follow-up 5.8 m). The authors concluded "In this small cohort, percutaneous RFA appears to be a safe and effective treatment for localized sites of progression. This procedure helps to manage limited IM-resistant GIST. Continuation of imatinib to control systemic sites of imatinib-sensitive GIST despite emergence of limited clonal resistance can be justified on the basis of this exploratory work." (49)

Evaluating the evidence about RFA for GIST. RFA appears to be a viable palliative option for patients with advanced GIST who develop focal progression of liver or peritoneal disease during imatinib therapy and who are not otherwise candidates for surgical resection. Alternatively, RFA offers a potentially curative option for patients who exhibit a partial response to imatinib and have focal residual disease that is not amenable to surgical resection .The guidelines (NCCN, 2010) also recommend the use of RFA for the treatment of gastrointestinal stromal tumors with limited progression. Progression is defined as a new lesion or increase in tumor size. The NCCN guidelines state that, for limited progressive disease that is potentially easily resectable, surgical resection should be considered. Other treatment options include RFA or embolization.

4.13. RFA of malignant biliary obstruction

In an open-label, pilot study, Steel et al in 2011 examined the safety of endobiliary bipolar RFA in patients with malignant biliary obstruction and reported the 90-day biliary patency of this novel procedure. Main outcome measures were immediate and 30-day complications as well as 90-day stent patency. A total of 22 patients (16 pancreatic, 6 cholangiocarcinoma) were includedin this study. Deployment of an RFA catheter was successful in 21 patients. Self-expandable metal stents (SEMSs) placement was achieved in all cases of successful RFA catheter deployment. One patient failed to demonstrate successful biliary decompression after SEMS placement and died within 90 days. All other patients maintained stent patency at 30 days. One patient had asymptomatic biochemical pancreatitis, 2 patients required percutaneous gallbladder drainage, and 1 patient developed rigors. At 90-day follow-up, 1 additional patient had died with a patent stent, and 3 patients had occluded biliary stents.

The authors concluded that endobiliary RFA treatment appears to be safe. They stated that randomized studies with prolonged follow-up are needed (50).

4.14. Role of hyperthermia in treatment of cervical cancer patients

Today, the technique is a standard treatment for patients with advanced cervical cancer, or patients with less advanced cervical cancer that cannot clinically tolerate chemotherapy. It is recommended and used as an alternative to the international gold standard of combined radiation therapy and cisplatin-based chemotherapy (51). The Dutch Deep Hyperthermia Trial, conducted between 1990 and 1996 and published in the Lancet in 2000, was a prospective, randomized trial that compared the outcomes of 358 patients with advanced bladder, cervical, and rectal tumors. Half of the patients received only radiation therapy and the other half received both radiation therapy and hyperthermia. Three-year outcomes revealed that hyperthermia improved both pelvic control and overall survival rates, but seemed to be most effective for patients with advanced cervical cancer (52). At 36 months, of an original cohort of 114 patients with advanced cervical cancer, the 58 patients receiving both treatments showed a complete response rate of 83%, compared with 57% for the 56 patients who only received radiation therapy. The survival rate was 51% for the combined treatment group, compared with 27% for the radiation therapy-only group. Furthermore, hyperthermia treatments did not enhance radiation toxicity and were reported to be cost-effective

However, long-term outcomes (**12-year follow-up**) was addressed by a follow-up study published in 2008 that tracked outcomes for both groups 12 years following treatment. The patients who received the combined treatment continued to have significantly better outcomes. The outcomes for the combined therapy group remained consistent. At the end of the study period, 37% of this group was still alive, compared with 20% who received radiation only. Of the combined therapy group, 56% retained pelvic tumor control, compared with 37% for the radiation therapy group. Pelvic recurrence developed in 25% of the combined therapy group and 31% of the radiation therapy group. Approximately one-third of both cohorts developed distant metastasis. Both groups experienced the same number of grades 3-5 radiation-induced toxicities (53).

4.15. Radiofrequency ablation therapy for varicose veins

Venous insufficiency resulting from superficial reflux because of varicose veins is a serious problem that usually progresses inexorably if left untreated. When the refluxing circuit involves failure of the primary valves at the saphenofemoral junction, treatment options for the patient are limited, and early recurrences are the rule rather than the exception. In the historical surgical approach, ligation and division of the saphenous trunk and all proximal tributaries are followed either by stripping of the vein or by avulsion phlebectomy. Proximal ligation requires a substantial incision at the groin crease. Stripping of the vein requires additional incisions at the knee or below and is associated with a high incidence of minor surgical complications. Avulsion phlebectomy requires multiple 2- to 3-mm incisions along the course of the vein and can cause damage to adjacent nerves and lymphatic vessels. Endovenous ablation has replaced stripping and ligation as the technique for elimination of saphenous vein reflux. One of the endovenous techniques is a radiofrequency-based procedure. Newer methods of delivery of radiofrequency were introduced in 2007. Endovenous procedures are far less invasive than surgery and have lower complication rates. The procedure is well tolerated by patients, and it produces good cosmetic results. Excellent clinical results are seen at 4-5 years, and the long-term efficacy of the procedure is now known with 10 years of experience (54-55).

The US Food and Drug Administration (FDA) cleared the original radiofrequency endovenous procedure in March 1999. Endovenous techniques (endovenous laser therapy, radiofrequency ablation, and endovenous foam sclerotherapy) clearly are less invasive and are associated with fewer complications compared with more invasive surgical procedures, with comparable or greater efficacy. The original radiofrequency endovenous ablation system worked by thermal destruction of venous tissues using electrical energy passing through tissue in the form of high-frequency alternating current. This current was converted into heat, which causes irreversible localized tissue damage. Radiofrequency energy is delivered through a special catheter with deployable electrodes at the tip; the electrodes touch the vein walls and deliver energy directly into the tissues without coagulating blood. The newest system, called ClosureFast, delivers infrared energy to vein walls by directly heating a catheter tip with radiofrequency energy. Published results show a high early success rate with a very low subsequent recurrence rate up to 10 years after treatment. Early and mid range results are comparable to those obtained with other endovenous ablation techniques. The authors' overall experience has been a 90% success rate, with rare patients requiring a repeat procedure in 6-12 months. Overall efficacy and lower morbidity have resulted in endovenous ablation techniques replacing surgical stripping. Patient satisfaction is high and downtime is minimal, with 95% of patients reporting they would recommend the procedure to a friend (56-58).

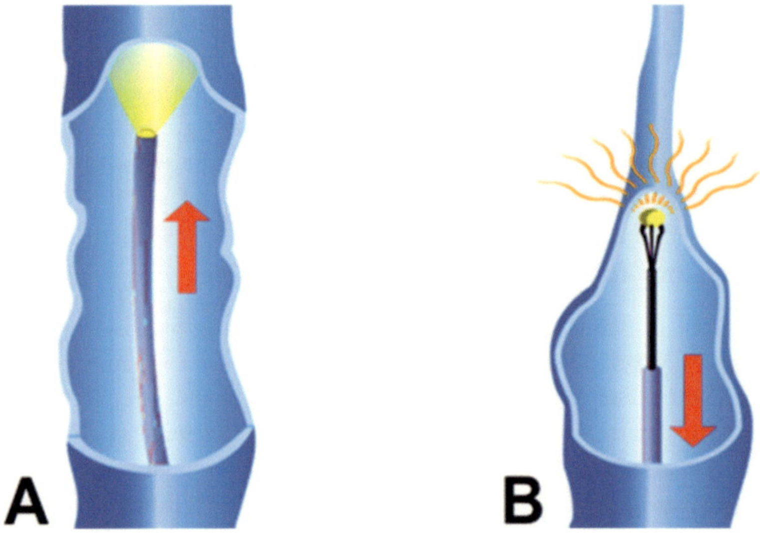

Figure 5. A diagram shows the technique of RFA for varicose veins .A. The catheter is inserted and advanced into the diseases vein through a small incision into the diseased vein under ultrasound guidance. B Then laser or radiofrequency energy is applied to the lining of the vein, heating and shrinking the vein walls, causing them to seal and as the catheter withdrawn the vein is closed

4.16. Catheter ablation for paroxysmal atrial fibrillation

Other diseases where ablation is used include cardiac catheter thermal ablation is now standard of care for a variety of cardiac arrhythmia types (irregular heart beat rhythm). Techniques are directed at cauterizing areas of high irritability that give rise to frequent ectopy and trigger paroxysmal atrial fibrillation (PAF), or cauterisation of the substrate that maintains PAF, (predominantly left atrial tissue), or both. Usually this is done with radiofrequency energy delivered percutaneously by steerable catheters. In the UK, recent Guidance from NICE approved catheter ablation for PAF on the NHS for patients who have failed treatment with two antiarrhythmic drugs. Similar guidelines exist in the USA. Success rates of 70-80% can be achieved, with multiple procedures being needed in many cases. RFCA for PAF carries significant risks. These are; stroke (<1%), cardiac tamponade (2-6%), pulmonary vein stenosis (0.5-1%), a small risk of arteriovenous fistula (<0.5%), and a very small but important risk of oesophago-atrial fistula. In older patients, (>70 years), patients with structural heart disease and patients with persistent or prolonged AF, there is significantly less chance of success with RFCA. Recently an electro-anatomic mapping systems" (a form of mini-"GPS", or "Sat-Nav" system), are becoming increasingly sophisticated at telling an electrophysiologist exactly where a catheter is within the heart, and exactly where anatomical structures are located relative to it. This is important for avoiding complications. A CT Scan or MRI scan of heart chambers is useful for obtaining the detailed anatomy of the heart for RFCA procedures (59-61).

RFA of the AV-junction followed by implantation of a pacemaker provides good control of symptoms, reduced drug and healthcare consumption, and reduced hospital admissions. However, AV-junctional ablation is not reversible, and allows atrial fibrillation to continue, albeit without allowing it to produce rapid, irregular ventricular rates, so that patients may be unaware of being in PAF. RFA of the AV-junction followed by implantation of a pacemaker is increasingly reserved for patients with established/chronic AF in whom ventricular rate-control cannot be achieved with AV-nodal blocking drugs. In these patients AF persists in spite of treatment anyway, and RFA of the AV-junction with permanent pacing can give excellent symptom control (NICE 2006) (62).

5. Combination of hyperthermia with radiotherapy in treatment of cancer

Hyperthermia is a heat cancer treatment FDA approved in combination with low-dose-radiation, applied to tumors, raising tumor temperature to about 42.5°C (108°F) for about 45 to 60 minutes. Heat improves blood circulation and makes tumor cells more susceptible to the low-dose- radiation therapy, killing them more efficiently and quickly. Hyperthermia can be compared with an artificial fever that attacks cancer cells. Starting in the late 1970s, a major focus of many researchers was on achieving focal, cytotoxic temperatures of 42-45 °C within tumors, a strategy which can sensitize tumors to radiation and/or chemotherapy. Remarkable progress in engineering and physics over the past 20 years has led to the implementation of clinical trials that are revealing the true potential of this strategy. Over the past decade, positive clinical data has emerged from trials utilizing HT in the treatment of recurrent chest wall breast cancer, melanoma, esophageal cancer, locally advanced head and neck cancer, locally advanced cervix cancer and gliomas. 1) Hyperthermia increases perfusion and oxygenation of neoplastic hypoxic cells, which are three times more resistant to ionizing radiation than normal cells. Consequently, the action of radiotherapy becomes 1.5-5 times more efficient. Hyperthermia has a direct cytotoxic action on cancer: due to the pathologic blood vessels, the thermal elevation persists inside the tumor, whereas neighboring normal tissues, adequately perfused, are cooled: at 43 °C, normal cells are not damaged, whereas tumor cells are damaged at the cell nucleus, plasmatic membrane and cytoskeleton, up to apoptosis. Hyperthermia acts mostly at an acid pH and in the S phase of the cell cycle, when cells are radioresistant. This means that radiotherapy and hyperthermia are complementary in their action: radiotherapy forms free radicals, which damage the DNA of tumor cells, whereas hyperthermia inhibits its reparation. 2) Hyperthermic inhibition of repairing radiation damage has been suggested as an essential factor causing the synergistic cell-killing effect of X-rays and hyperthermia. Heating cells before X-irradiation has been shown to inhibit the repair of DNA strand breaks as well as the excision of base damage1. There are several DNA repair pathways involved in restoration of damage after ionizing irradiation and the kinetics of all of them are affected by heat shock. However, this does not imply that the inhibition of each of these pathways is relevant to the effect of heat on cellular radiosensitivity. Data reported by Kampinga et al showed that thermal inhibition of the non-homologous end-joining pathway plays a role in heat radiosensitization. Furthermore, limited data suggest that the homologous recombination pathway may not be a major heat target. The inhibition of base-excision damage repair could be, by deduction, the crucial step in the mechanism of radiosensitization by heat (63). 3) Hyperthermia enhances the sensitivity of cells to radiation and drugs and this sensitization is not directly related to altered heat-shock proteins (HSP) expression. Elevating HSP prior to heating makes cells thermo- tolerant and altering their expression will affect the extent of thermal action because the HSP will attenuate the heat-induced protein damage, responsible for radiation and drug sensitization. Nuclear protein damage is considered to be responsible for hyperthermic effects on DNA repair, especially base-excision damage repair (64).

In an effort to provide a clearer picture of the interaction between hyperthermia and radiation, asynchronous CHO cell survivals for a matrix of doses of radiation and hyperthermia were determined· The survival matrix was then analyzed by fitting a survival function that was the product of survivals due to hyperthermia alone, to radiation alone and to the interaction of hyperthermia and radiation. This survival function is an expression for the survival surface, a surface in the space defined by the three axes of logarithm of cell survival, hyperthermia dose and radiation dose. The survival surface is a three dimensional extension of the two-dimensional survival curve (65).

The two principal rationales for applying hyperthermia in cancer therapy are that: (a) the S phase, which is relatively radioresistant, is the most sensitive phase to hyperthermia, and can be selectively radiosensitized by combining hyperthermia with x-irradiation; the cycling tumor cells in S phase which would normally survive an x-ray dose could thus be killed by subjecting these cells to hyperthermia; and (b) the relatively radioresistant hypoxic cells in the tumor may be selectively destroyed by combinations of hyperthermia and x-irradiation. Both of these rationales have been mentioned as reasons for using high LET irradiation in cancer therapy; therefore where such irradiation may be of use, hyperthermia may also be advantageous.

It is a **heat cancer treatment FDA approved** in combination with low-dose-radiation, applied to tumors, raising tumor temperature to about 42.5°C (108°F) for about 45 to 60 minutes. Heat improves blood circulation and makes tumor cells more susceptible to the low-dose- radiation therapy, killing them more efficiently and quickly As a result of these and other clinical applications, combined with a rapidly expanding research base, interest in thermal medicine is rapidly growing, attracting the attention of laboratory and clinical researchers, physicians, engineers, physicists and biotechnologists.

6. Rationale for chemotherapy and hyperthermia association

Hyperthermia can also be used to activate cytotoxic effects of chemotherapy within tumors, thereby sparing normal tissue, when the drugs are encapsulated in thermally sensitive nanoparticles. Hyperthermic drug sensitization can be seen for several anti-cancer drugs, in particular alkylating agents. The combined action between heat and drugs arises from multiple events such as drug accumulation, drug detoxification pathways and repair of drug-induced DNA adducts. Cells with acquired drug resistance can be made responsive to the same drugs again by combining drugs with heat. Hyperthermia, which increases tumor tissue perfusion, facilitates the absorption of chemotherapeutic drugs through cell membrane. The heat accelerates chemical reactions, so that chemotherapy becomes more effective, without being more toxic. Hyperthermia allows the response of tumors resistant to various chemotherapeutic drugs: doxorubicin, cisplatin, bleomycin, mitomycin c, nitrosoureas, cyclophosphamide. Use of liposomes, including adriamycin (Caelyx®) administered i.v., hyperthermia fuses and frees their content inside the heated tumor bed, thus obtaining a target chemotherapy, with reduction of side effects.

On March 18, 2010, the Celsion Corporation (http://www.celsion.com, accessed 17 November 2010) announced that an abstract about the phase I/II trial of ThermoDox® in recurrent chest wall cancer has been accepted for presentation at the American Society of Clinical Oncology (ASCO) 2010 Annual Meeting. The abstract presents the background, rationale and design of the DIGNITY study which is ongoing and evaluating ThermoDox® in combination with hyperthermia in women with recurrent breast cancer on their chest wall (66).

In a separate trial with a similar design being conducted at Duke University Medical Center, researchers are reporting convincing evidence of clinical activity. The DIGNITY clinical trial is a phase I/II, open label, dose- escalating trial to evaluate the safety and efficacy of ThermoDox® with hyperthermia for the treatment of recurrent chest wall breast cancer, an aggressive form of cancer with a poor prognosis and limited treatment options. The primary end point in the DIGNITY trial is durable complete local response at the tumor site. Once the safe dose is determined, Celsion intends to enroll up to 100 patients to establish efficacy. The results from the DIGNITY trial are expected to build on the promising data from the phase I dose-escalation study currently being conducted at Duke University Medical Center. ThermoDox® has also demonstrated evidence of efficacy in a phase I study for primary liver cancer. Celsion has been granted FDA orphan drug designation for ThermoDox® and is conducting a pivotal 600 patient global phase III study in primary liver cancer under an FDA special protocol assessment, thus obtaining a target chemotherapy, with reduction of side effects. It has been demonstrated that hyperthermia also has an anti-angiogenic action and an immunotherapeutic role, due to thermal shock proteins, which are produced by stressed tumor cells. Finally, hyperthermia substains the action of genic therapy (67).

The immunotherapeutic role of hyperthermia is not yet completely understood. Especially, the effects on natural killer (NK) cell cytotoxicity against tumor cell targets have not been fully demonstrated. At treatment temperatures above 40 °C, both enhancing and inhibitory effects of cytotoxic activity of NK cells against tumor cells have been reported. In particular, an enhancement of human NK cytotoxicity against tumor cell targets has been demonstrated using a temperature of 39.5 °C10. Data in the literature indicate a strong potential for heat-induced enhancement of NK cell activity in mediating the improved clinical response. A better understanding in this field should be achieved in order to maximize the clinical benefits obtained by using hyperthermia for cancer therapy (68).

7. Heat-activated drug delivery

An exciting new generation of clinical trials is now harnessing drug-containing thermosensitive liposomes, and other nanoparticle drug carriers, that release contained chemotherapy agents upon heating above ~40 °C. Combined with localized heating methods as described above, this allows for targeted chemotherapy delivery to tumors. Thermal ablation or hyperthermia can be combined with heat-activated drug carriers to selectively deposit chemotherapy in the heated area. Initial clinical trial results suggest patient benefits from this combination and thus there is considerable excitement among members of our Society in this approach.

8. Conclusions

Hyperthermia, thanks to the improved systems for achieving an optimal distribution of heat inside the tumor and precise and noninvasive thermometry, is today an important treatment modality in the treatment of cancer, and its results are strongly supported by criteria of evidence-based medicine. Hyperthermia is an important treatment modality in cancer treatment and its results are strongly supported by criteria of evidence-based medicine. Hyperthermia is a therapeutic modality that, employing nonionizing radiations, can be used not only by radiation oncologists but also by clinical oncologists. Its addition to radiotherapy with or without chemotherapy is important when it is necessary to treat advanced or high-risk tumors, or to retreat a relapse in a pre-irradiated area. Hyperthermia appears to be the fourth pillar besides surgery, radiotherapy and chemotherapy.

Author details

Ragab Hani Donkol
Department of Radiology, Faculty of Medicine, Cairo University, Cairo, Egypt
Aseer Central Hospital, Abha, Saudi Arabia

Ahmed Al Nammi
Aseer Central Hospital, Abha, Saudi Arabia

9. References

[1] Moulvi Azimuddin Ahmad: Catalogue of Arabic and Persian Manuscripts in the Oriental Public Library, Bankipur, Patna, India. Calcutta, 1910, p. 30

[2] Nikfarjam M, Muralidharan V, Christophi C. Mechanisms of focal heat destruction of liver tumors. J Surg Res. 2005; 127:208–23.

[3] Stauffer PR, Goldberg SN. Introduction: thermal ablation therapy. Int J Hyper-®thermia. 2004;7:671–7.

[4] Stauffer PR. Evolving technology for thermal therapy of cancer. Int J Hyperther- mia. 2005; 21:731–44.

[5] Ahar K (2004) The role and limitations of radiofrequency ablation in treatment of bone and soft tissue tumors. Curr Oncol Rep 6:315–320

[6] Rosenthal DI, Hornicek FJ, Wolfe MW et al (1998) Percutaneous radiofrequency coagulation of osteoid osteoma compared with operative treatment. J Bone Joint Surg Am 80:815–821

[7] Towbin R, Kaye R, Meza M et al (1995) Osteoid osteoma: percutaneous excision using a CT-guided coaxial technique. AJR 164:945–949

[8] Sans N, Galy-Fourcade D, Assoun J et al (1999) Osteoid osteoma: CT-guided percutaneous resection and follow-up in 38 patients. Radiology 212:687–692

[9] Rosenthal DI, Springfield DS, Gebhardt MC et al (1995) Osteoid osteoma: percutaneous radio-frequency ablation. Radiology 197:451–454

[10] Gebauer B, Tunn PU, Gaffke G et al (2006) Osteoid osteoma: experience with laser- and radiofrequency-induced ablation. Cardiovasc Intervent Radiol 29:210–215

[11] Kjar RA, Powell GJ, Schilcht SM et al (2006) Percutaneous radiofrequency ablation for osteoid osteoma: experience with a new treatment. Med J Aust 184:563–565 406

[12] Donkol RH, Al-Nammi A, Moghazi K. Efficacy of percutaneous radiofrequency ablation of osteoid osteoma in children. Pediatr Radiol. 2008 Feb;38(2):180-5. Epub 2007 Nov 27

[13] Le QT, Petrik DW. Nonsurgical therapy for stages I and II non-small cell lung cancer. Hematol Oncol Clin N AM, 2005,19:237-261.

[14] National Institute of Health and Clinical Excellence. Lung cancer: the diagnosis and treatment of lung cancer. Clinical Guideline CG24. 2005 (review expected February 2009).

[15] U.S. Food and Drug Administration. FDA Public Health Notification: Radiofrequency Ablation of Lung Tumors - Clarification of Regulatory Status. September 24, 2008 Available at: http://www.fda.gov/cdrh/safety/092408-ablation.html. Accessed on March 28, 2011.

[16] Girelli, R.; et al. (2010) Feasibility and safety of radiofrequency ablation for locally advanced pancreatic cancer. Brit J Surg. 97(2). 220-225.

[17] Wood BJ, Ramkaransingh JR, Fojo T, Walther MM, et al. Percutaneous tumor ablation with radiofrequency. Cancer 2002; 94(2):443–51. BJ,

[18] Atkins, M.; Choueiri, T. (2011). Epidemiology, pathology, and pathogenesis of renal cell carcinoma. In: UpToDate, Basow, DS (Ed), UpToDate, Waltham, MA.

[19] National Institute for Clinical Excellence, Interventional Procedures Programme. Interventional procedures overview of percutaneous radiofrequency ablation of renal tumors, 2010 http://www.nice.org.uk/page.aspx?o=ip215overview

[20] Hailey D. Radiofrequency ablation in the treatment of kidney cancer. Canadian Coordinating Office for Health Technology Assessment (CCOHTA); 2006
[21] Hinshaw JL, Lee FT Jr. Image-guided ablation of renal cell carcinoma. Magn Reson Imaging Clin NAm 2004;12(3):429 –47
[22] Mahnken JAH. Percutaneous radiofrequency ablation of renal cell cancer. Radiologe. 2004; 44:358–363.
[23] Kutikov A, Guzzo TJ, Canter DJ, Casale P. Initial experience with laparoscopic enucleation of renal cell carcinoma with ablation of the tumour base in patients with renal cell carcinoma. Journal of Urology 181(2): 486-491, Feb. 200.
[24] Nabi G, Cleves A, Shelley M. Surgical management of localised renal cell carcinoma. Cochrane Database Syst Rev. 2010;(3):CD006579
[25] Sooriakumaran P, Gibbs P, Coughlin G, Attard V, Elmslie F, Kingswood C, Taylor J, Corbishley C, Patel U, Anderson C. Angiomyolipomata: challenges, solutions, and future prospects based on over 100 cases treated. BJU int, 2009 June
[26] Wood, B. (2002). Feasibility of Thermal Ablation of Lytic Vertebral Metastases with Radiofrequency Current. The Cancer Journal, 8(1): 26-29.
[27] Rhim H, Dodd GD III, Chintapalli KN, Wood BJ, Dupuy DE, Hvizda JL, Sewell PE and Goldberg SN: Radiofrequency thermal ablation of abdominal tumors: lessons learned from complications. Radiographics 24: 41-52, 2004.
[28] Hilger I, Andrä W, Hergt R, Hiergeist R, Schubert H, Kaiser WA. Electromagnetic heating of breast tumors in interventional radiology: in vitro and in vivo studies in human cadavers and mice. Radiology. 2001 Feb;218(2):570-5.
[29] Agnese DM, Burak WE Jr. Ablative approaches to the minimally invasive treatment of breast cancer. Cancer J 2005;11:77–82
[30] van der Ploeg I M, van Esser S, van den Bosch M A, Mali W P, van Diest P J, Borel Rinkes I H, van Hillegersberg R. Radiofrequency ablation for breast cancer: a review of the literature. European Journal of Surgical Oncology 2007; 33(6): 673-677
[31] .Carrafiello G, Laganà D, Mangini M, et al. Treatment of secondary hyperparathyroidism with ultrasonographically guided percutaneous radiofrequency thermoablation. Surg Laparosc Endosc Percutan Tech 2006; 16:112 -116
[32] .Hänsler J, Harsch IA, Strobel D, Hahn EG, Becker D. Treatment of a solitary adenoma of the parathyroid gland with ultrasound-guided percutaneous Radio-Frequency-Tissue-Ablation (RFTA)]. Ultraschall Med. 2002 Jun;23(3):202-6
[33] Gary J. R. Cook, Ignac Fogelman and John F. Reidy Successful repeat transcatheter ablation of a mediastinal parathyroid adenoma 6 years after alcohol embolization. Cardiovascular and interventional radiology. Volume 20, Number 4 (1997), 314-316, DOI: 10.1007/s002709900157
[34] Feagins LA, Souza RF. Molecular targets for treatment of Barrett`s esophagus. Dis Esophagus. 2005; 18(2): 75-86
[35] Johnston, MH, Eastone, JA, Horwhat, JD, Cartledge, J, Mathews, JS, Foggy, JR. Cryoablation of Barrett's esophagus: a pilot study. Gastrointest Endosc. 2005 Dec;62(6):842-8. PMID: 16301023
[36] Hubbard N, Velanovich V.Endoscopic endoluminal radiofrequency ablation of Barrett's esophagus in patients with fundoplications. Surg Endosc 2007;21:625-8.

[37] Ganz RA, Utley DS, Stern RA, et al. Complete ablation of esophageal epithelium with a balloon-based bipolar electrode; a phased evaluation in the porcine and in the human esophagus. Gastrointest Endosc 2004;60:1002-10.
[38] Shaheen NJ, Sharma P, Overholt BF, et al .Radiofrequency ablation in Barrett's esophagus with dysplasia.. N Engl J Med 2009;360:2277-88
[39] Bergman JJ, Zhang YM, He S, Weusten B, Xue L, Fleischer DE, Lu N, Dawsey SM, Wang GQ Outcomes from a prospective trial of endoscopic radiofrequency ablation of early squamous cell neoplasia of the esophagus. Gastrointest Endosc. 2011 Dec;74(6):1181-90. Epub 2011 Aug 15. PMID: 21839994
[40] Wang KK, Sampliner RE. Updated guidelines 2008 for the diagnosis, surveillance and therapy of Barrett's esophagus. Am J Gastroenterol 2008;103:788-797
[41] Yeh R, Triadafilopoulos G. Endoscopic therapy for Barrett's esophagus. Gastrointest Endosc Clin North Am 2005; 15:377–397.
[42] Pedrazzani C, Catalano F, Festini M, Zerman G, Tomezzoli A, Ruzzenente A, Guglielmi A, de Manzoni G. Endoscopic ablation of Barrett's esophagus using high power setting argon plasma coagulation: A prospective study. World J Gastroenterol 2005; 11(12): 1872-1875
[43] Hage M, Siersema PD, Vissers KJ, et al. Molecular evaluation of ablative therapy of Barrett`s oesophagus. J Pathol. 2005; 205(1): 57- 64.
[44] National Comprehensive Cancer Network. NCCN Clinical Practice Guidelines in Oncology: Thyroid Cancer. Version 1.2011
[45] Monchik JM, Donatini G, Iannuccilli J, Dupuy D: Radiofrequency ablation and percutaneous ethanol injection treatment for recurrent local and distant well differentiated thyroid cancer. Ann Surg 244:296, 2006.
[46] George D. Demetri; Scott Antonia; Robert S. Benjamin; Marilyn M. Bui; Ephraim S. Casper; Ernest U. Conrad III; Thomas F. DeLaney; Kristen N. Ganjoo; Martin J. Heslin; et al. Soft tissue sarcoma .JNCCN Journal of the National Comprehensive Cancer Network 2010;8(6):630-674.
[47] Pawlik TM, Vauthey JN, Abdalla EK, et al. Results of a single-center experience with resection and ablation for sarcoma metastatic to the liver. Arch Surg 2006;141:537–43
[48] Avritscher R, Gupta S. Gastrointestinal stromal tumor: role of interventional radiology in diagnosis and treatment. Hematol Oncol Clin North Am. 2009 Feb;23(1):129-37, ix. PubMed PMID: 19248976.
[49] Dileo P, Randhawa R, Vansonnenberg E, et al. Safety and efficacy of percutaneous radio-frequency (RFA) in patients with metastatic gastrointestinal stromal tumor (GIST) with clonal evolution of lesions refractory to imatinib mesylate. J Clin Oncol 2004;22:9024
[50] Steel, Alan W.; Postgate, Aymer J.; Khorsandi, Shirin; Nicholls, Joanna; Jiao, Long; Vlavianos, Pangiotis; Habib, Nagy; Westaby, David. Endoscopically applied radiofrequency ablation appears to be safe in the treatment of malignant biliary obstruction.Gastrointestinal Endoscopy vol. 73 issue 1 January, 2011. p. 149-153
[51] Franckena M, Fatehi D, de Bruijne M, Canters RA, van Norden Y, Mens JW, van Rhoon GC, van der Zee J. Long-term improvement in treatment outcome after radiotherapy and hyperthermia in locoregionally advanced cervix cancer: an update of the Dutch Deep Hyperthermia Trial. Int J Radiat Oncol Biol Phys. 2008 Mar 15; 70(4):1176-82. Epub 2007.
[52] van der Zee J, González González D, van Rhoon GC, van Dijk JD, van Putten WL, Hart AA. Comparison of radiotherapy alone with radiotherapy plus hyperthermia in locally

advanced pelvic tumours: a prospective, randomised, multicentre trial. Dutch Deep Hyperthermia Group. Lancet. 2000 Apr 1; 355(9210):1119-25.

[53] Franckena M, Lutgens LC, Koper PC, Kleynen CE, van der Steen-Banasik EM, Jobsen JJ, Leer JW, Creutzberg CL, Dielwart MF, van Norden Y, et al .Radiotherapy and hyperthermia for treatment of primary locally advanced cervix cancer: results in 378 patients. Int J Radiat Oncol Biol Phys. 2009 Jan 1; 73(1):242-50. Epub 2008

[54] Sadick NS. Advances in the treatment of varicose veins: ambulatory phlebectomy, foam sclerotherapy, endovascular laser, and radiofrequency closure. Dermatol Clin. Jul 2005;23(3):443-55

[55] Nael R, Rathbun S. Treatment of varicose veins. Curr Treat Options Cardiovasc Med. Apr 2009;11(2):91-103.

[56] Merchant RF, Pichot O, Myers KA. Four-year follow-up on endovascular radiofrequency obliteration of great saphenous reflux. Dermatol Surg. Feb 2005;31(2):129-34.

[57] Nicolini P. Treatment of primary varicose veins by endovenous obliteration with the VNUS closure system: results of a prospective multicentre study. Eur J Vasc Endovasc Surg. Apr 2005;29(4):433-9.

[58] Helmy ElKaffas K, ElKashef O, ElBaz W. Great saphenous vein radiofrequency ablation versus standard stripping in the management of primary varicose veins-a randomized clinical trial. Angiology. Jan 2011;62(1):49-54.

[59] Brugada J, Berruezo A, Cuesta A, Osca J, Chueca E, Fosch X, Wayar L, Mont L. Nonsurgical transthoracic epicardial radiofrequency ablation: an alternative in incessant ventricular tachycardia. J Am Coll Cardiol. 2003; 41: 2036

[60] Segal OR, Chow AW, Markides V, Schilling RJ, Peters NS, Davies DW. Long-term results after ablation of infarct-related ventricular tachycardia. Heart Rhythm. 2005; 2: 474–482.

[61] Sosa E, Scanavacca M. Percutaneous pericardial access for mapping and ablation of epicardial ventricular tachycardias. Circulation. 2007: 115: e542–e544.

[62] NICE. Percutaneous radiofrequency ablation for atrial fibrillation. National Institute for Health and Clinical Excellence/www.nice.org/IPG168 2006; Guidance 168.

[63] Kampinga HH, Dynlacht JR, Dikomey E: Mechanism of radiosensitization (43 °C) as derived from studies with DNA repair defective mutant cell lines. Int J Hyperthermia, 20: 131-139, 2004.

[64] Kampinga HH: Cell biological effects of hyperthermia alone or combined with radiation or drugs: A short introduction to newcomers in the field. Int J Hyperthermia, 22: 191-196, 2006.

[65] Borys N: Phase I/II study evaluating the maximum tolerated dose, pharmacokinetics, safety, and efficacy of approved hyperthermia and lyso-thermosensitive liposomal doxorubicin in patients with breast cancer recurrence at the chest wall. ASCO abstracts book, 2010.

[66] Wahl ML, Bobyock SB, Leeper DB, Owen CS: Effects of 42 degrees C hyperthermia on intracellular pH in ovarian carcinoma cells during acute or chronic exposure to low extracellular pH. Int J Radiat Oncol Biol Phys, 39: 205-212, 1997.

[67] Nakano H, Kurihara K, Okamoto M, Toné S, Shinohara K: Heat-induced apoptosis and p53 in cultured mammalian cells. Int J Radiat Oncol Biol Phys, 71: 519-529, 1997.

[68] Coss RA, Sedar AW, Sistrun SS, Storck CW, Wang PH, Wachsberger PR: Hsp27 protects the cytoskeleton and nucleus from the effects of 42 degrees C at pH 6.7 in CHO cells adapted to growth at pH 6.7. Int J Hyperthermia, 18: 216-232, 2002

Chapter 6

Principles and Application of RF System for Hyperthermia Therapy

Timothy A. Okhai and Cedric J. Smith

Additional information is available at the end of the chapter

http://dx.doi.org/10.5772/55108

1. Introduction

In recent times, different strategies for thermal ablation therapy have been in use. They include radiofrequency ablation, cryoablation therapy, laser ablation therapy, microwave ablation and high intensity focused ultrasound ablation, among others. *Radiofrequency ablation (RFA)* is used to destroy pathological tissue by inducing tissue necrosis through the heating of targeted tissue [1]. While ablation is currently used in the treatment of different diseases, tumour ablation is considered here, i.e. the treatment of cancerous tumours. Apart from RFA, thermal ablation therapy involves other strategies employed in the destruction of cancerous tumours. *Cryoablation therapy (or cryotherapy)* uses liquid nitrogen (or the expansion of argon gas) to freeze and kill abnormal tissue. After numbing the tissue around the mass, a cryoprobe, which is shaped like a large needle, is inserted into the middle of the lesion. An ice ball forms at the tip of the probe and continues to grow until the images confirm that the entire tumour has been engulfed, killing the tissue [2], [3]. The whole process involved in cryotherapy takes about 10 – 20 minutes to complete. The temperature and duration of freezing necessary to induce complete killing and necrosis are based on numerous in vivo and in vitro animal studies, some of which have been reviewed by Gage & Baust [4]. Generally, it has been accepted that a minimum freezing temperature of -40°C must be reached for at least 3 minutes for complete eradication of the tumour [5]. A rapid freeze followed by a slow thaw is the most damaging to cells, and a minimum of two freeze-thaw cycles (freeze-thaw-freeze-thaw) was necessary for effective cryonecrosis to take place than a single cycle [6]. The cost of a cryoablation unit ranges upwards from $190,000, and each multi-use cryoprobe costs approximately $3,750 [7]. *Laser Ablation (or interstitial laser photocoagulation)* uses a highly concentrated beam of light to penetrate the cancerous tissue. The laser energy is emitted from an optical fibre placed within a needle positioned at the centre of the tumour using either stereotactic guidance or Magnetic Resonance Imaging (MRI) [8], [9]. Two methods for delivery of light have been described to produce larger volumes of necrosis: multiple bare fibres in an array and cooled-tip diffuser fibres. The major drawback to this technique is its cost, requiring $30,000 to $75,000 for a portable, solid-state laser and $3,000 per set of multiple (50) user fibres [10]. *Microwave ablation (MWA) or microwave coagulation* uses microwave tissue coagulator for irradiation. Ultra-high frequency (2450 MHz) microwaves are emitted from a percutaneously placed microwave electrode inserted into the target tissue under ultrasonographic guidance. Microwave irradiation is carried out for about 60 seconds at a power setting of 60W per pulse. During irradiation, the ultrasonographic probe is placed adjacent to the microwave electrode to monitor the effectiveness of the tumour coagulation [11], [12]. A typical microwave generator costs approximately $65,000 [13]. *High Intensity Focused Ultrasound (HIFU) ablation* is a non-invasive treatment modality that induces complete coagulative necrosis of a deep tumour through the intact skin. HIFU uses sound energy to produce heat [14]-[16]. HIFU treatments are usually carried out in a single session, often as a day case procedure in the doctor's office, with the patient either fully conscious, lightly sedated or under light general anaesthesia. One major advantage of HIFU over other thermal ablation techniques is that the transcutaneous insertion of probes into the target tissue is not necessary. The high powered focused beams employed in the procedure are generated from sources placed either outside the body (for treatment of tumours of the liver, kidney, breast, uterus, pancreas and bone) or in the rectum (for treatment of the prostate), and are designed to enable rapid heating of a target tissue volume, while leaving tissue in the ultrasound propagation path relatively unaffected [17]. Numerous extra-corporeal, transrectal and interstitial devices have been designed to optimise application-specific treatment delivery for HIFU procedures.

This chapter focuses on the discussion of principles and application of the radiofrequency ablation therapy system as a minimally invasive treatment modality for hyperthermia therapy. Detailed work completed in the use of radiofrequency (RF) energy in cancer management by developing and testing an economical and effective thermal probe that will effectively destroy volumes of pathological tumours by means of hyperthermia is presented.

2. Radiofrequency energy and the RF ablation system

Basically, the term *radio-frequency* refers not to the emitted waves, but rather to the alternating electric current that oscillates in the high frequency range. Radiofrequency is a form of electromagnetic energy. This energy is formed from waves of electromagnetic energy moving together (or radiating) through space at the speed of light. Unlike ionizing radiation (e.g. gamma rays and x-rays), which affects the chemical makeup of cells and alters their genetic code, electromagnetic energy is non-ionizing. This means that it is not strong enough to ionize atoms and molecules in cells or alter their genetic makeup. Radiofrequency energy is safer than many cancer therapies because it is absorbed by living tissue as simple heat. Regardless of the heat source, cells die when they reach a certain temperature. The main tumoricidal effect of RF ablation occurs because the absorption of electromagnetic energy induces thermal injury to the tissue. But RF energy and the heat it generates does not alter the basic chemical structure of cells. A very important part of the RF ablation system is the RF signal generator. This is where the energy deposited by the needle-like active electrode is generated. The system comprises of a closed circuit consisting of a radiofrequency generator circuit, a power amplifier circuit, and the control circuit. A power supply circuit is also included to meet the power supply requirements of the system. The energy generated by the system is delivered to the tissue by the active electrode, whereas a dispersive electrode that acts as a patient plate provides a return part to complete the circuit. A simplified block diagram of the whole system is shown in figure 1 below.

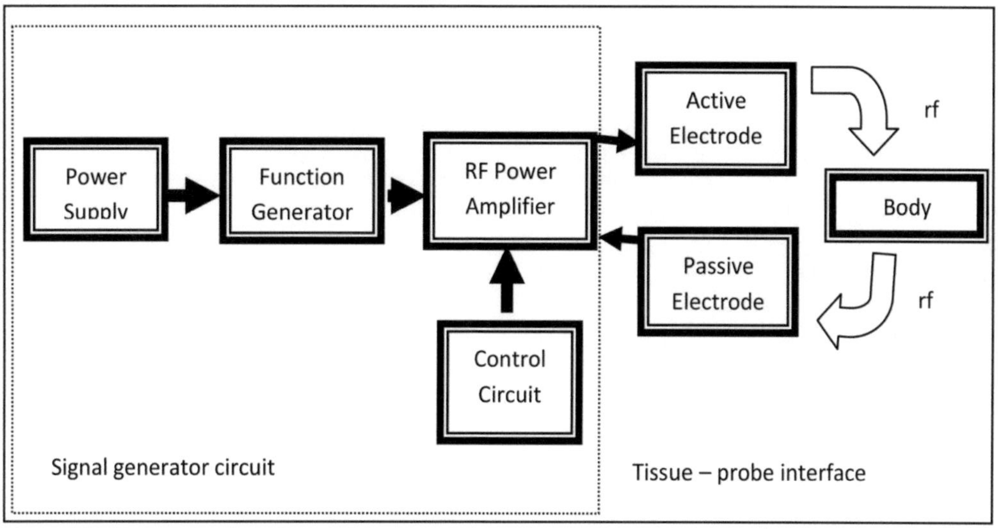

Figure 1. Block diagram of the RF ablation circuits

2.1. Hyperthermic (thermal) coagulation necrosis

Coagulation necrosis denotes "irreversible thermal damage to cells even if the ultimate manifestations of cell death do not fulfill the strict histological criteria of coagulative necrosis" [18]. The nature of the thermal damage caused by radiofrequency heating is dependent on both the tissue temperature achieved and the duration of heating. Here is what happens at various temperatures:

- At 42°C, cells die but it may take a significant amount of time (approximately 60 min).
- Between 42°C and 45°C, cells are more susceptible to damage by other agents like chemotherapy and radiation.
- Over 46°C irreversible damage occurs depending on the duration of heating.
- Between 50°C and 55°C, the duration necessary to shorten irreversible damage to cells is shortened to 4 – 6 minutes.
- Between 50°C and 100°C there is near immediate coagulation of tissue, almost instantaneous protein denaturation, melting of lipid bilayers, irreversible damage to mitochondrial and cytosolic (key cellular) enzymes of the cells, DNA and RNA.
- From 100°C to 110°C, tissue vaporizes and carbonizes, all of which decrease energy transmission and impede ablation.

Figure 2 shows tissue reaction to thermal injury at different temperatures [19]. For successful ablation, the tissue temperature should be maintained in the ideal range (50 – 100°C) to ablate tumour adequately and avoid carbonization around the tip of the electrode due to excessive heating. For adequate destruction of tumour tissue, the entire volume of a lesion must be subjected to cytotoxic temperatures. Hence effective heating throughout the target volume (i.e. the tumour and about 5mm thickness around normal tissue) is required as shown in figure 3. Thus, the main objective of radiofrequency ablation therapy is to reach and maintain a temperature range of 50° – 100°C throughout the entire target volume for at least 4 – 6 minutes. However, the relatively slow thermal conduction from the electrode surface through the tissues increases the duration of application to 10 – 30 minutes.

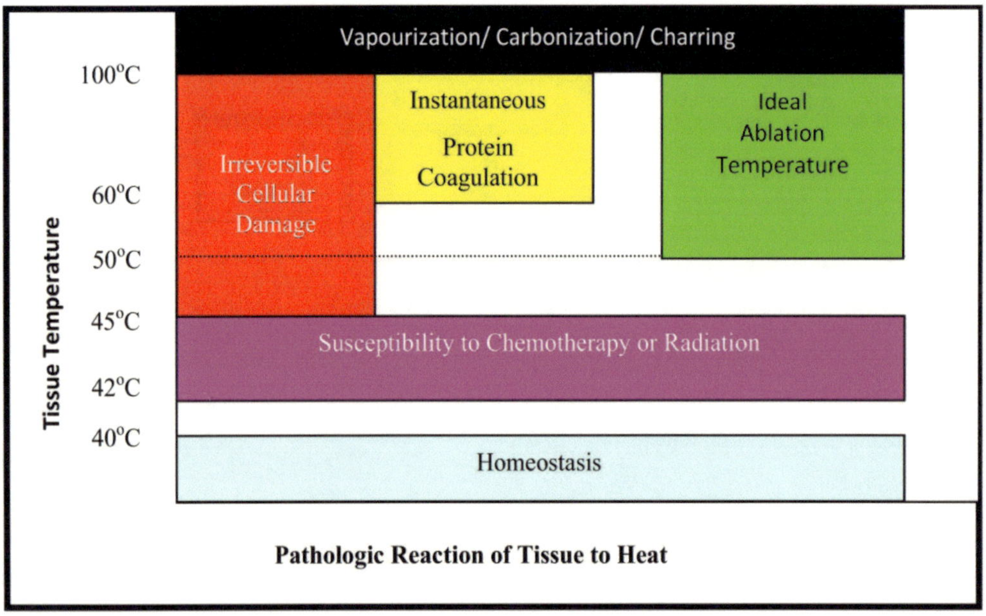

Figure 2. Tissue reaction to thermal injury at different temperatures

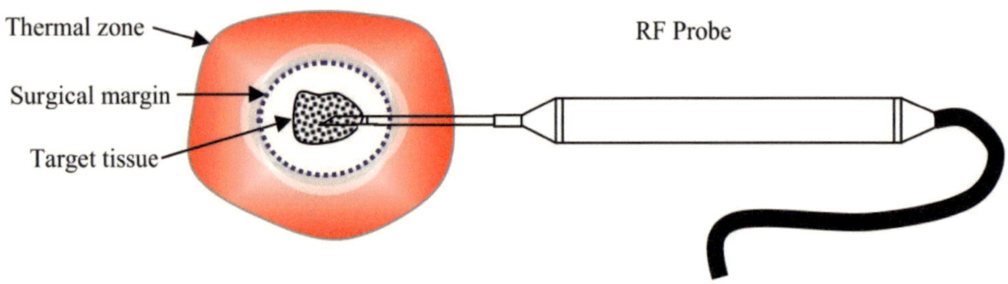

Figure 3. Schematic diagram illustrating RF ablation

Recommendations of heating for these extended durations are based on experimental and clinical data suggesting that thermal equilibrium and, hence, complete induction of coagulation are not achieved for a given radiofrequency application until these thresholds are achieved. The development of a radiofrequency ablation system in this study is aimed at producing a device that is able to satisfy the minimum requirement for effective tumour ablation at the ideal (cytotoxic) ablation temperature.

2.2. Principles of radiofrequency ablation

Radiofrequency ablation is physically based on radiofrequency current (about 460 kHz) that passes through the target tissue from the tip of an active electrode (RF thermal probe) towards a dispersive electrode which serves as the grounding pad. These two electrodes are connected to a radiofrequency generator. The active electrode has a very small cross-sectional area (a few square millimetres) with respect to the passive electrode. The active electrode is usually fashioned into the form of a needle-like probe that is inserted into the tumour. The dispersive electrode has a much larger area than the active electrode, on the order of $100cm^2$ or larger, and is usually placed firmly behind the right shoulder or the thigh of the subject, depending on the location of the tumour in the body. Current flowing into the dispersive electrode is the same as the current flowing into the active electrode. But since the active electrode has a far smaller cross-sectional area than the dispersive electrode, the current density in amperes per square meter (A/m^2) is far greater. As a result of the difference in current density between the two electrodes, the energy at the tip of the probe leads to ionic agitation with subsequent conversion of friction into heat. The tissue ions are agitated as they attempt to follow the changes in direction of alternating electric current as shown in figure 4 below.

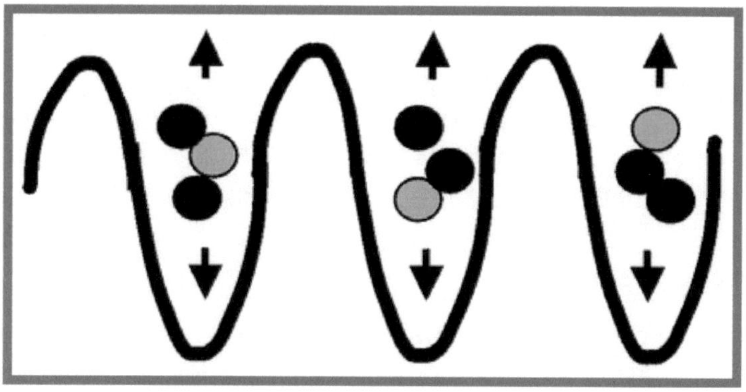

Figure 4. Ionic agitation by alternating electric current

The agitation results in frictional heat around the electrode. The marked discrepancy between the surface area of the needle electrode and the dispersive electrode causes the generated heat to be tightly focused and concentrated around the needle electrode. The use of a large grounding pad ensures maximum surface area for dispersion of current from the needle electrode. The grounding pad also maximizes dispersion of equal amounts of energy and heat at the grounding pad sites, thereby minimizes the risk of burns. The tissue underneath the passive electrode heats up only slightly, while the tissue in contact with the active electrode is resistively heated to elevated temperatures sufficient for tumour ablation (coagulative necrosis). The strategy of RF ablation is to create a closed-loop circuit including the RF generator, the needle electrode, the patient (tissue) and the passive electrode (grounding pad) in series. The heating of tissue is due to the power dissipated in the tissue, which is found from the expression

$$P = \rho V I_d^2 \quad (1)$$

where P is the power in watts (W), ρ is the resistivity of the tissue in Ohm-metres (Ω-m), V is the tissue volume in cubic metres (m^3), and I_d is the current density in amperes per square metre (A/m^2).

Appreciable advances have been made over the past decade to produce application devices for RFA. The *Radionics probe* is an internally cooled device that also uses pulsing sequences to improve heating. It is available in one size (17Ga) and 10, 15, and 25cm lengths. It comes with a single electrode with a tip exposure of 2-4cm, or cluster electrode [20]. The *RITA probe* is a 15Ga device that comes with various arrays. It has a thermocouple at the tip of the probe that registers the tissue temperature, and that is used to monitor its effect. The *LeVeen probe* has multiple (36, 37) tines. There are 2.0, 3.0, 3.5 and 4.0cm diameter needles from which the tines are deployed. The LeVeen needle electrode is designed to deliver a consistent pattern of heat throughout the lesion [21]. These and other application devices for RFA are available for use in the USA and some parts of Europe. In spite of technical progress in the development of various application devices for radiofrequency ablation therapy, most patients with malignant tumours, especially in Sub-Saharan Africa, have not yet benefitted from this technology due to their limited availability and exhorbitant cost. A typical RF generator costs $25,000 and each single use probe costs approximately $800 to $1200 [22]. This paper presents the structure and experimental results of a low cost minimally invasive radiofrequency thermal probe developed for hyperthermia therapy. The probe developed is effective and economical, and represents more than 70% in cost reduction compared to commercially available reusable RF thermal probes reviewed.

3. Materials and methods

The RF thermal probe developed was designed on a SolidWorks platform and manufactured according to design specifications. The device consists of an RF shielded insulated handle with a needle probe. The shaft of the needle is also insulated except for the tip which makes physical contact with the tumour or volume to be treated. A coaxial cable connects the device to the RF power unit. The RF thermal probe uses a stainless steel needle (size 14G x 3-1/4) with a diameter and length of 2.1 x 80 mm, connected to the conducting coaxial cable in one end, and housed in an epoxy resin holder (probe handle) that is 120 mm long and 15 mm in diameter. The stainless steel needle is insulated, except for the exposed 20 mm tip that makes direct contact with tissue. The insulation prevents normal tissue from being destroyed along with cancerous tissue during thermal ablation treatment. The probe (as shown in figure 5) is reusable and is made of epoxy-resin material that can be easily steam-cleaned.

An essential objective of radiofrequency ablation therapy is to achieve and maintain a temperature range of 50 – 100°C throughout the entire target volume for at least 4 – 6 minutes [23-25]. From equation (1), power dissipated (P) is directly proportional to volume (V). Tumour is usually treated as a sphere, and volume of a sphere is given by,

$$V = (4/3)\pi r^3 \tag{2}$$

where r is the radius of the sphere. It follows that, power dissipated is directly proportional to the cube of the radius. The temperature rise follows the accepted cube root heating function. This means that the outer limit of critical cell temperature where cell necrosis takes place is reasonably well-defined by the applied power and will be spherical around a point source if the impedance remains constant. In practice, we have a short cylindrical contact volume in the tumour with non linear impedances. This results in an egg shaped volume being treated.

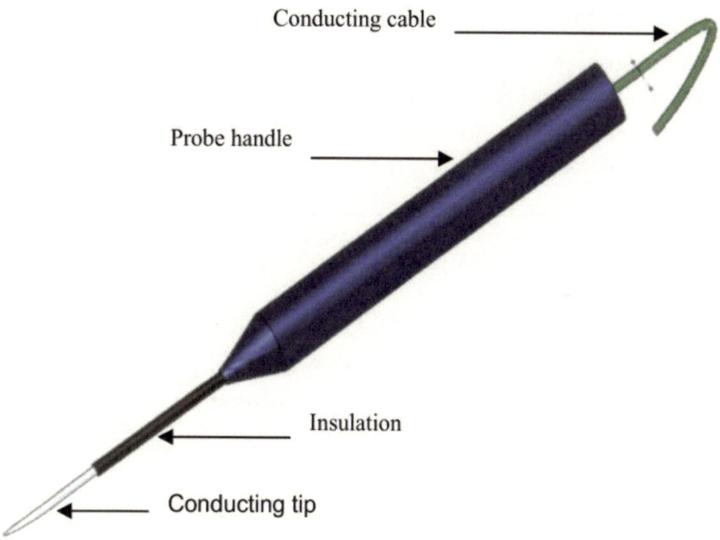

Figure 5. RF thermal probe

To verify that the radiofrequency thermal probe developed is a device that is able to satisfy this minimum requirement for effective tumour ablation at the ideal cytotoxic temperature, experimental tests were done with different tissues types to determine how each tissue type responds to RF energy by observing and recording the temperature change at the probe tip. Liver, lung, brain, kidney and soft tissue were tested at different power settings to determine which power setting gives the best results with each tissue type in terms of the minimum time to reach the ideal temperature range, and the maximum time to remain within this range without charring or vapourizing. An RF generator (460 KHz) was connected in a closed circuit with the RF thermal probe, tissue sample, and dispersive electrode in series. Each tissue type was tested with different power settings, and each test was done for about 15 minutes.

4. Results and discussion

The extent of coagulation necrosis is dependent on the energy deposited, local tissue interaction minus the heat lost.

$$\textit{Coagulation necrosis} = \textit{energy deposited} \times \textit{local tissue interactions} - \textit{heat loss}$$

Heat efficacy is defined as the difference between the amount of heat produced and the amount of heat lost. Therefore, effective ablation can be achieved by optimizing heat production and minimizing heat loss within the area to be ablated. The relationship between these factors has been well characterized as the "bio-heat equation." Heat production is correlated with the intensity and duration of the radio-frequency energy deposited. Heat conduction or diffusion is usually explained as a factor of heat loss in regard to the electrode tip. Heat is lost mainly through convection by means of blood circulation. Therefore, the cooling tissue by perfusion can limit the reproducible size of the ablation lesion in vivo.

Macroscopic and microscopic examination of tissue samples tested show clear evidence of coagulation necrosis. A tissue volume of up to 20 mm diameter was necrosed with the single-tine probe developed. The plots of temperature versus time for different tissue types tested using different power settings are presented in the following figures:

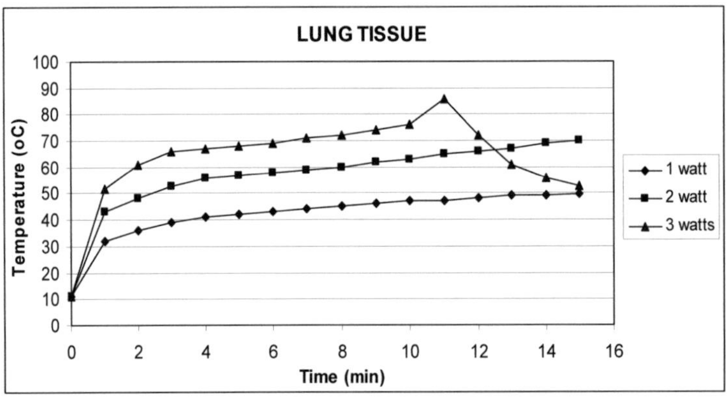

Figure 6. Lung tissue results.

From figure 6, it is seen that, while 1 watt was inadequate for coagulation necrosis in lung tissue, 3 watts showed evidence of carbonization, leading to a drop in temperature as further conduction is inhibited. The best result was achieved with 2 watts, which showed a steady rise in temperature maintained within the ideal ablation temperature range.

The plot in figure 7 shows that, while 2 watts was below the ideal temperature range, and therefore inadequate for effective tissue necrosis, 4 watts was too high and showed evidence of carbonization, resulting in a drop in temperature due to inhibition in conduction. The best result in terms of effective tissue necrosis was achieved with the 3 watts power setting.

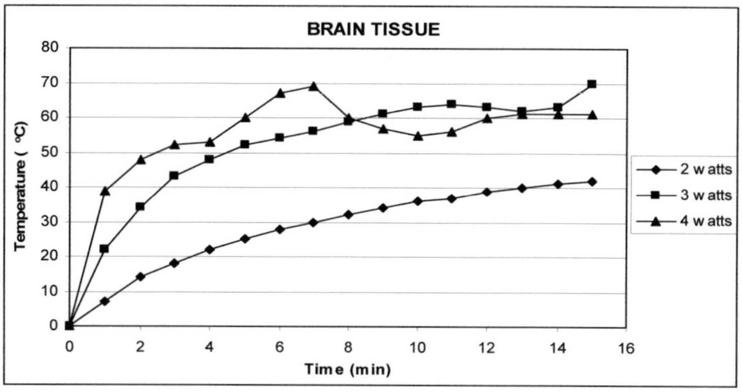

Figure 7. Brain tissue results.

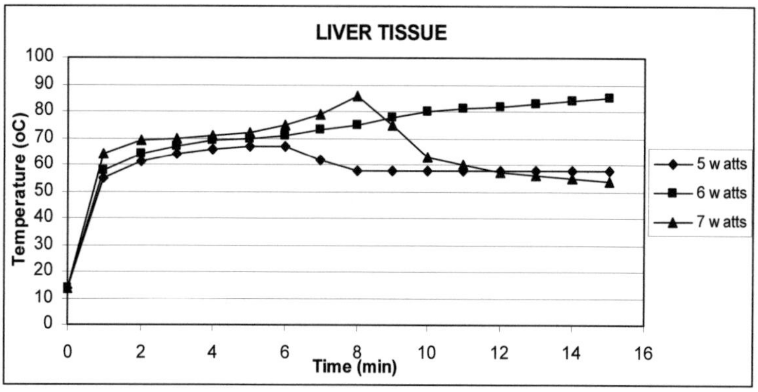

Figure 8. Liver tissue results.

In figure 8, the plot shows that, while 5 watts and 6 watts are within the ideal ablation zone, the 7 watts setting is too high for liver tissue as it produced carbonization resulting in temperature drop. The best result however was recorded with the 6 watts setting which shows a steady rise in temperature without carbonization or charring.

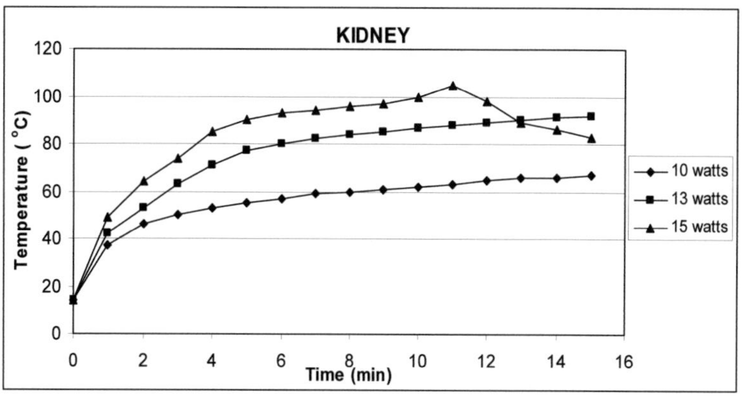

Figure 9. Kidney tissue results.

In figure 9, the results show that 15 watts produced temperature above the ideal ablation range, leading to carbonization and consequently a drop in temperature. Both 10 watts and 13 watts are suitable for ablating kidney tissue as seen, with 13 watts giving the best results since it allows the use of a higher temperature.

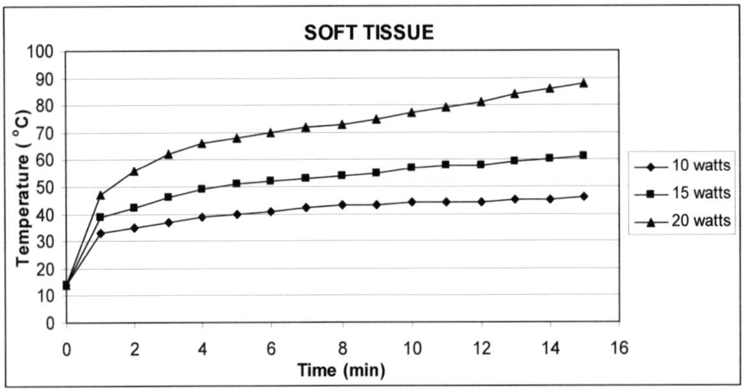

Figure 10. Soft tissue test results.

In figure 10, the results show that, while 15 watts produced temperature within the ideal ablation range, the best result was obtained with the 20 watts power setting since the temperature is higher. This means that the ideal temperature range for treatment will be reached quicker with 20 watts. The 10 watts power setting produces temperature below the ideal range, and was therefore inadequate for ablating soft tissue.

5. Summary of results

The above results have been summarized in table 2 below showing the different tissue types, the best power settings suitable for each tissue type, the minimum and maximum time required to keep the temperature within the ideal ablation range of 50 to 100^{0}C, and the total duration. The total duration is the difference between the maximum time and minimum time.

Tissue Type	Power (w)	Min. Time (min)	Max. Time (min)	Duration (min)
Brain	3.0	4.30	15.0	10.30
Kidney	13.0	1.30	15.0	13.30
Liver	6.0	0.30	15.0	14.30
Lung	2.0	2.30	15.0	12.30
Soft tissue	20.0	1.30	15.0	13.30

Table 1. Summary of results

6. Conclusion

The search for less morbid and less invasive techniques for cancer treatment has led to a strong drive within the global oncology community to develop and implement even more minimally invasive diagnostic and therapeutic procedures. The goals of these minimally invasive therapies for the treatment of cancerous tumours that have made them attractive to both patients and physicians are summarized as:

- Viable and effective treatment options and eradicate in situ local disease
- They are minimally invasive and less traumatic
- Real-time imaging guidance is possible
- Most procedures require only local anaesthesia, and recovery time is faster
- Procedure can be repeated in case of cancer recurrence
- They are safer, with minimal side effects, and limit postoperative morbidities and mortality
- Real-time imaging guidance is possible
- Non-surgical candidates can benefit from these treatment modalities
- They can be performed as an outpatient procedure, or with only a short hospital stay
- Shorten the time to return to daily function and work, and
- Their low-cost make them cheaper and ultimately reduce the overall cost of cancer treatment.

With several ablation techniques available, the ablation characteristics and method of application will differentiate one ablation method from another. Though RF ablation is more widely used, it has its limitations. Most thermo-ablative procedures could be performed in the doctor's office as an outpatient procedure with mild or no sedation. With RF ablation, it requires an increase in temperature to induce necrosis (tissue death). The heat needed for this necrosis requires that large amount of local anaesthetic be infused around the treatment site. This excess fluid blurs the ultrasound visualization of RFA and other heat-based ablation techniques. Though all the available literature agree that thermal ablation therapy is relatively safe and much less traumatic than radical surgical procedures, some complications and side effects have been reported. Some of these complications and side effects have been associated with probe design, probe placement, or the use of multiple probes. The use of both single and multiple probe placements have been described in many studies. Both have their advantages and disadvantages. Though multiple probes appear to be more successful in destroying larger tissue volumes, their use increases the risk of complications in the procedure. Finally, the high cost of RF ablation equipment, coupled with their limited availability has placed these treatment procedures above the reach of most patients and physicians in Sub-Saharan Africa. This project work which aims to investigate the design and development of a minimally invasive thermo-active oncology probe, will narrow this price gap and make treatment more affordable, and readily available to the ordinary patient in Sub-Saharan Africa.

Author details

Timothy A. Okhai
Clinical Engineering Department, Faculty of Engineering and The Built Environment, Tshwane University of Technology, Pretoria, South Africa

Cedric J. Smith
Centurion Academy, Pretoria, South Africa

7. References

[1] Singleton SE. 2003. "Radiofrequency ablation of breast cancer", American journal of surgery, vol. 69, pp. 37-40.

[2] Cowan BD., Sewell PE., Howard JC., Arriola RM., and Robinette LG. 2002. "Interventional Magnetic Resonance Imaging Cryotherapy of Uterine Fibroid Tumours: Preliminary Observation", American journal of obstetricians and gynecologists, vol.186, no. 6, pp. 1183-1187.

[3] Anonymous. 2002. "Ablation therapy destroys breast cancer without scarring", Radiological Society of North America. http://www.rsna.org/ (Last accessed: 10 June 2008).

[4] Gage AA. & Baust J, 1998. "Mechanism of tissue injury in cryosurgery", Cryobiology, 37:171-186.

[5] Moore Y., Sofer P., & Ilovich M., 2001. "The science and technology behind cryosurgery. Technical notes, [Online]. Available from: http://www.galilmedical.com/Prostate/The%20science%20and%20technology%20behind%20cryosurgery.pdf (Accessed: 10 May 2005).

[6] Larson TR., Robertson DW., Corica A., & Bostwick DG., 2000. "In vivo interstitial temperature mapping of the human prostate during cryosurgery with correlation to histopathologic outcomes", Urology, 55: 547-552.

[7] Dodd III GD., Soulen MC., Kante RA. et al, 2000. "Minimally invasive treatment of malignant hepatic tumors: At the threshold of a major breakthrough", Radiographics, vol. 20, pp. 9-27.

[8] Bloom KJ., Dowlat K., and Assad L., 2001. "Pathologic changes after interstitial laser therapy of infiltrating breast carcinoma", American journal of surgery, vol. 182, pp. 384-388.

[9] Sabel MS. 2001. "In Situ Ablation of Breast Tumors. What is The State of the Art?", Cancernews, [Online], Available from: http://www.cancernews.com/articles/breastcancer therapies.htm (Last accessed: 19 August 2008).

[10] Shah A. 2000. "Recent developments in the chemotherapeutic management of colorectal cancer", BC Medical Journal, vol. 42, pp. 180-182.

[11] Gardner RA., Vargas HI., and Block JB. 2002. "Focused microwave phased array thermotherapy for primary breast cancer", Annals of surgical oncology, vol. 9, pp. 326-332.

[12] Ishikawa T., Kohno T., Shibayama T., Fukushima Y, Obi T., Teratani T., Shiina S., Shiratori Y., and Omata M. 2001. "Thoracoscopic thermal ablation for hepatocellular carcinoma located beneath the diaphragm", Endoscopy, vol. 33(8), pp. 697-702.

[13] Ho SG., Munk PL., Legiehn GM., Chung SW., Scudamore CH., and Lee MJ., 2002. "Minimally invasive treatment of colorectal cancer metastasis: Current status and new directions", BC Medical Journal, vol. 42, no. 10, pp. 461-464.

[14] Hynynen K., Pomeroy O., and Smith DN. 2001. "MR Imaging-guided focused ultrasound surgery of fibroadenomas in the breast: a feasibility study", Radiology, vol. 219, pp. 176-185.

[15] Wu F, Wang ZB., Cao YD, Chen WZ, Bai J., Zou JZ., and Zhu H. 2003. "A randomized clinical trial of high-intensity focused ultrasound ablation for the treatment of patients with localized breast cancer", British journal of cancer, vol. 89, pp. 2227-2233.

[16] Wu F., Wang Z., Chen W., Zhu H., Bai J., Zou J., Li K., Jin C., Xie F., and Su H., 2004. "Extracorporeal high intensity focused ultrasound ablation in the treatment of patients with large hepatocellular carcinoma", Annals of surgical oncology, vol. 11, pp. 1061-1069.

[17] Haar GT, and Coussios C, 2007. "High intensity focused ultrasound: Physical principles and devices", International Journal of Hyperthermia, Vol. 23, No. 2, pp 89-104.

[18] Caridi, J. (comp.), "Radio-frequency ablation", University of Florida, Florida, 2004.

[19] Rhim, H., Goldberg, S.N., Dodd, G.D., Solbiati, L., Lim, K. L., Tonolini, M., & Cho, O.N. 2001. Helping the hepatic surgeon: Essential techniques for successful radio-frequency thermal ablation of malignant hepatic tumours. *Radiographics*, 21:S17-S35.
http://radiographics.rsnajnls.org/cgi/content/full/21/suppl_/1/S17
(Accessed: 26/07/2005).

[20] Anonymous, *RadiologyInfo.*
http://www.radiologyinfo.org/en/photocat/photos_pc.cfm?image=ri-rfa-devices.jpg&pg=rfa, 2007. (Accessed: 15 September 2008).

[21] Anonymous, *Boston Scientific Company.* http://tinyurl.com/d2dbt4e, 2007. (Accessed: 27 June 2008).

[22] Dodd III GD., Soulen MC., Kante RA.et al. "Minimally invasive treatment of malignant hepatic tumors: At the threshold of a major breakthrough", *Radiographics, 2000, vol.* 20, pp. 9-27.

[23] Rhim H., Goldberg SN., Dodd GD, Solbiati L., Lim KL., Tonolini M., and Cho ON. "Helping the hepatic surgeon: Essential techniques for successful radio-frequency thermal ablation of malignant hepatic tumours", *Radiographics*, 2007, vol. 21, pp. S17-S35.

[24] Goldberg SN., Solbiati L., Gazelle GS., Tanabe KK., Compton CC., and Mueller PR. "Treatment of intrahepatic malignancy with radio-frequency ablation: radiologic-

pathologic correlation in 16 patients" (abstr), *American journal of roentgenology, 168. [American Roentgen Ray Society 97th Annual Meeting Program Book suppl], 1997, pp. 121.*

[25] Goldberg SN., Gazelle GS., and Mueller PR. "Thermal ablation therapy for focal malignancy. A unified approach to underlying principles, techniques, and diagnostic image guidance", *American journal of roentgenology,* 2000, vol. 174, pp. 323-331.

Chapter 7

Effects of Low-Dose Radon Therapy Applied Under Hyperthermic Conditions (RnHT) on Inflammatory and Non-Inflammatory Degenerative Disease Conditions

Angelika Moder, Heidi Dobias and Markus Ritter

Additional information is available at the end of the chapter

http://dx.doi.org/10.5772/51401

1. Introduction

Low dose radon therapy is a traditional treatment in Central and Eastern Europe typically applied to alleviate chronic pain derived from inflammatory and non-inflammatory disorders of the musculoskeletal system. Additionally it has also been reported to be effective for the treatment of chronic airway inflammation and inflammatory conditions of the skin.

Radon (^{222}Rn) is a radioactive alpha particle emitting inert gas, present in natural soil and water at several European, Japanese and American health resorts and is administered either transcutaneously by balneotherapy or per inhalationem by balneotherapy or per inhalationem by speleotherapy either at „cold" ambient temperature of 20° to 23° C (RnT) or at „hot" ambient temperatures between 37° and 41.5° C (RnHT). Speleotherapy is performed in curative caves and tunnels where radon emanation occurs due to the presence of uranium containing soil. Low dose ^{222}Rn - balneotherapy is performed in bath tubs filled with ^{222}Rn containing thermal water at a concentration typically found in the respective region but usually between 370 and 1600 Bq/L. Whereas ^{222}Rn-containing water is typically applied at 37.0° C, speleotherapeutic administration is performed either as RnT [1] or RnHT. The latter treatment regime is uniquely performed at the Gasteiner Heilstollen in Bad Gastein, Austria, which offers an average ^{222}Rn concentration of 44000 Bq/m^3 in a hyperthermic atmosphere between 37.0° and 41.5° C with high humidity between 70 and 100% that facilitates a mild increase of the body's core-temperature of 0.5 - 1° Cdue to prevention of heat loss via evaporation confirmed by rectal measurement. A typical low-dose ^{222}Rn-therapy consists of nine to ten treatment units within a period of three weeks and an effective dose of 0.05 to 2 mSv for balneotherapeutic and speleotherapeutic regimen, respectively [2]. ^{222}Rn has a half-life of 3.8 days and decays via several short-lived daughters into the beta-emitting ^{210}Plumbum with a half-life of 22.3 years. In general, radionuclide-based therapy has a long history in the management of rheumatic diseases and has been proven to alleviate pain and inflammation upon intraarticular or intravenous injection. Apart from conventional corticoid or cytostatic based therapy, radiosynoviorthesis is an alternative approach for the management of synovitis in course of chronic inflammatory arthropathies. The intraarticular injection of colloidal beta-emitters, e.g. ^{90}Yttrium, ^{186}Rhenium or ^{169}Erbium, lead to reduction of pain and joint swelling via abrogation of synovia hypertrophy by radiation-induced inhibition of the proliferative activity of synovial cells. The applied dose depends on the magnitude of the affected joint(s) and the severity of inflammation, whereas factors like intraarticular distribution of the radionuclide and thickness of the synovia dictate the absorbed dose. Therapeutic benefits in terms of pain and reduction of the inflammatory symptoms occur in 40 to 80% of the patients and manifest several months after therapy. However, numerous side effects like headache, fatigue, nausea and sometimes lymphedema, radiation-induced synovitis and periarticular necrosis due to aberrant injections have been reported [3].

Positive therapeutic effects of ^{224}Radiumchloride-injections for patients suffering from ankylosing spondylitis were reported from Koch and Reske in 1952[4], after this therapy had been abolished due to the high incidence of malignant bone tumours and leukaemia in children and young adults previously treated for tuberculosis. Until now several studies have been conducted with a reduced dose regimen of 10 weekly injections with 1 MBq each resulting in an effective dose of 2.5 Sv [5] and a cumulative bone dose of 0.6 Gy [6]. The short-lived ^{224}Radium has a half-life of 3.6 days and preferentially accumulates in the bone and in recently formed tissue calcifications when introduced into the body. In 2000 it was re-approved in Germany by the German Federal Institute for Drugs and Medical Devices (Bundesinstitut für Arzneimittel und Medizinprodukte) as a pharmaceutical product for patients suffering from ankylosing spondylitis with stage II and III spinal ossification, provided that other therapy options had either failed or been contraindicated. However, recent findings clearly demonstrated an increased incidence of leukaemia and other malignant diseases in patients that were treated between 1948 and 1975 [6]. Despite the analgesic effects elicited by ^{224}Radiumchloride-injections, the risk for malignant diseases exceeds the benefit and therefore, the committee for quality assurance of the German Society for Rheumatology no longer recommends this kind of therapy. Compared to a ^{222}Rn-speleotherapy regimen according to dosimetric calculations by Hofmann [7], the average dose to bone achieved by ^{224}Radiumchloride injection regimen is approximately a factor $3x10^5$ higher. In contrast to the bone-seeking ^{224}Radiumchlorid, inhalation of ^{222}Rn and its daughters lead to a dose distribution that predominantly affects the bronchial epithelium in the upper tracheobronchial tree. When administered balneotherapeutically, diffusion of ^{222}Rn through the skin results in a uniform dose distribution throughout the organism [7]. To the best knowledge of the authors up to date no evidence points to an increased risk for the development of malignant diseases in context with RnHT [1, 2, 8].

Hyperthermia treatment (HT) has been reported to exert analgesic effects in rheumatoid disorders, to reduce systemic levels of the pro-inflammatory cytokines TNF-alpha, IL-1beta, and IL-6 [9, 10] and to accelerate the healing of sport injuries [11]. The postulated mechanisms include increased blood perfusion of the affected tissues and relaxation of muscle tissue. Given the fact, that combined RnHT or hyperthermia alone has been reported to alleviate pain in rheumatic conditions, presently, it cannot clearly be distinguished to which extent each of the active components – ^{222}Rn and/or hyperthermia – are efficient for achieving the clinical-therapeutic benefits. According to empirical observations described below, these two agents may rather act in a synergistic manner.

Apart from clinical observations, evidence from several controlled trials, one meta-analysis and numerous clinical observational studies further substantiate the beneficial effects of intermediate up to long term pain relief and functional improvement in patients suffering from rheumatic disorders of inflammatory or degenerative etiology. From a health economic point of view, cost effective therapies in the prevention or management of rheumatic diseases are of great importance since rheumatic disorders state a relevant cost factor due to the need for long term medication, frequent hospitalizations, joint arthroplasty and loss of productivity. The dramatically increasing proportion of aged individuals further aggravates the health economic issue of rheumatic diseases since at least the prevalence of non-inflammatory, degenerative rheumatic disorders increases with progressing age [12].

The long term intake of typically employed corticosteroids and non-steroidal anti-inflammatory drugs (NSAID) for the treatment of rheumatic disorders are reported to cause severe side effects that - apart from the primary disease - result in additional medical interventions and dramatically reduce the life quality of the affected individual. Some years ago, the mortality rate caused by gastrointestinal side effects due to NSAID intake was about 2000 per year in Germany [13] and 16.500 per year in the USA [14]. Despite the additional intake of gastro-protective drugs, the ratio of NSAID-consumers suffering from gastrointestinal ulcers was 1 in 400 and the ratio of those who died was 1 in 8000 [15]. The generation of cyclooxygenase-2 inhibitors diminished the risk for gastrointestinal complications, however, the elevated risk for cardio-vascular events remained [16-18]. Taken together, from the patient´s as well as from the socio-economic point of view there is an urgent need for therapeutic strategies that allow either a reduction or discontinuation of medicament intake [19]. Combined RnHT can be regarded as a promising candidate in addressing these issues. Lind-Albrecht et al. demonstrated a long term reduction of analgesics during a 12-years follow-up in patients suffering from ankylosing spondylitis, who regularly received combined RnHT [20].

A recently published meta-analysis including 338 patients suffering from rheumatic disorders showed a superior effect of combined RnHT compared to hyperthermia therapy in terms of pain reduction [21]. Although there was no difference between the treatment groups immediately after the therapeutic regimen, the group receiving the combination of ^{222}Rn and hyperthermia showed a significantly lower pain score during the three - and six - months follow-up. Prospective, randomized studies comparing the effect of combined RnTT with either HT or no treatment were included in the meta-analysis and are described along with more recently published findings in detail below.

Franke et. al demonstrated an intermediate to long term pain reduction in patients suffering from rheumatoid arthritis during a nine month follow-up after combined RnHT. This randomized, double-blinded study included 134 patients and compared the efficacy of balneotherapeutic regimen applied at 37° C either with or without ^{222}Rn. Although both groups showed a beneficial effect immediately after therapy, the radon group predominated significantly at the three and six months follow up. Similar results were obtained concerning cut-down in NSAID and corticosteroid intake [22]. Consistent with these findings, a previous study including 60 patients with rheumatoid arthritis clearly demonstrated pain reduction and functional improvement of affected joints after a typical regimen of thermal water baths. However, patients receiving ^{222}Rn thermal water showed a significantly pronounced effect on the analyzed parameters [23].

Van Tubergen et al. investigated in course of a randomized, controlled study the efficacy of speleotherapeutically applied RnHT combined with a complex rehabilitation program including gymnastics, hydro – and sport therapy. 120 patients suffering from ankylosing spondylitis were enrolled in the study and randomized in two treatment and one control group. Whereas the control group maintained its regular physiotherapeutic program at home, the intervention groups received the complex rehabilitation program either concomitantly with hyperthermia treatment in form of sauna regimen or concomitantly with speleotherapeutic combined RnHT. Bath Ankylosing Spondylitis Functional Index (BASFI), quality of life assessment score, pain score on a visual analogue scale and duration of morning stiffness were taken together to a Pooled Index of Change (PIC) as primary endpoint. Immediately after therapy both intervention groups showed a 20 to 30% improvement in contrast to the control group that remained unaffected. In the six to nine months follow up only the ^{222}Rn group significantly prevailed [24, 25].

In line with these results, Lind-Albrecht demonstrated a significant long-term pain reduction, improved mobility of the spine and reduced drug intake of patients with ankylosing spondylitis receiving a rehabilitation program combined with speleotherapeutic RnHT compared to those, who exclusively received the rehabilitation program [26, 27].

According to two double-blinded randomized studies by Pratzel et al., an intermediate-term pain reduction could be achieved by serially applied thermal water baths with or without ^{222}Rn in patients with non-inflammatory cervical syndrome and degenerative disorders of spine or joints, respectively. Immediately after therapy both treatment groups benefitted from an elevated threshold of pressure-provoked pain in the paravertebral muscles. A sustainable and significant pain reduction lasting until the two and four months follow-up could be demonstrated only in the ^{222}Rn group [28, 29].

A recent prospective study including 222 patients suffering from non-inflammatory, degenerative rheumatoid disorders investigated the sustainability of beneficial effects achieved by serially applied ^{222}Rn containing thermal water baths. Compared to baseline levels, pain score and functional restriction of affected joints were significantly reduced up to twelve or six months, respectively. The fraction of patients with sickness absence was significantly reduced within one year after versus one year prior to therapy [30].

Although the clinical benefit of combined RnHT has been investigated, to date little is known about the underlying cellular and molecular mechanisms of action. According to findings of Reinisch et al., suppression of the oxidative burst in neutrophil granulocytes of patients suffering of ankylosing spondylitis may be at least one key element explaining the therapeutic efficacy of speleotherapeutically applied combined RnHT. Reactive oxygen species (ROS) are released from activated phagocytes in course of inflammation and play a major role in tissue destruction in rheumatoid disorders. Neutrophil granulocytes isolated from peripheral blood of patients produced significantly less superoxide anions when restimulated *ex vivo* after a regimen of ten to twelve units of combined RnHT [31].

According to a previous study by Shehata et al., pain alleviation in ankylosing spondylitis correlates to an elevation in post-treatment serum levels of the anti-inflammatory cytokine TGF-beta [32].

Apart from its role as an immune-modulator, TGF-beta1 also plays a crucial role in bone homoeostasis, particularly by acting as differentiation factor for osteoclasts and via stimulation of osteoblast and downregulation of osteoclast activity [33]. TGF-beta1 exerts its effects in concert with other cytokines and hormones by influencing the OPG/RANKL/RANK system, which is crucial in the control of osteoblast and osteoclast interplay. Receptor activator of nuclear factor κB-ligand (RANKL) is a potent stimulator of osteoclast-mediated bone resorption and promotes osteolysis. It acts via binding to receptor activator of nuclear factor-κB (RANK) on osteoclasts. Osteoprotegerin (OPG) is the functional antagonist of RANKL as it acts as a soluble RANKL decoy receptor that, upon engagement with RANKL, abrogates the interaction with RANK and consequently inhibits maturation and activation of osteoclasts and their precursors. The relative concentrations of OPG and RANKL determine the status of bone metabolism and thus, the OPG/RANKL ratio has become an important marker to assess the prevailing metabolic bone turnover situation. An increased OPG/RANKL ratio indicates an anabolic and a decreased ratio a katabolic bone metabolism state. Chronic inflammatory processes give rise to increased bone resorption, which frequently results in secondary osteoporosis, a typical complication in rheumatic diseases. Moreover, osteoporosis is further aggravated by functional and pain-related disuse bone atrophy and frequently employed glucocorticoid medication hence, predisposing the patient to a high risk of bone fracture [34]. In line with the results of Shehata et al. and the osteoimmunologic context explained above, a recently published pilot study confirmed the elevation of TGF-beta1 and demonstrated an increase of the OPG/RANKL ratio, thus indicating a shift of bone metabolism towards anabolic processes after speleotherapeutically applied RnHT [35, 36].

2. Conclusions

Numerous studies have demonstrated a sustaining beneficial effect of combined low-dose RnHT when serially applied either by speleotherapy or balneotherapy to patients suffering from inflammatory or non-inflammatory degenerative disorders of the musculo-skeletal-system. Of note, the most dominant effect is recognized several months rather than immediately after therapy. Combined RnHT represents a cost effective method that alleviates pain and, thus, allows reducing drug intake which, in turn, may contribute to the prevention of adverse events caused by NSAIDs and glucocorticoids. As mentioned above, radionuclide-based therapy has been employed in the management of rheumatic disorders for decades. However, the poor benefit-risk ratio led to severe limitations or complete discontinuation in clinical use. RnHT poses doses to the patients which are in magnitude 10^{-5} lower in respect to the bone dose compared to ^{224}Radiumchloride-injection regimens. However, further studies are necessary to evaluate potential risks of low-dose RnHT. Although some studies implicate a beneficial effect of hyperthermia therapy for rheumatic diseases, combined RnHT turned out to be more effective than sauna or balneotherapy at an ambient temperature of 37° C lacking ^{222}Rn. As combined RnHT may also exert beneficial effects in other disease entities, further studies are necessary to prove its place among the current treatment options.

Author details

Angelika Moder, Heidi Dobias and Markus Ritter*
Institute of Physiology and Pathophysiology,
Gastein Research Institute, Paracelsus Medical University, Salzburg, Austria

3. References

[1] Erickson B. E., Radioactive pain relief: health care strategies and risk assessment among elderly persons with arthritis at radon health mines. J Altern Complement Med, 2007. 13(3): p. 375-79.

[2] Kaul A., Strahlenbedingtes Risiko, in Radon als Heilmittel, Deetjen P., et al., Editors. 2005, Verlag Dr. Kovac: Hamburg. p. 57-71.

[3] Bahous I., Radiosynoviorthesis: local treatment of rheumatoid arthritis, in Biological Effects of 224-Ra, Müller W.A. and Ebert H.G., Editors. 1978, Martinus Nijhoff Medical Division the Hague / Boston for The Commission of the European Communities: Boston. p. 71-78.

[4] Koch W. and Reske W., Die Ergebnisse der intravenösen Thorium X-Behandlung bei der Spondylarthritis ankylopoetica (M. Bechterew). Strahlenther, 1952. 87: p. 439-457.

[5] Lassmann M., Nosske D., and Reiners C., Therapy of ankylosing spondylitis with 224Ra-radium chloride: dosimetry and risk considerations. Radiat Environ Biophys, 2002. 41(3): p. 173-8.

[6] Wick R., Atkinson M.J., and Nekolla E.A., Incidence of leukaemia and other malignant diseases following injections of the short-lived α-emitter ^{224}Ra into man. Radiat Environ Biophys, 2009. 48: p. 287-294.

[7] Hofmann W., Radon doses compared to X-ray doses, in Radon in der Kurortmedizin, Pratzel H.G. and Deetjen P., Editors. 1997, ISMH Verlag: Geretsried. p. 57-67.

* Corresponding author

[8] Falkenbach A., Radon und Gesundheit. Dt Ärztebl, 1999. 96(23): p. A1576 - A1577.

[9] Tarner I. H., et al., The effect of mild whole-body hyperthermia on systemic levels of TNF-alpha, IL-1beta, and IL-6 in patients with ankylosing spondylitis. Clin Rheumatol, 2009. 28(4): p. 397-402.

[10] Oosterveld F. G., et al., Infrared sauna in patients with rheumatoid arthritis and ankylosing spondylitis. A pilot study showing good tolerance, short-term improvement of pain and stiffness, and a trend towards long-term beneficial effects. Clin Rheumatol, 2009. 28(1): p. 29-34.

[11] Giombini A., et al., Hyperthermia induced by microwave diathermy in the management of muscle and tendon injuries. Br Med Bull, 2007. 83: p. 379-96.

[12] Nowossadeck E., Population aging and hospitalization for chronic disease in Germany. Dtsch Arztebl Int, 2012. 109(9): p. 151-7.

[13] Singh G., Gastrointestinal complications of prescription and over-the-counter nonsteroidal anti-inflammatory drugs: a view from the ARAMIS database. Arthritis, Rheumatism, and Aging Medical Information System. Am J Ther, 2000. 7(2): p. 115-21.

[14] Koelz H.R. and Michel B., Nichtsteroidale Antirhematika: Magenschutztherapie oder COX-2-Hemmer? Dt Arztebl, 2004. 101(45): p. A3041-A3046.

[15] Laine L., et al., Stratifying the risk of NSAID-related upper gastrointestinal clinical events: results of a double-blind outcomes study in patients with rheumatoid arthritis. Gastroenterology, 2002. 123(4): p. 1006-12.

[16] Topol E. J., Failing the public health--rofecoxib, Merck, and the FDA. N Engl J Med, 2004. 351(17): p. 1707-9.

[17] Topol E. J. and Falk G. W., A coxib a day won't keep the doctor away. Lancet, 2004. 364(9435): p. 639-40.

[18] Fitzgerald G. A., Coxibs and cardiovascular disease. N Engl J Med, 2004. 351(17): p. 1709-11.

[19] Bolten W.W., et al., Konsequenzen und Kosten der NSA-Gastropathie in Deutschland. Aktuelle Rheumatol, 1999. 24: p. 127-134.

[20] Lind-Albrecht G., Ergebnisse der Langzeitbeobachtung von Morbus-Bechterew-Patienten nach wiederholter Radonstollenbehandlung, in Tagungsband: Herbsttagung der Arbeitsgemeinschaften Europäischer Radonheilbäder 2004: Bad Kreuznach.

[21] Falkenbach, A., et al., Radon therapy for the treatment of rheumatic diseases--review and meta-analysis of controlled clinical trials. Rheumatol Int, 2005. 25(3): p. 205-10.

[22] Franke A., Reiner L., and Resch K. L., Long-term benefit of radon spa therapy in the rehabilitation of rheumatoid arthritis: a randomised, double-blinded trial. Rheumatol Int, 2007. 27(8): p. 703-13.

[23] Franke, A., et al., Long-term efficacy of radon spa therapy in rheumatoid arthritis--a randomized, sham-controlled study and follow-up. Rheumatology, 2000. 39(8): p. 894-902.

[24] Van Tubergen A., et al., Cost effectiveness of combined spa-exercise therapy in ankylosing spondylitis: a randomized controlled trial. Arthritis Rheum, 2002. 47(5): p. 459-67.

[25] Van Tubergen A., et al., Combined spa-exercise therapy is effective in patients with ankylosing spondylitis: a randomized controlled trial. Arthritis Rheum, 2001. 45(5): p. 430-8.

[26] Lind-Albrecht G., Einfluss der Radonstollentherapie auf Schmerzen und Verlauf bi Spondylitis ankylosans., in Dissertation 1994: Johannes Gutenberg-University: Mainz.

[27] Lind-Albrecht G., Radoninhalation bei Morbus Bechterew, in Radon und Gesundheit, Deetjen P., Editor 1999, Verlag Peter Lang: Frankfurt am Main. p. 131-137.

[28] Pratzel H., Wirksamkeitsnachweis von Radonbädern im Rahmen einer kurortmedizinischen Behandlung des zervikalen Schmerzsyndroms. Phys Rehab Kurmed, 1993. 3: p. 76-82.

[29] Pratzel H., Schmerzstillender Langzeiteffekt durch Radonbäder bei nicht-entzündlichen rheumatischen Erkrankungen, in Radon und Gesundheit, Deetjen P., Editor 1999, Verlag Peter Lang: Frankfurt/Main.

[30] Moder A., et al., Schmerz, Krankenstände, Befindlichkeit, Medikamentenverbrauch und Funktionsverbesserung im Jahr vor und nach einer kombinierten Radonthermalkur. Phys Med Rehab Kuror, 2011. 21: p. 215-219.

[31] Reinisch N., et al., Decrease of respiratory burst in neutrophils of patients with ankylosing spondylitis by combined radon-hyperthermia treatment. Clin Exp Rheumatol, 1999. 17(3): p. 335-8.

[32] Shehata M., et al., Effect of combined spa-exercise therapy on circulating TGF-beta1 levels in patients with ankylosing spondylitis. Wien Klin Wochenschr, 2006. 118(9-10): p. 266-72.

[33] Fox S. W. and Lovibond A. C., Current insights into the role of transforming growth factor-beta in bone resorption. Mol Cell Endocrinol, 2005. 243(1-2): p. 19-26.

[34] Sambrook P. and Lane N. E., Corticosteroid osteoporosis. Best Pract Res Clin Rheumatol, 2001. 15(3): p. 401-13.

[35] Moder A., et al., Effect of combined Low-Dose Radon- and Hyperthermia Treatment (LDRnHT) of patients with ankylosing spondylitis on serum levels of cytokines and bone metabolism markers: a pilot study. Int J Low Radiation, 2010. 7(6): p. 423-435.

[36] Lange U., Müller-Ladner U., and Kürten B., Einfluss einer seriellen niedrig dosierten Radonstollen-Hyperthermie auf zentrale Zytokine des Knochenmetabolismus bei ankylosierender Spondylitis, in Osteologie 2011, Schattauer: Fürth. p. 54.

Chapter 8

Histaminergic Modulation of Body Temperature and Energy Expenditure

Iustin V. Tabarean

Additional information is available at the end of the chapter

http://dx.doi.org/10.5772/52400

1. Introduction

The role of histamine signaling in the brain in thermoregulation has been unraveled in various organisms. The preoptic area/ anterior hypothalamus (PO/AH), region which contains thermoeregulatory neurons, is the main locus in which histamine affects body temperature. Histamine has a complex influence on thermoregulation and its circadian cycle and appears to be involved also in numerous pathological responses that involve changes in core body temperature. The neurotransmitter activates several signaling pathways involving H1, H2 and H3 subtype receptors and recruits distinct neuronal networks to modulate body temperature. In this review we describe the mechanism involved in the hypothalamic control of thermoregulation, the signaling mechanisms activated by histamine in the brain, the evidence for its role in thermoregulation as well as recent advances in the understanding of the cellular and neural network mechanisms involved.

2. Hypothalamic control of thermoregulation

Homeothermia is present in mammals and birds and enables them to maintain their deep-body temperature (Tcore) at stable levels. Tcore can physiologically deviate from its normal value (the value at rest in thermoneutral environment) under the influence of the day-night cycle, the menstrual cycle, or seasonal cycles, such as hibernation. Pathophysiological changes in Tcore include fever (a hyperthermic response to infections), dehydration hyperthermia, and starvation-induced hypothermia. The key role played by the preoptic area/anterior hypothalamus (PO/AH) in the regulation of Tcore was recognized more than a 100 years ago, based on experiments using experimental brain lesions, and selective hypothalamic cooling and heating with chronically implanted thermodes (reviewed in [1]). Sustained or alternating PO/AH cooling and heating induce thermoregulatory activities (physiological or behavioral), causing Tcore to change in the direction opposite to that of the hypothalamic temperature (T_{hy}). Hammel and collegues proposed that a particular net thermoregulatory response was proportional to (T_{hy} $-T_{set}$), where T_{set} was conceived as a hypothetical set reference, a complex parameter representing the state of activity of thermosensitive neuronal populations [2].

Since the first extracellular single-unit study [3], which found that some PO/AH neurons, termed "warm-sensitive", increase their firing rates when T_{hy} increases, it has been considered that they represent the central thermoreceptors. The other PO/AH neurons, which display little temperature-dependent changes in firing rate, are considered temperature-insensitive. PO/AH thermosensitive neurons respond not only to changes in local and peripheral temperature, but also to hormones, osmolarity and glucose concentration (reviewed in [1]). These findings suggest that these neurons, or a subgroup of them, also play a role in the integration of thermoregulation with other homeostatic processes such as control of metabolic rate (glucose sensing). The thermosensitivity of PO/AH neurons is a plastic property both *in vivo* and *in vitro*. It has been found that the thermosensitivity can change rapidly in the presence of the pyrogens PGE2 [4] or IL-1 [5,6]. Slower changes are observed in some warm-sensitive PO/AH neurons which decrease their thermosensitivity during NREM sleep [7].

The mechanism of intrinsic thermosensitivity of PO/AH neurons is controversial. Boulant and colleagues consider that the increased firing rate is solely due to an increased rate of rise of the prepotential which precedes an action potential (reviewed in [8]. Other studies describe strong depolarizations (10 mV or larger) in response to heating which cause the increased firing rate in warm-sensitive neurons ([9]). In cultured PO/AH neurons both phenomena are present, however they occur also in temperature-insensitive neurons [10]. Finally, the warming-activated inward current was found to be tetrodotoxin (TTX)-insensitive in some studies [9,10,11] and TTX-sensitive (i.e. mediated by voltage-gated Na channels) in others [12]. The question remains open as to whether all warm-sensitive PO/AH neurons have some intrinsic thermosensitivity or if they can also display thermosensitive firing that is synaptically-driven [10]. We have shown that prostaglandin E2 (PGE2), a well established endogenous pyrogen, increases the thermosensitivity and firing rates of PO/AH neurons by decreasing the frequency of IPSPs [4]. In contrast, IL-1β hyperpolarizes a different set of PO/AH neurons and reduces their thermosensitivity by increasing the frequency of IPSPs and of miniature IPSPs [5,13].

3. Thermoregulatory neuronal networks comprising PO/AH thermosensitive neurons

The neuronal network controlling brow adipose tissue (BAT) thermogenesis and the fever response has been studied extensively. Thermal and chemical stimulation in the PO/AH combined with selective hypothalamic transections have shown that warm-sensitive PO/AH neurons send efferent signals to loci involved in the control of BAT thermogenesis) [14,15]. PO/AH warming or injection of glutamate suppressed BAT thermogenesis thus suggesting that it is controlled by warm-sensitive neurons ([14]). Studies using combined retrograde labeling and immunocytochemistry revealed that EP3 prostanoid receptor-positive GABAergic PO/AH neurons project to the sympathetic premotor neurons in the rostral raphe pallidus (rRPA). The projections are either direct or via the dorsomedial hypothalamus (DMH) [16,17]. Bilateral microinjections of GABA-A receptor agonists or antagonists into the rRPa or DMH, blocked the fever induced by intra-PO/AH PGE2 applications. The central role of EP3-receptors in PO/AH neurons in the fever response was demonstrated also by local knockdown of its expression [18]. The role of the DMH in the control of BAT thermogenesis was proven also by direct chemical or electrical stimulation [19]. These studies clearly revealed a tonic GABAergic inhibition of the DMH and rRPA by the PO/AH as crucial for basal thermoregulation and hyperthermic responses.

Recent studies have established also the existence of direct glutamatergic projections from the PO/AH [20,21] as well as from the lateral hypothalamus [22] to the rRPA that control thermoregulation. Some glutamatergic PO/AH neurons projecting to rRPa are also peptidergic [20].

Shivering, a different mechanism of thermogenesis, is also controlled by the PO/AH.

Injections of excitatory amino acids as well as PO/AH warming inhibited cold-induced shivering suggesting that this mechanism, similar to BAT thermogenesis, is controlled by PO/AH warm-sensitive neurons [15]. In contrast, cooling of the PO/AH had little effect on cold-induced shivering. The efferent signals mediating shivering descend in the medial forebrain bundle [23].

Evaporative heat loss is also controlled by a network originating in the PO/AH since it is the only brain region that induces salivary secretion when warmed [23]. Preoptic warming, glutamate injections as well as electrical stimulation facilitate salivary secretion [5,13,15] as well as body extension [24], another aspect of evaporative heat loss.

The neuronal network controlling cutaneous blood flow also originates in the PO/AH.

Warming the PO/AH elicits skin vasodilation [25], by activation of warm-sensitive neurons [15]. The efferent pathway descends through the medial forebrain bundle [23]. It is believed that warm-sensitive neurons in PO/AH send excitatory signals to vasodilator neurons and inhibitory signals to vasoconstrictor neurons. PO/AH neurons controlling cutaneous blood flow project to the rostral medullary raphe region directly [26], suggesting that distinct populations of PO/AH neurons control thermogenesis and cutaneous vasomotion. This concept is supported by the observation that the two thermoregulatory mechanisms are activated at different threshold temperatures [27].

Little is known about the local networks comprising warm-sensitive and temperature-insensitive neurons. One study found little thermosensitivity in the frequency of spontaneous IPSPs and EPSPs recorded in either warm-sensitive or temperature-insensitive PO/AH neurons, suggesting that the former do not send local projections [28]. This study also compared the morphologies of w-s and t-i PO/AH neurons filled with Lucifer yellow or biocytin. The dendritic arbors were characterized, however the axonal projections could not be described. This finding may reflect technical limitations or the fact that PO/AH neurons send few local projections [28]. Our studies in mice have not found evidence for local projections of PO/AH GABAergic neurons but have revealed reciprocal connections of PO/AH glutamatergic neurons [21].

4. Histamine signaling in the brain

Histamine is synthesized in the tuberomammilary nucleus (TMN) neurons from histidine by the specific enzyme histidine decarboxylase (HDC). After release histamine is methylated by histamine N-methyl-transferase (which is located postsynaptically and in glia). The turnover of neuronal histamine is high, with its half-life being ~ 30 min. The histaminergic TMN neurons project their axons throughout the brain and they control arousal, attention, energy expenditure, feeding, and thermoregulation. Histaminergic fibers are especially dense in the cortex, hypothalamus, amygdala and striatum (reviewed in [29]). In the hypothalamus the histaminergic fibers are particularly dense in the anterior part [30]. Another source of histamine in the brain is represented by resident mast cells [31].

Four histamine receptors, which are GPCRs, have been cloned (H1-H4R). The H1R, H2R and H3R are expressed in distinctive patterns in the brain [32] and all three receptor types are highly expressed in the hypothalamus. The H1Rs mediate excitatory actions on central neurons. At the cellular level, excitation is achieved by activation of $G_{q/11}$ and PLC, which leads to the formation of the two second messengers, diacylglycerol (DAG) and inositol-1,4,5-triphosphate (Ins(1,4,5)P3). Ins(1,4,5)P3 releases Ca^{2+} from internal stores, and this activates at least four Ca^{2+}-dependent processes. First, the opening of a cation channel, which causes depolarization [33]. Second, activation of the electrogenic Na-Ca exchanger in supraoptic neurons, which also causes depolarization [34]. Third, formation of nitric oxide and cyclic GMP [35]. And finally, opening of K^+ channels, resulting in hyperpolarization [36]. Furthermore, blocking a leak potassium conductance through direct G-protein action, or through PLC, DAG and PKC, can cause excitation in the thalamus [37], and in the striatum [38].

The H2Rs are coupled to G_s, adenylyl cyclase (AC) and PKA, which phosphorylates proteins and activates the transcription factor cyclic-AMP-response element (CRE)-binding protein (CREB). The direct action on neuronal membranes is usually excitatory or potentiates excitation. Like other transmitters that use this signaling pathway histamine blocks the small Ca^{2+}-dependent K^+ conductance ([39]). This conductance causes a long-lasting afterhyperpolarization and affects the accommodation of firing. A cortical neuron under active histaminergic input remains quiescent until it is reached by a sensory stimulus, which will then cause an enhanced and long-lasting response. Activation of H2Rs, by increasing cyclic AMP concentration, shifts the activation of the inwardly rectifying I_h towards a more positive voltage and contributes to a depolarization that modifies the thalamic relay of sensory input [37].

The H3Rs are located on histaminergic and other cell somata, dendrites and axons (varicosities), where they provide negative feedback to restrict histamine synthesis and release. They also provide negative feedback on the release of other transmitters, such as glutamate [40], acetylcholine and noradrenaline [41]. H3Rs are coupled to $G_{i/o}$ and inhibit high voltage activated Ca^{2+} channels, a typical mechanism for the regulation of transmitter release. In rat, there are three functional splice variants of the H3R. In mouse, both RNase protection assay experiments and PCR results indicate that only one isoform of the H3R is present [42] which is coupled negatively to cAMP. H3Rs also activated the phospholipase A2 (PLA2) via the Gi/o proteins which results in production of arachidonic acid [43].

In summary, H1Rs and H2Rs have mostly excitatory actions on neurons or potentiate excitatory inputs. By contrast, H3-receptor activation causes autoinhibition of TMN neurons and inhibition of neurotransmitter release. Recent morphological and physiological studies suggest the presence of H3 receptors also postsynaptically [21,44,45].

5. Central histaminergic modulation of core body temperature

The role of CNS histamine in thermoregulation has been established in various organisms from invertebrates [46] to lower vertebrates [47] as well as mammals. Early studies in mammals have reported a role of hypothalamic histamine in the control of body temperature [48]. The preoptic area/ anterior hypothalamus (PO/AH), region which contains temperature-sensitive neurons and regulates the thermoregulation setpoint, is the main locus in which histamine affects body temperature [49]. Histamine injected in the medial preoptic nucleus (MPON) induces hyperthermia. Similarly, intra-MPON injection of a histamine-N-methyltransferase inhibitor (which results in a local increase of histamine concentration) also produces hyperthermia [50]. Behavioral temperature selection studies suggest that preoptic histamine signaling affects both the set point of the hypothalamic thermostat, as well as heat loss mechanisms [51]. Both H1 and H2 receptors have been implicated in these responses.

Some studies suggest a hyperthermic tone due to histamine signaling. Thus, premedication with a H2R antagonist before general anesthesia augments core hypothermia during this procedure [52]. In pathological conditions histamine appears to mediate hypothermic responses. Ionizing radiation induces hypothermia that can be blocked by H1R and H2R antagonists applied centrally [53]. Exposure of the head to ionizing radiation appers to stimulate histamine release from brain-resident mast-cells [53].

Peripherally, histamine is involved in the rise of skin blood flow during whole body heating [54]. Similarly, combined H1R and H2R antagonists diminish the alcohol-induced flushing in individuals of Oriental origin [55].

More recent observations using transgenic models further indicate a role of histamine signaling in thermoregulation are. Thus H3R-/- transgenic mice display a lowered core body temperature suggesting that these receptors mediate a tonic hyperthermic action [56]. Other studies point to a hypothermic action of histamine, mediated by H1 subtype receptors. Thus, anaphylaxis induced hypothermia is not observed in HDC(-/-) mice or in the presence of H1R antagonists [57]. Also, IL-1β-induced thermogenesis is potentiated by depletion of hypothalamic histamine [58].

Our studies have established that in mice histamine induces hyperthermia when administered in either the medial or the median preoptic nuclei [59]. Similarly, when the endogenous concentration of histamine was raised in either nucleus by local injection of histamine *N*-methyl transferase inhibitor a hyperthermia of similar amplitude was observed [59]. H1R and H3R specific agonists were equally potent in inducing a hyperthermia when infused in the median preoptic nucleus [21]. In contrast, H2R specific agonists mimicked the histamine effect when administered intra-MPON, while H1R specific agonists had little effect [60]. Surprisingly, H3R specific agonists were without effect in this nucleus [60].

Our experiments have also revealed that histamine modulation of the activity of GABAergic PO/AH neurons provides a mechanism for selective modulation of body temperature at the beginning of the active phase of the circadian cycle [61]. Thus, injection of a H3 antagonist in the MnPO induces a delay in the onset of the rise of the body temperature associated with the active phase of the circadian cycle [61].

6. Histaminergic control of energy expenditure

Maintenance of core body temperature represent a major energy expenditure of a homeothermic organism. Uncoupling proteins (UCPs) are inner mitochondrial membrane transporters of free fatty acids, which dissipate the proton gradient by releasing stored energy as heat, without coupling to other energy consuming processes [62]. UCP1 in brown adipose tissue (BAT) plays a crucial role in regulating energy expenditure and thermogenesis in rodents and neonates of larger mammalian species, including humans. UCP2 and UCP3 are not involved in adaptive thermogenesis, however their activation *in vivo* by physiological activators or pharmacological intervention has the capacity to be significantly thermogenic [63]. The hypothalamus controls UCP1 and UCP3 expression in BAT and white adipose tissue (WAT) via the sympathetic neuron system. Infusion of histamine in the third ventricle or in the preoptic area (POA) produces similar increases in BAT sympathetic nerve activity (SNA) and in the UCP1 mRNA expression [64]. By contrast injections of histamine in the lateral hypothalamus or the ventromedial hypothalamic nucleus were without effect ([64]), suggesting that the POA is the principal hypothalamic site which mediates the stimulatory effect of histamine of this efferent pathway. Histamine-deficient animals (HDC-/-) have an impaired ability to express UCP1 in BAT [65] further suggesting a role of histamine signaling in the control of energy expenditure. Similarly, the upregulation of UCP1 mRNA expression induced by central infusion of leptin is attenuated in H1R-/- mice [66] suggesting a role of this receptor subtype in mechanisms regulating energy expenditure. The role of the other histamine receptor subtypes also present in the PO/AH in this effect remains to be determined. Increased hypothalamic histamine also results in a decreased respiratory quotient, which indicates increased lipid oxidation [67].

In our study [59] we have determined the effects of activation of histamine receptors in the preoptic area by increasing the concentration of endogenous histamine or by local injection of specific agonists. Both approaches induce an elevation of core body temperature and decreased respiratory exchange ratio (RER). The hyperthermic effect is associated with a rapid increase in mRNA expression of uncoupling proteins in thermogenic tissues, the most pronounced being that of uncoupling protein (UCP) 1 in brown adipose tissue and of UCP2 in white adipose tissue. In diet-induced obese mice histamine had much diminished hyperthermic effects as well as reduced effect on RER. Similarly, the ability of preoptic histamine signaling to increase the expression of uncoupling proteins was abolished. We also found that the expression of mRNA encoding the H1 receptor subtype in the preoptic area was significantly lower in obese animals [59].

Several H1R and H2R antagonists are clinically used in the treatment of several diseases. H1R antagonists (e.g. diphenhydramine hydrochloride, trade name Benadryl) are clinically used in the treatment of histamine-mediated allergic conditions. Clinically-relevant histamine H2R antagonists (e.g. ranitidine and cimetidine, trade names Zanatac and Tagamet, respectively) are used to reduce the secretion of gastric acid by acting on H2 receptors found principally in the parietal cells of the gastric mucosa. Interestingly, few side effects related to thermoregulation have been reported, due probably to the fact that these compounds cross the blood-brain barrier to a small extent. More recently, H3R antagonists have received a great interest from the pharmaceutical industry, with some drugs being in phase I or phase II of clinical trials [68]. Some projects have proposed H3R antagonists for the treatment of narcolepsy and/or cognitive disorders while others are trying H3R antagonists for the treatment of obesity and diabetes mellitus. All these drugs act at central H3Rs and produce increased levels of histamine in the brain, in particular in the hypothalamus. Since these compounds are designed to work centrally, the possibility of thermoregulatory side effects is significantly enhanced.

H1R antagonists have been reported to increase seizure susceptibility in patients with febrile seizures [69,70]. These observations strengthen the idea that these drugs can act centrally to influence body temperature and other centrally regulated functions. Thus, H1R antagonists in most cases should not be prescribed to patients, particularly young infants, with febrile seizures and epilepsy. Drug-induced fever due to H2R blockers was also encountered, however the effect appears to be mediated by an allergic reaction to the drugs, characterized by a marked increase in IgE [71].

7. Cellular mechanisms involved in histamine induced hyperthermia

An early extracellular recording study found that most rat PO/AH neurons, irrespective to their thermosensitivities were excited by histamine, effect which was blocked by a H1 antagonist in most neurons [72]. In few neurons the excitation was blocked also by an H2 antagonist [72]. Our recent studies have revealed that histamine acts differentially on neurons of the median and medial preoptic nuclei (MnPO and MPON respectively). The neurotransmitter reduced the spontaneous firing rate of thermoregulatory GABAergic MnPO neurons by activating H3 subtype histamine receptors [21]. This effect involved a decrease in the level of phosphorylation of the extracellular signal-regulated kinase

(ERK1/2) and was not dependent on synaptic activity. Single-cell reverse transcription-PCR analysis revealed expression of H3 receptors in the histamine responsive population of GABAergic MnPO neurons. Histamine applied in the MnPO nucleus induced a robust, long-lasting hyperthermia effect that was mimicked by H3 histamine receptor subtype-specific agonists [21]. We have also established that an increase in the A-type K^+ current in GABAergic MnPO neurons in response to activation of H3 histamine receptors results in decreased firing rate and hyperthermia in mice [61]. The Kv4.2 subunit is required for these actions since Kv4.2-/- preoptic GABAergic neurons are not affected by histamine or H3 agonists. Moreover, Kv4.2-/- mice develop much reduced hyperthermias in response to histamine or H3 agonists. Dynamic clamp experiments demonstrate that enhancement of the A-type current by a similar amount to that induced by histamine is sufficient to mimic its robust effect on firing rates. These experiments reveal a central role played by the Kv4.2 subunit in histamine regulation of body temperature and its interaction with pERK1/2 downstream of the H3 receptor.

Our studies have also established that a population of non-GABAergic MnPO preoptic neurons was depolarized, and their firing rate was enhanced by histamine acting at H1 subtype receptors [21]. In our experiments, activation of the H1R receptors was linked to the phospholipase C pathway and Ca^{2+} release from intracellular stores. This depolarization persisted in TTX or when fast synaptic potentials were blocked, indicating that it represents a postsynaptic effect. Single-cell reverse transcription-PCR analysis revealed the expression of H1 receptors in these putative glutamatergic cells. The inward current is activated in a Ca-dependent manner. At high histamine (20 μM) concentration the excitation elicited by histamine in glutamatergic MnPO neurons has also a persistent component that can last for at least 40 min after the removal of the bioamine. TRPC1 and TRPC5 channels appear to be the channels that contribute most to the inward current activated downstream of H1Rs. H1 agonists also induced long-lasting hyperthermia when injected intra-MnPO. These studies have shown that histamine modulates the core body temperature by acting at two distinct populations of preoptic neurons that express H1 and H3 receptor subtypes, respectively.

The mechanisms activated by histamine in the MPON are different. Histamine activates H2 subtype receptors in the MPON and induces hyperthermia [60]. We also found that a population of glutamatergic MPON neurons express H2Rs and are excited by H2R specific agonists. The agonists decreased the input resistance of the neuron and increased the depolarizing "sag" observed during hyperpolarizing current injections. Activation of H2Rs induced an inward current that was blocked by ZD7288, a specific blocker of the hyperpolarization activated cationic current (Ih). In voltage-clamp experiments, activation of H2R receptors resulted in increased Ih amplitude in response to hyperpolarizing voltage steps and a depolarizing shift in its voltage-dependent activation. The neurons excited by H2 specific agonism expressed the HCN1 and HCN2 channel subunits. Our data indicate that at the level of the MPON histamine influences thermoregulation by increasing the firing rate of glutamatergic neurons that express H2Rs [60].

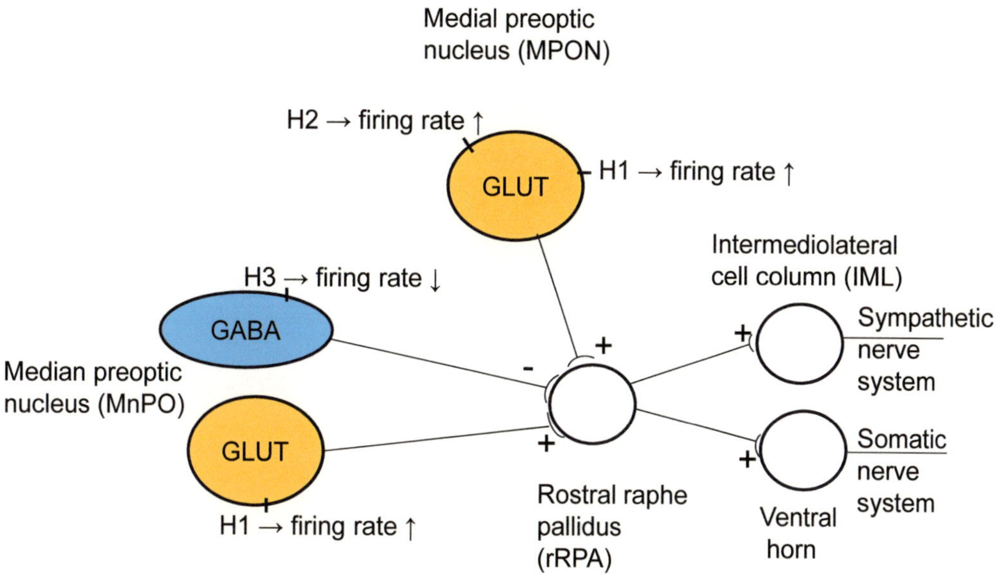

Figure 1. Simplified diagram of the neural pathways controlling thermoeffector mechanisms (Morrison and Nakamura, 2011). The diagram also illustrates the proposed cellular mechanisms activated by histamine. GABAergic neurons in the MnPOA tonically inhibit sympathetic premotor neurons in the rostral raphe pallidus. Histamine reduces the firing rates of GABAergic MnPO neurons. This results in stimulation of the sympathetic output system. Activation of H1 and H2 receptors expressed by MnPO and MPON neurons, respectively, increased firing rates and stimulates the sympathetic neuron system. The dashed lines indicate that the respective projections have been suggested by physiological studies but have not been demonstrated directly.

8. Conclusion

Histamine has a complex influence on thermoregulation and its circadian cycle and appears to be involved in numerous pathophysiological responses that involve changes in core body temperature. At the level of the MnPO and MPON histamine induces potent hyperthermia and an increase in energy expenditure by activating several signaling pathways and neuronal networks.

Author details

Iustin V. Tabarean
The Department of Molecular and Integrative Neurosciences, The Scripps Research Institute, La Jolla, USA

Acknowledgement

This work was supported by the National Institutes of Health Grant NS060799.

9. References

[1] Simon E (2000) The enigma of deep-body thermosensory specificity. Int J Biometeorol 44: 105-120.

[2] Hammel HT, Jackson DC, Stolwijk JA, Hardy JD, Stromme SB (1963) Temperature Regulation by Hypothalamic Proportional Control with an Adjustable Set Point. J Appl Physiol 18: 1146-1154.

[3] Nakayama T, Eisenman JS, Hardy JD (1961) Single unit activity of anterior hypothalamus during local heating. Science 134: 560-561.

[4] Tabarean IV, Behrens MM, Bartfai T, Korn H (2004) Prostaglandin E2-increased thermosensitivity of anterior hypothalamic neurons is associated with depressed inhibition. Proc Natl Acad Sci U S A 101: 2590-2595.

[5] Sanchez-Alavez M, Tabarean IV, Behrens MM, Bartfai T (2006) Ceramide mediates the rapid phase of febrile response to IL-1{beta}. Proc Natl Acad Sci U S A.

[6] Vasilenko VY, Petruchuk TA, Gourine VN, Pierau FK (2000) Interleukin-1beta reduces temperature sensitivity but elevates thermal thresholds in different populations of warm-sensitive hypothalamic neurons in rat brain slices. Neurosci Lett 292: 207-210.

[7] Alam MN, McGinty D, Szymusiak R (1995) Preoptic/anterior hypothalamic neurons: thermosensitivity in rapid eye movement sleep. Am J Physiol 269: R1250-1257.

[8] Boulant JA (1998) Cellular mechanisms of temperature sensitivity in hypothalamic neurons. Prog Brain Res 115: 3-8.

[9] Kobayashi S, Takahashi T (1993) Whole-cell properties of temperature-sensitive neurons in rat hypothalamic slices. Proc Biol Sci 251: 89-94.

[10] Tabarean IV, Conti B, Behrens M, Korn H, Bartfai T (2005) Electrophysiological properties and thermosensitivity of mouse preoptic and anterior hypothalamic neurons in culture. Neuroscience 135: 433-449.

[11] Zhao Y, Boulant JA (2005) Temperature effects on neuronal membrane potentials and inward currents in rat hypothalamic tissue slices. J Physiol 564: 245-257.

[12] Kiyohara T, Hirata M, Hori T, Akaike N (1990) Hypothalamic warm-sensitive neurons possess a tetrodotoxin-sensitive sodium channel with a high Q10. Neurosci Res 8: 48-53.

[13] Tabarean IV, Korn H, Bartfai T (2006) Interleukin-1beta induces hyperpolarization and modulates synaptic inhibition in preoptic and anterior hypothalamic neurons. Neuroscience 141: 1685-1695.

[14] Chen XM, Hosono T, Yoda T, Fukuda Y, Kanosue K (1998) Efferent projection from the preoptic area for the control of non-shivering thermogenesis in rats. J Physiol 512 (Pt 3): 883-892.

[15] Zhang YH, Yanase-Fujiwara M, Hosono T, Kanosue K (1995) Warm and cold signals from the preoptic area: which contribute more to the control of shivering in rats? J Physiol 485 (Pt 1): 195-202.

[16] Nakamura K, Matsumura K, Kaneko T, Kobayashi S, Katoh H, et al. (2002) The rostral raphe pallidus nucleus mediates pyrogenic transmission from the preoptic area. J Neurosci 22: 4600-4610.

[17] Nakamura Y, Nakamura K, Matsumura K, Kobayashi S, Kaneko T, et al. (2005) Direct pyrogenic input from prostaglandin EP3 receptor-expressing preoptic neurons to the dorsomedial hypothalamus. Eur J Neurosci 22: 3137-3146.
[18] Lazarus M, Yoshida K, Coppari R, Bass CE, Mochizuki T, et al. (2007) EP3 prostaglandin receptors in the median preoptic nucleus are critical for fever responses. Nat Neurosci 10: 1131-1133.
[19] Zaretskaia MV, Zaretsky DV, DiMicco JA (2003) Role of the dorsomedial hypothalamus in thermogenesis and tachycardia caused by microinjection of prostaglandin E2 into the preoptic area in anesthetized rats. Neurosci Lett 340: 1-4.
[20] Dimitrov E, Kim Y, Usdin TB (2011) Tuberoinfundibular peptide of 39 residues modulates the mouse hypothalamic-pituitary-adrenal axis via paraventricular glutamatergic neurons. J Neurosci 518: 4375-4394.
[21] Lundius EG, Sanchez-Alavez M, Ghochani Y, Klaus J, Tabarean IV (2010) Histamine influences body temperature by acting at H1 and H3 receptors on distinct populations of preoptic neurons. J Neurosci 30: 4369-4381.
[22] Tupone D, Madden CJ, Cano G, Morrison SF (2011) An orexinergic projection from perifornical hypothalamus to raphe pallidus increases rat brown adipose tissue thermogenesis. J Neurosci 31: 15944-15955.
[23] Kanosue K, Yanase-Fujiwara M, Hosono T (1994) Hypothalamic network for thermoregulatory vasomotor control. Am J Physiol 267: R283-288.
[24] Tanaka H, Kanosue K, Nakayama T, Shen Z (1986) Grooming, body extension, and vasomotor responses induced by hypothalamic warming at different ambient temperatures in rats. Physiol Behav 38: 145-151.
[25] Ishikawa Y, Nakayama T, Kanosue K, Matsumura K (1984) Activation of central warm-sensitive neurons and the tail vasomotor response in rats during brain and scrotal thermal stimulation. Pflugers Arch 400: 222-227.
[26] Rathner JA, Madden CJ, Morrison SF (2008) Central pathway for spontaneous and prostaglandin E2-evoked cutaneous vasoconstriction. Am J Physiol Regul Integr Comp Physiol 295: R343-354.
[27] Ootsuka Y, McAllen RM (2006) Comparison between two rat sympathetic pathways activated in cold defense. Am J Physiol Regul Integr Comp Physiol 291: R589-595.
[28] Griffin JD, Saper CB, Boulant JA (2001) Synaptic and morphological characteristics of temperature-sensitive and -insensitive rat hypothalamic neurones. J Physiol 537: 521-535.
[29] Haas H, Panula P (2003) The role of histamine and the tuberomamillary nucleus in the nervous system. Nat Rev Neurosci 4: 121-130.
[30] Wada H (1992) [From biochemistry to pharmacology: the histaminergic neuron system in the brain]. Nippon Yakurigaku Zasshi 99: 63-81.
[31] Ulugol A, Karadag HC, Dokmeci D, Baldik Y, Dokmeci I (1996) The role of histamine H1 receptors in the thermoregulatory effect of morphine in mice. Eur J Pharmacol 308: 49-52.
[32] Arrang JM, Drutel G, Garbarg M, Ruat M, Traiffort E, et al. (1995) Molecular and functional diversity of histamine receptor subtypes. Ann N Y Acad Sci 757: 314-323.

[33] Smith BN, Armstrong WE (1993) Histamine enhances the depolarizing afterpotential of immunohistochemically identified vasopressin neurons in the rat supraoptic nucleus via H1-receptor activation. Neuroscience 53: 855-864.

[34] Smith BN, Armstrong WE (1996) The ionic dependence of the histamine-induced depolarization of vasopressin neurones in the rat supraoptic nucleus. J Physiol 495 (Pt 2): 465-478.

[35] Richelson E (1978) Histamine H1 receptor-mediated guanosine 3',5'-monophosphate formation by cultured mouse neuroblastoma cells. Science 201: 69-71.

[36] Weiger T, Stevens DR, Wunder L, Haas HL (1997) Histamine H1 receptors in C6 glial cells are coupled to calcium-dependent potassium channels via release of calcium from internal stores. Naunyn Schmiedebergs Arch Pharmacol 355: 559-565.

[37] McCormick DA, Williamson A (1991) Modulation of neuronal firing mode in cat and guinea pig LGNd by histamine: possible cellular mechanisms of histaminergic control of arousal. J Neurosci 11: 3188-3199.

[38] Munakata M, Akaike N (1994) Regulation of K+ conductance by histamine H1 and H2 receptors in neurones dissociated from rat neostriatum. J Physiol 480 (Pt 2): 233-245.

[39] Haas HL, Konnerth A (1983) Histamine and noradrenaline decrease calcium-activated potassium conductance in hippocampal pyramidal cells. Nature 302: 432-434.

[40] Brown RE, Haas HL (1999) On the mechanism of histaminergic inhibition of glutamate release in the rat dentate gyrus. J Physiol 515 (Pt 3): 777-786.

[41] Schlicker E, Behling A, Lummen G, Gothert M (1992) Histamine H3A receptor-mediated inhibition of noradrenaline release in the mouse brain cortex. Naunyn Schmiedebergs Arch Pharmacol 345: 489-493.

[42] Chen J, Liu C, Lovenberg TW (2003) Molecular and pharmacological characterization of the mouse histamine H3 receptor. Eur J Pharmacol 467: 57-65.

[43] Leurs R, Traiffort E, Arrang JM, Tardivel-Lacombe J, Ruat M, et al. (1994) Guinea pig histamine H1 receptor. II. Stable expression in Chinese hamster ovary cells reveals the interaction with three major signal transduction pathways. J Neurochem 62: 519-527.

[44] Lazarov NE, Gratzl M (2006) Selective expression of histamine receptors in rat mesencephalic trigeminal neurons. Neurosci Lett 404: 67-71.

[45] Zhou FW, Xu JJ, Zhao Y, LeDoux MS, Zhou FM (2006) Opposite functions of histamine H1 and H2 receptors and H3 receptor in substantia nigra pars reticulata. J Neurophysiol 96: 1581-1591.

[46] Hong ST, Bang S, Paik D, Kang J, Hwang S, et al. (2006) Histamine and its receptors modulate temperature-preference behaviors in Drosophila. J Neurosci 26: 7245-7256.

[47] Leger JP, Mathieson WB (1997) Development of bombesin-like and histamine-like innervation in the bullfrog (Rana catesbeiana) central nervous system. Brain Behav Evol 49: 63-77.

[48] Green MD, Cox B, Lomax P (1975) Histamine H1- and H2-receptors in the central thermoregulatory pathways of the rat. J Neurosci Res 1: 353-359.

[49] Colboc O, Protais P, Costentin J (1982) Histamine-induced rise in core temperature of chloral-anaesthetized rats: mediation by H2-receptors located in the preopticus area of hypothalamus. Neuropharmacology 21: 45-50.

[50] Gatti PJ, Gertner SB (1984) The effect of intrahypothalamic injection of homodimaprit on blood pressure. Neuropharmacology 23: 663-670.
[51] Bugajski J, Zacny E (1981) The role of central histamine H1- and H2-receptors in hypothermia induced by histamine in the rat. Agents Actions 11: 442-447.
[52] Hirose M, Hara Y, Matsusaki M (1995) Premedication with famotidine augments core hypothermia during general anesthesia. Anesthesiology 83: 1179-1183.
[53] Kandasamy SB, Hunt WA (1988) Involvement of histamine H1 and H2 receptors in hypothermia induced by ionizing radiation in guinea pigs. Life Sci 42: 555-563.
[54] Wong BJ, Wilkins BW, Minson CT (2004) H1 but not H2 histamine receptor activation contributes to the rise in skin blood flow during whole body heating in humans. J Physiol 560: 941-948.
[55] Miller NS, Goodwin DW, Jones FC, Gabrielli WF, Pardo MP, et al. (1988) Antihistamine blockade of alcohol-induced flushing in orientals. J Stud Alcohol 49: 16-20.
[56] Toyota H, Dugovic C, Koehl M, Laposky AD, Weber C, et al. (2002) Behavioral characterization of mice lacking histamine H(3) receptors. Mol Pharmacol 62: 389-397.
[57] Kang M, Yoshimatsu H, Kurokawa M, Ogawa R, Sakata T (1999) Prostaglandin E2 mediates activation of hypothalamic histamine by interleukin-1beta in rats. Proc Soc Exp Biol Med 220: 88-93.
[58] Sakata T, Kang M, Kurokawa M, Yoshimatsu H (1995) Hypothalamic neuronal histamine modulates adaptive behavior and thermogenesis in response to endogenous pyrogen. Obes Res 3 Suppl 5: 707S-712S.
[59] Sethi J, Sanchez-Alavez M, Tabarean IV (2012) Loss of histaminergic modulation of thermoregulation and energy homeostasis in obese mice. Neuroscience.
[60] Tabarean IV, Sanchez-Alavez M, Sethi J (2012) Mechanism of H2 histamine receptor dependent modulation of body temperature and neuronal activity in the medial preoptic nucleus Neuropharmacology (in press).
[61] Sethi J, Sanchez-Alavez M, Tabarean IV (2011) Kv4.2 mediates histamine modulation of preoptic neuron activity and body temperature. PLoS One 6: e29134.
[62] Nicholls DG, Locke RM (1984) Thermogenic mechanisms in brown fat. Physiol Rev 64: 1-64.
[63] Brand MD, Esteves TC (2005) Physiological functions of the mitochondrial uncoupling proteins UCP2 and UCP3. Cell Metab 2: 85-93.
[64] Yasuda T, Masaki T, Sakata T, Yoshimatsu H (2004) Hypothalamic neuronal histamine regulates sympathetic nerve activity and expression of uncoupling protein 1 mRNA in brown adipose tissue in rats. Neuroscience 125: 535-540.
[65] Fulop AK, Foldes A, Buzas E, Hegyi K, Miklos IH, et al. (2003) Hyperleptinemia, visceral adiposity, and decreased glucose tolerance in mice with a targeted disruption of the histidine decarboxylase gene. Endocrinology 144: 4306-4314.
[66] Masaki T, Chiba S, Yasuda T, Noguchi H, Kakuma T, et al. (2004) Involvement of hypothalamic histamine H1 receptor in the regulation of feeding rhythm and obesity. Diabetes 53: 2250-2260.

[67] Malmlof K, Zaragoza F, Golozoubova V, Refsgaard HH, Cremers T, et al. (2005) Influence of a selective histamine H3 receptor antagonist on hypothalamic neural activity, food intake and body weight. Int J Obes (Lond) 29: 1402-1412.

[68] Celanire S, Wijtmans M, Talaga P, Leurs R, de Esch IJ (2005) Keynote review: histamine H3 receptor antagonists reach out for the clinic. Drug Discov Today 10: 1613-1627.

[69] Takano T, Sakaue Y, Sokoda T, Sawai C, Akabori S, et al. (2010) Seizure susceptibility due to antihistamines in febrile seizures. Pediatr Neurol 42: 277-279.

[70] Zolaly MA (2012) Histamine H1 antagonists and clinical characteristics of febrile seizures. Int J Gen Med 5: 277-281.

[71] Hiraide A, Yoshioka T, Ohshima S (1990) IgE-mediated drug fever due to histamine H2-receptor blockers. Drug Saf 5: 455-457.

[72] Tsai CL, Matsumura K, Nakayama T, Itowi N, Yamatodani A, et al. (1989) Effects of histamine on thermosensitive neurons in rat preoptic slice preparations. Neurosci Lett 102: 297-302.